Gerard Chiche / Alain Pinault

Esthetics of Anterior Fixed Prosthodontics

Esthetics of Anterior Fixed Prosthodontics

Gerard Chiche, DDS, FACD
Professor
Department of Fixed Prosthodontics
School of Dentistry
Louisiana State University
New Orleans, Louisiana

Alain Pinault, MDT
Paris, France
Visiting Lecturer
Department of Fixed Prosthodontics
School of Dentistry
Louisiana State University
New Orleans, Louisiana

Quintessence Publishing Co, Inc
Chicago, Berlin, London, Tokyo, Moscow, Prague, Sofia, and Warsaw

To Lynn and Monique
for their love and understanding

Library of Congress Cataloging-in-Publication Data

Chiche, Gerard J.
   Esthetics of anterior fixed prosthodontics / Gerard Chiche, Alain Pinault.
       p.   cm.
   Includes bibliographical references and index.
   ISBN 0-86715-258-3
   1. Crowns (Dentistry) 2. Bridges (Dentistry) 3. Dentistry—Aesthetics.
I. Pinault, Alain. II. Title.
   [DNLM: 1. Crowns 2. Dentures, Partial, Fixed. 3. Esthetics, Dental.
4. Dental Restoration, Permanent. WU 515 C533e 1993]
RK666.C55   1994
617.6'92—dc20
DNLM/DLC
for Library of Congress   93-25776
                                                CIP

quintessence
books

Composition: Focus Graphics, St Louis, MO
Printing and Binding: Toppan Printing Co (S) Pte, Ltd, Singapore
Printed in Singapore

Contents

Contributors

James D Harrison, DDS, MSc, MA, FACD, FICD
Chairman
Department of Fixed Prosthodontics
School of Dentistry
Louisiana State University
New Orleans, Louisiana

Edmund E Jeansonne, DDS, FACD
Dean Emeritus
School of Dentistry
Louisiana State University
New Orleans, Louisiana

Vincent G Kokich, DDS, MSD
Professor and Director of Orthodontic Research
Department of Orthodontics
School of Dentistry
University of Washington
Seattle, Washington

**John W McLean, OBE, FDS, RCS (Eng), MDS,
  DSc (London), DOdont (Lund)**
Consultant in Biomaterials
School of Dentistry
Louisiana State University
New Orleans, Louisiana

Richard F Caudill, DMD
Private Practice
West Palm Beach, Florida
Formerly Associate Professor
Department of Periodontics
School of Dentistry
Louisiana State University
New Orleans, Louisiana

Ronald R Lemon, DMD
Chairman
Department of Endodontics
School of Dentistry
Louisiana State University
New Orleans, Louisiana

Foreword

Esthetic dentistry is finding an expanding place in dental school curriculums. The challenge we face as educators, however, is to teach this abstract discipline in a practical and methodical way.

Dr Gerard Chiche and Mr Alain Pinault have demonstrated their outstanding artistic and scientific expertise by writing this easy-to-read book on esthetics in fixed prosthodontics. Their refreshing approach to anterior esthetics provides the dental practitioner and laboratory technician with definitive information on the "hows" and "whys" of the subject.

In a well-organized format, the first three chapters cover the artistic and scientific principles of esthetics, diagnosis and treatment planning, and remaking deficient crowns. The next three chapters orient the reader to metal ceramic crowns, all-ceramic and foil crowns, and communication with the dental technician. To round out this informative book, the final three chapters deal most importantly with tissue management, impression procedures, and the necessity of establishing a healthy gingival appearance.

Readers will be most impressed with the overall organization of the text, the clarity of each chapter, and the outstanding photography that clearly demonstrates the clinical application of this material by its authors. Our department is proud to have been involved in this exciting project, and we hope that it will contribute to a better understanding of the challenging discipline of esthetic dentistry.

James D Harrison, DDS, MSc, MA, FACD, FICD
Professor and Chairman
Department of Fixed Prosthodontics
School of Dentistry
Louisiana State University
New Orleans, Louisiana

Preface

Esthetic dentistry, like other disciplines, adheres to rules and techniques. When we perceive some scheme of harmony or balance, we react to an interaction of form, light, and contour. In all fields of art, the artist appeals to the senses of the observer through a conscious and calculated effort using principles and techniques. Likewise, in dentistry, the clinician and technician must move beyond intuitive appraisal and use fundamental esthetic principles to help achieve an esthetically pleasing smile. To think that an artistic predisposition is necessary in esthetic dentistry is a misconception: as in any other discipline, a knowledge of certain principles is more important than intuition alone.

In his book *Drawing the Head and Hands*, Loomis[1] states "as artists, we only see, analyze and set down. . . . Creating beauty is not a matter of 'soul searching,' but primarily interpreting form in its proportion, perspective and lighting." For example, with objective criteria, the clinician can easily develop an analytical and critical appraisal of elements such as proportion, symmetry, and pleasing variation.

In this contemporary era of fitness and elegance, patients' expectations and self-image are forcing ever-improving standards in dentistry, placing increasing demands upon the dental practitioner to produce lifelike restorations. Christensen[2] sums up well the importance of improving esthetic skills: "Most dental schools do not offer significant predoctoral courses in Aesthetic Dentistry. However, this portion of one's practice is one of the major growth areas in Dentistry, and it has enormous importance to new dentists as they initiate their careers."

This text outlines esthetic principles that can be applied clinically for creating esthetic fixed restorations. The first three chapters emphasize diagnosis. The following two chapters address tooth preparations as well as solving the problems that may jeopardize the esthetic rendition of anterior restorations. Communication between the clinician and the technician, which is paramount in achieving predictable and desirable results, is the subject of the longest chapter in this text. Finally, the gingival aspects of anterior restorations are discussed in three chapters on gingival preparation, the final impression, and plastic periodontal surgery.

It is impossible to write any material on esthetic dentistry without borrowing from the pioneering work of master clinicians and technicians whose impact is constantly felt in this field. We are deeply indebted to Dr John McLean, Dr Ronald Goldstein, Dr David Garber, Dr Harold Shavell, Dr Lloyd Miller, Dr Jack Preston, and Dr Peter Dawson for contributing so significantly to the field of esthetic dentistry. We would also like to acknowledge the invaluable contributions of Dr Leonard Abrams, Dr Frank Spear, Dr Vincent Kokich, and Dr Pat Allen to the knowledge of the interaction between the facial, gingival, and dental elements. Finally, the ultimate artistry of Willi Geller, MDT, and Makoto Yamamoto, MDT, remains a constant source of inspiration in this ever-expanding and exciting field.

References

1. Loomis A. *Drawing the Head and Hands*. New York: Viking, 1956.
2. Christensen GJ. Achieving and maintaining skills in esthetic dentistry. *Aesthet Chron* 1991;3;32.

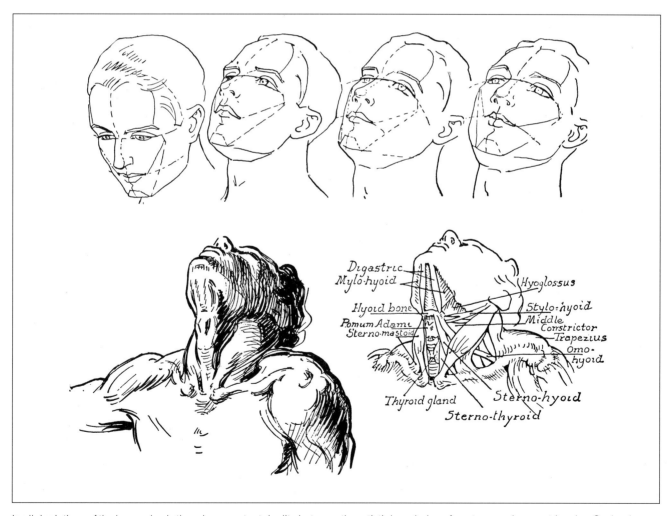

In all depictions of the human body there is a constant duality between the artist's knowledge of anatomy and geometric rules. Such rules are not meant to restrict the imagination of the artist, but simply to serve as a reference. (From V. Perard *Anatomy and Geometry*. New York: Crown Publishers, 1989.)

Acknowledgments

Louisiana State University has always demonstrated a strong commitment to teaching dental ceramics, thanks to the unselfish dedication of Dr Edmund E Jeansonne, Dean Emeritus, and Dr John W McLean, OBE. Their principles and techniques remain a constant source of reference in our work. Dr James D Harrison, Professor and Chairman of the Department of Fixed Prosthodontics, Louisiana State University, has been throughout these past ten years our most inspiring mentor; without his unending support and guidance, this book would not exist. We feel most indebted to our coauthors, Dr Richard Caudill, Dr James Harrison, Dr Edmund Jeansonne, Dr Vincent Kokich, Dr Ron Lemon, and finally Dr John McLean. We would like to acknowledge their invaluable contributions in sharing their unique expertise in this text.

The graphic illustrations are a testimony of the talent of Mrs Kathy Martello, to whom we want to express our deepest gratitude for her persistence and constant attention to details. We would also like to thank those who kindly provided slide materials that serve as a most useful complement to this text: Dr David Garber, Dr John Kent, Dr Kenneth Malament, Dr Michelle de Rouffignac, Dr Harold Shavell, Mr Jacques de Cooman, MDT, Mr Kyle Hale, CDT, Mr Romeo Pascetta, MDT, and Mr Asami Tanaka, CDT.

This project also owes much to the ever-useful technical assistance of Larry LaHoste, CDT, head of the Dental Ceramics Laboratory, and Ron Elliott, CDT, Clinical Instructor of the Dental Technology Program at Louisiana State University. We would also like to extend our gratitude to Dr Israel Finger, Coordinator of the Prosthodontic Graduate Program at Louisiana State University, and his students, Dr D Palmisano, Dr J Ortiz, and Dr R Rooney, for their collaboration. Finally, the editing of the book benefitted from the most helpful assistance and advice of Mrs Maureen Raymond, word processing supervisor at Louisiana State University, School of Dentistry.

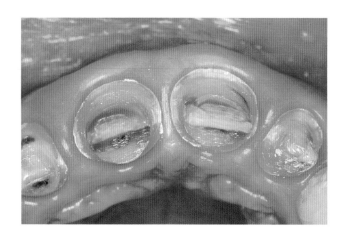

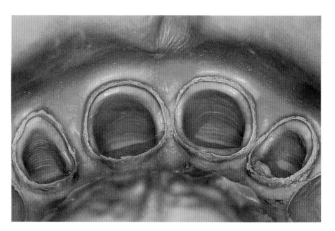

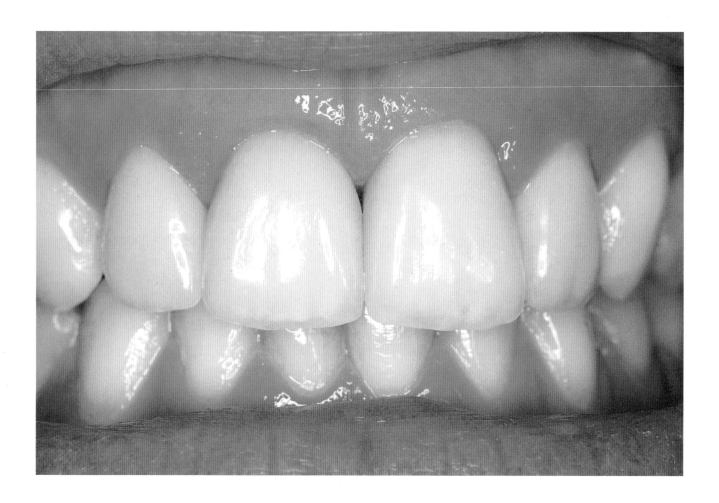

Chapter 1

Artistic and Scientific Principles Applied to Esthetic Dentistry

Gerard Chiche and Alain Pinault

An organized and systematic approach is required to evaluate, diagnose, and resolve esthetic problems predictably. Tooth color is obviously essential in the final result, but esthetic treatment planning should never be devised around shading improvements alone. Our ultimate goal as clinicians is to achieve a pleasing composition in the smile—to create an arrangement of the various esthetic elements to proper proportion or relation according to known principles.[1-3]

Four factors of esthetic composition can be simply and effectively applied to the smile. They serve to assist the clinician in determining adequate tooth display, tooth size, tooth arrangement, and orientation to the face during esthetic diagnosis and during treatment. They are:

- *Frame and reference*[4]: the constructional system that gives shape; a standard for measuring or constructing.
- *Proportion and idealism*[4]: the relation of one part to another or to the whole with respect to magnitude, quantity, or degree; a standard of perfection, beauty, or excellence.
- *Symmetry*[4]: the correspondence in size, shape, and relative position of parts on opposite sides of a dividing line or median plane or around a center or axis.
- *Perspective and illusion*[4]: The technique or process of representing on a plane or curved surface the spatial relation of objects as they might appear to the eye.

The two main objectives in dental esthetics are *(1)* to create teeth of pleasing inherent proportions and of pleasing proportions to one another, and *(2)* to create a pleasing tooth arrangement in harmony with the gingiva, lips, and face of the patient. These two objectives are established by using references and are reinforced with perspective and illusion.

Frame and reference

Artists draw within a measured general frame that is square, rectangular, or circular. This formula is subsequently refined with inner frames and imaginary reference points in order to relate parts to each other and to the original frame.[1-3] In a similar fashion, teeth interact and must harmonize with three frames: face, lips, and gingiva. Esthetic dental diagnosis and treatment are based on the interrelationship between these four elements (Figs. 1-1 and 1-2). These frames themselves may need to be enhanced before dental reconstruction through orthognathic surgery, cosmetic surgery, or gingival surgery.[5]

Horizontal reference lines

An artist drawing a face first establishes a "T" from the central midline and the interpupillary line or the ophriac line.[1-3] From this reference frame, he draws the face from the midline in a purely symmetrical fashion, emphasizing the "T" effect the closer he draws to the midline. Attractiveness results from a general sense of parallelism and symmetry between structural facial features, because parallelism is the most harmonious relationship between two lines.[6] The interpupillary line, the ophriac line, and the commissural line impart an overall sense of harmony and horizontal perspective in the esthetically pleasing face.

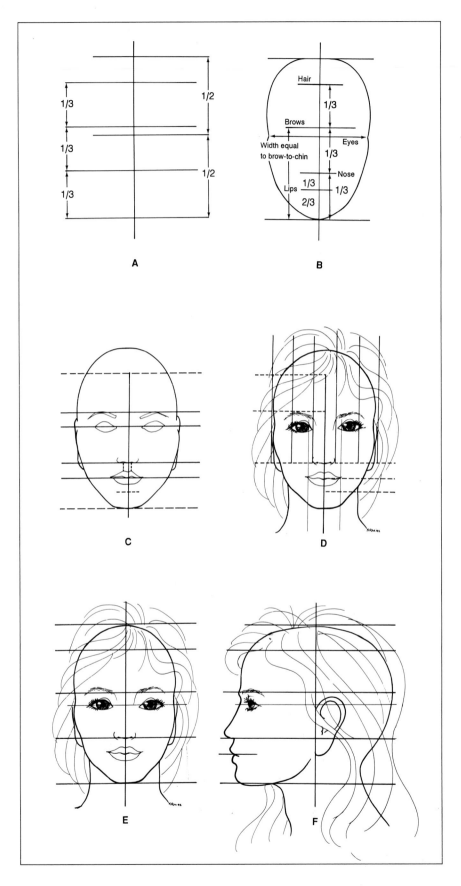

Fig. 1-1 Facial Proportions
A and B, An artist begins drawing a face with a measured general frame that incorporates horizontal and vertical reference lines.

C and D, This formula is subsequently refined with inner frames and imaginary reference points in order to relate parts to each other and to the original frame.

E and F, Vertically, the face is organized around the facial midline. Horizontally, several reference lines perpendicular to the midline create an organized network: the hairline, the ophriac line (eyebrows), the interpupillary line, the interalar line, and the commissural line. Several of these lines are used as reference in esthetic dentistry.

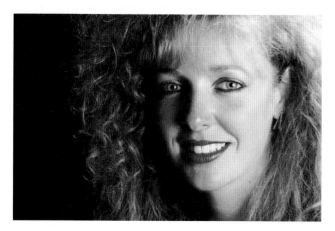

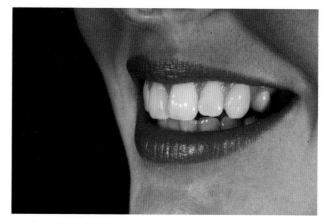

Fig. 1-2a and b   A pleasing natural smile is in harmony with the lips and the face. Objective parameters must be used in esthetic diagnosis to achieve a similar relationship in esthetic rehabilitation.

Interpupillary line

From a dental standpoint, the general direction of the incisal plane of the maxillary teeth and the gingival margin outline must parallel the interpupillary line mainly,[7] whereas the ophriac and commissural lines serve as accessory lines. This harmony must be further reinforced by the incisal plane following the lower lip line during smiling. Achieving a general sense of alignment is more important than focusing on one preconceived line and basing an entire diagnosis on it (Fig. 1-3).

Fig. 1-3   An esthetically pleasing incisal plane has a general horizontal orientation that is parallel to the interpupillary line.

The Interpupillary Line

The Interpupillary Line Serves to Evaluate the Orientation of the:

- Incisal plane
- Gingival margins
- Maxilla

Even though strict parallelism between these elements is not required, it must be determined whether they conflict or not with the general horizontal perspective of the face. Many individuals exhibit some degree of canting of the maxilla, which can be easily demonstrated by drawing an imaginary line across the gingival margins or the cusp tips of the canines or first premolars.

For most patients, mild canting is not conspicuous and requires little or no correction. Moderate canting results in some pleasing irregularity in the dental reconstruction, but the gingival plane may have to be partially corrected to achieve pleasing symmetry of the central incisors (Fig. 1-4).

Other patients place greater importance on perfect alignment and symmetry of the dentition and the gingiva because their expectations are based on a media image.[8] Full correction of the gingival plane may be required for such patients before crown reconstruction. Severe canting of the maxilla involves more aggressive treatment with various combinations of surgery, orthodontics, or crown restorations[9] (Fig. 1-5).

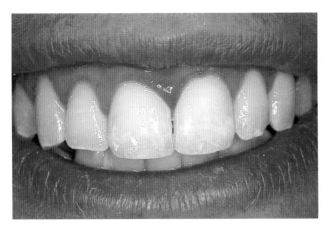

Fig. 1-4 The slant of the incisal plane in this patient is caused by the inclination of the maxilla. The gingival plane follows the direction of the maxilla and should be surgically altered before cosmetic or restorative corrections. A partial realignment of the gingival margins of the central incisors and of the left lateral incisor with the interpupillary line is indicated.

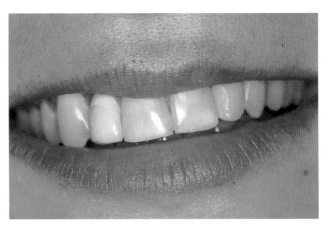

Fig. 1-5 This patient shows severe misalignment of the incisal plane in relation to the upper lip and the interpupillary line. Correction may require orthognathic surgery, orthodontics or periodontics, and restorative dentistry in various combinations.

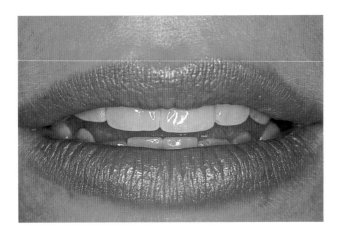

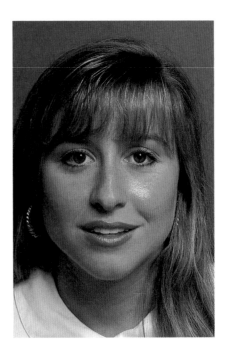

Fig. 1-6a and b At rest the incisal display varies according to the length of the upper lip and the age and sex of the patient. This patient has a display of approximately 3.5 mm, which falls within the expected average for a young female patient.

Lip lines

The length and curvature of the lips significantly influence the amount of tooth exposure at rest and in function. For example, full concave lips are often associated with a prominent display of the maxillary teeth. From a cultural standpoint, a prominent smile with bright teeth is synonymous with youth and dynamism.[5] The clinician should be aware that many middle-aged and older patients prefer, consciously or not, the benefits of a youthful appearance, with prominent tooth display.[10] Vig and Brundo[11] demonstrated

that the average maxillary incisor display with the lips at rest is 1.91 mm in men and 3.40 mm in women. Short upper lips generally display more maxillary tooth structure (3.65 mm) than do long lips (0.59 mm). Younger patients (up to 29 years) display more maxillary tooth structure (3.37 mm) than middle-aged (30 to 50 years) patients (1.26 mm) (Figs. 1-6 and 1-7). These findings invalidate the standard practice of establishing an average tooth display of 1 to 2 mm regardless of lip length.

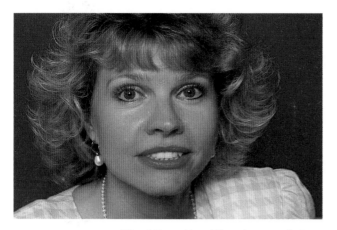
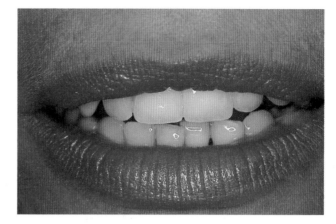

Fig. 1-7a and b When the upper lip is concave, more incisal display is expected, especially in young female patients. The incisal length achieved with this three-unit fixed partial denture replacing the left central incisor is critical for harmony with the lips and the face.

Lip Lines

The Upper Lip Line Serves to Evaluate:
- The length of maxillary incisor exposed at rest and during smile
- The vertical position of the gingival margins during smile

The Lower Lip Line Serves to Evaluate:
- The buccolingual position of the incisal edge of maxillary incisors
- The curvature of the incisal plane

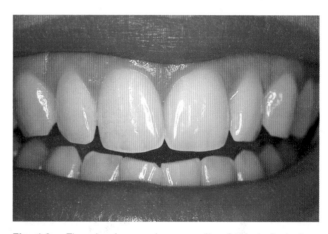

Fig. 1-8 The pleasing regular convexity of this incisal plane results in a progression of the size of the incisal embrasures from the central incisors to the canines.

In unrestored dentitions, a straight smile line is usually caused by attrition,[12] therefore, a correlation between wear of the incisal edge and patient's age is logical. When the incisal edges of the canines and the central incisors are aligned on a convexity, the incisal plane is convex (Fig. 1-8). When the incisal edges of the canines and the central incisors are aligned but are longer than the lateral incisors, the incisal plane has a "gull wing" configuration[13] (Fig. 1-9). Finally, a combination of these two pleasing arrangements is also often observed in the same mouth. Youth is expressed with prominent and well-developed central incisors, well-defined incisal embrasures, and a convex or "gull wing" smile line. Age is associated with reduced incisal embrasures, leveling of the "gull wing" effect, and a straight smile line (Fig. 1-10).[5,13] Currently most patients are more interested in enhancing their self-esteem with the benefits of youthful

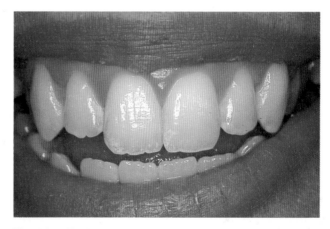

Fig. 1-9 The incisal plane assumes a "gull wing" configuration where the incisal edges of the lateral incisors are apical to the level of the central incisors and canines. The gull wing, convex, and combination pattern (convex and gull wing on either side of the midline) represent esthetically pleasing configurations.

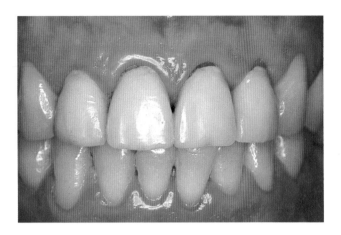

Fig. 1-10 Deficient anterior crowns typically include a straight incisal plane, closed incisal embrasures, and a lack of progression of incisal embrasures from the central incisors to the canines. This implies that the central incisors may be too short and the convexity of the incisal plane must be accentuated, or that the lateral incisors may be too long and the "gull wing" of the incisal plane must be emphasized, or possibly a combination of both modifications.

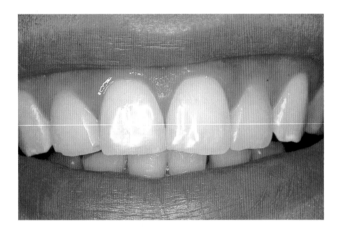

Fig. 1-11a The concave configuration of the incisal plane may be displeasing. This patient requested correction of the irregularities in her smile as well as crowning of the left lateral incisor, which had been devitalized and was fractured lingually.

Fig. 1-11b and c Cosmetic and restorative correction that included an all-ceramic crown helped reduce the concavity of the incisal plane and create a moderate convexity in harmony with the lower lip line.

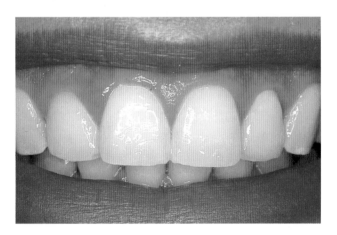

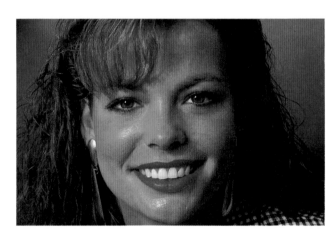

smiles rather than in obtaining realistic and aged smiles.[5] Therefore, esthetic reconstruction of middle-aged and older patients must often incorporate unworn, prominent central incisors and a convex smile line normally expected in young individuals (Fig. 1-11).

A straight smile line is a common mistake found in previously restored dentitions for young or middle-aged patients and results in lack of progression of the incisal embrasures from central incisor to canine. This either means that the central incisors were shortened or that the lateral incisors were elongated in comparison with the original.

The exposure of the gingival margins must be evaluated at various smile positions. During a "moderate"

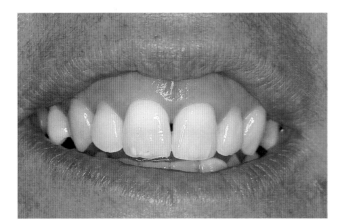

Fig. 1-12 This patient shows an excessive display of gingival tissue or a "gummy smile." Esthetic correction is preferably achieved with orthognathic surgery. Periodontal treatment consisting of surgical elongation would likely expose the cementoenamel junctions excessively and result in elongated teeth. Full crowns would then be required to restore the teeth to a normal size and would create difficulty in maintaining a correct anterior guidance and harmony with the posterior plane of occlusion.

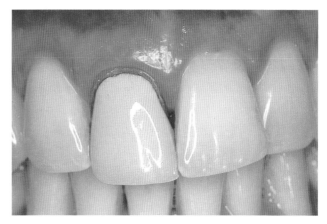

Fig. 1-13 The orientation of the gingival plane is evaluated in relation to the interpupillary line and the upper lip line. Severe gingival asymmetry between the maxillary central incisors must be surgically or orthodontically corrected before prosthetic treatment. Bilateral asymmetry between the lateral incisors or canines does not automatically require realignment.

smile, the upper lip border may cover the cervical aspect of the maxillary incisors with no gingival display or may expose up to 3 mm of gingival tissue. There is thus a wide range of acceptability. A smile can be termed "gummy" when more than 3 mm of gingival tissue is exposed during a "moderate" smile.[14] Various smile positions, including a strained smile, must be used to confirm the initial impression (Fig. 1-12).

Gingival asymmetry of the maxillary central incisors requires special attention. No correction is required if the lip line is low. With medium-to-high lip lines, obvious cervical disharmony between the maxillary central incisors requires either surgical or orthodontic correction (Fig. 1-13 and 1-14). Gingival symmetry between the lateral incisors or between the canines is not mandatory, and unilateral display of the free gingival margin of a lateral incisor or a canine in various smile positions is also esthetically acceptable.

Vertical reference lines

The "T" effect created by the interpupillary line perpendicular to the facial midline is emphasized in a pleasing face, with horizontal elements such as the ophriac line and the commissural line, and with vertical elements such as the bridge of the nose and the philtrum. This sense of harmony must be reinforced with the direction of the incisal plane, the gingival plane, and the position and axis of the dental midline. According to Golub,[15] the dental midline perpendicular to the interpupillary line offers one of the most striking facial contrasts, serving to anchor the smile on the face.

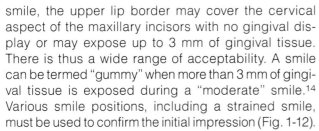

Facial Midline

The Facial Midline Serves to Evaluate:
- The location and axis of the dental midline
- Mediolateral discrepancies in tooth position

Logically, the maxillary central incisal midline should coincide with the midline of the face. However, daily observation reveals that a lack of coincidence between location and direction of the two midlines is no esthetic liability unless the dental midline is conspicuously oblique or distinctly off to one side (Fig. 1-15). In the latter case, the verticality of the dental midline appears to be much more critical than its mediolateral position.[16]

A distinct discrepancy between the maxillary central incisal midline and the facial midline indicates a mediolateral abnormality in tooth position usually caused by the absence of a single anterior tooth. A severe discrepancy may require orthodontic therapy to restore coincidence of the midlines by providing space for the missing tooth prior to prosthetic replacement.[17] In milder deviations, no treatment may be indicated. Golub[15] cautions against achieving a perfectly centered dental midline with the face because it creates too much uniformity. Conversely, a vertical and centered dental midline may be used to avert attention from asymmetrical facial features.

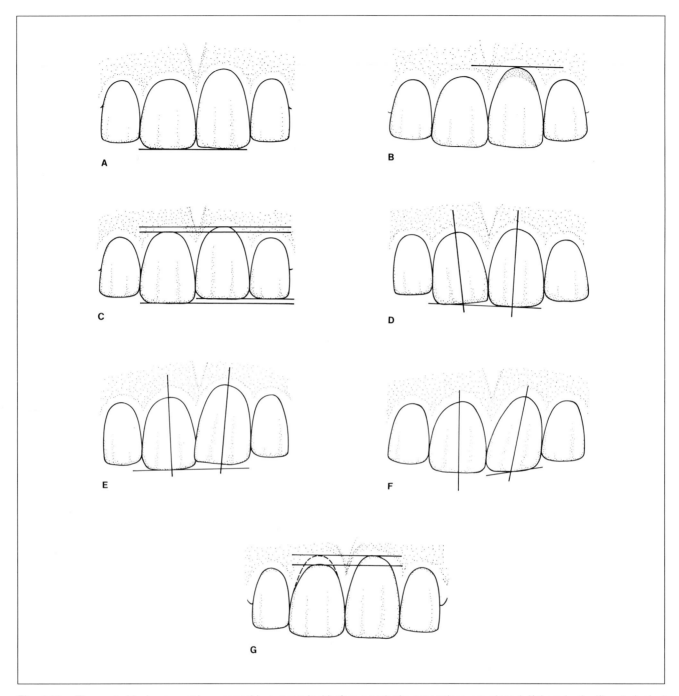

Fig. 1-14 The central incisors must be reasonably symmetrical before prosthetic restorations are placed. If there is significant gingival asymmetry between the central incisors, several restorative options are available according to the patient's preference:

A, Restore the central incisors at the same incisal level. This option is indicated with a low lip line.

B, Restore the central incisors at the same incisal level but create a root effect on the long crown to align its cervical convexity with the shorter crown.

C, Restore the central incisors with equal crown length so that the gingival discrepancy is reproduced at the incisal level.

D, Restore the shorter incisor with a mesial tilt for additional length.

E, Rotate the longer incisor mesially and shorten its distal incisal aspect to shorten it slightly.

F, Bevel the distal incisal aspect of the longer crown so that it is significantly shorter than the mesial aspect (Geller modification).

G, Correct the gingival discrepancy surgically before restoring the two crowns with the same length. This option is preferred when the patient objects to significant irregularities in the smile.

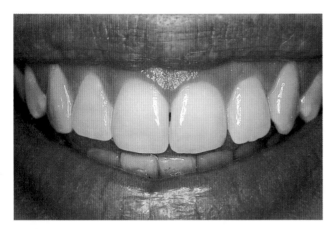

Fig. 1-15 In a pleasing natural smile, the dental midline is frequently inclined, imparting a mild pleasing asymmetry. When the midline is centered with the philtrum, it may be restored with a slight oblique inclination. If it is deviated in relation to the center of the philtrum, it should preferably be restored vertical. Bilateral asymmetry between the shape and rotation of the lateral incisors and between the facial-lingual inclination of the canines is frequently encountered in natural dentition.

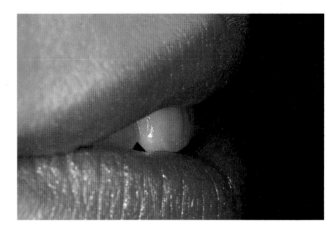

Fig. 1-16 Normal central incisor–lower lip relationship during "f" or "v" sounds. The incisal third contacts the mucous part of the lower lip, allowing for a smooth path of closure of the lower lip.

Sagittal references

The contours of the upper and lower lips are part of the profile analysis and should be used as a guide to tooth position. Various soft tissue analyses are available[18–21] for the assessment of the profile convexity, the amount of lip protrusion or retrusion, and the amount of chin recession or prominence. For more complex situations, and especially with skeletal abnormalities, an orthodontic consultation with cephalometric analysis is strongly recommended.

Upper lip support

Upper lip support is controlled to a certain extent by the position of the maxillary teeth. According to Pound,[22] tooth position more significantly affects thinner and protruded lips than lips that are thick, retruded, or vertical.

Lip support is a better guide of tooth position than of incisal edge position, as suggested on cephalometric studies by Maritato and Douglas[23]: in 70% of the subjects they investigated, the gingival two thirds rather than the incisal one third of the maxillary central incisors contributed the main support of the lip.

Lower lip relation

The relationship of the maxillary incisal edges to the lower lip is a guide for a general assessment of incisal edge position and length. The "F" or "V" position is defined as the position at which the incisal edges of the maxillary anterior teeth permit the most fluent pronunciation of the "F" or "V" sounds.[24] When these consonants are pronounced, the incisal edges should make a definite contact at the inner vermilion border of the lower lip (Fig. 1-16).

These positions are valuable in determining the facial position of the incisal third of the maxillary central incisor, which must conform to the path of closure of the lower lip.[25] The lips must slide smoothly without interference from the teeth, but according to Dawson,[25] the failure to properly contour the incisal third is a common mistake seen in anterior restorations, in which case the incisal edge frequently contacts the cutaneous part of the lip.

The occlusal plane

The occlusal plane is the common plane established by the incisal and occlusal surfaces of the teeth and conventionally coincides (with minor variations[26]) with Camper's plane, which is a plane extending from the inferior border of the ala of the nose to the superior border of the tragus of the ear.[27]

The incisal plane may not correspond to the posterior plane of occlusion in case of supraeruption of maxillary anterior teeth, and if the posterior plane of occlusion is correctly aligned, it may serve to diagnose faulty incisal length.[28]

Phonetic references

Four separate phonetic references aid esthetic diagnosis. The "M" sound is used to achieve a relaxed rest position. Between "M" sounds repeated at slow intervals, the clinician can evaluate the amount of incisal display in the rest position.[14] The "F" or "V" sounds are used to determine the lingual tilt of the incisal third of the maxillary central incisors and whether they are abnormally elongated.[24,25] The "S" sound determines the vertical dimension of speech.[29] In this position,

Fig. 1-17a–c   Excessive length of the central incisors is diagnosed in relation to: *(1)* the upper lip, *(2)* the level of the posterior plane of occlusion, and *(3)* tooth length (ie, 13 mm) that is above average. When planning modifications in incisal length, it is best not to rely solely on a single diagnostic clue. When in the "s"-sound position, the central incisors are in near contact, but there is approximately 4 to 6 mm of posterior speaking space between the premolars and molars. If it were required for esthetic improvement and/or restorative purposes, it would be possible to restore the vertical dimension of occlusion by an additional 3 mm and still not violate the closest speaking space between the teeth necessary to make an "s" sound.

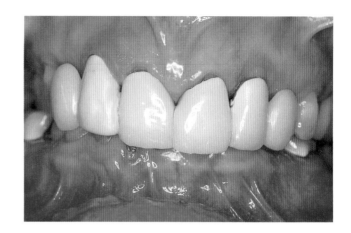

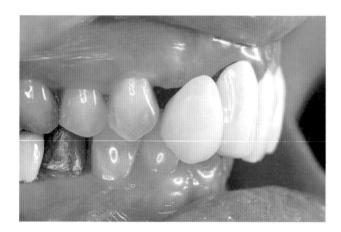

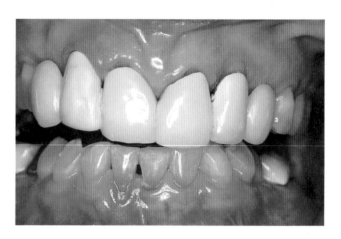

the incisal edges of the maxillary and mandibular anterior teeth come in near contact and determine the "anterior speaking space." The amount of posterior speaking space varies with the amount of mandibular protrusion necessary to bring the anterior teeth in near contact for the "S" sound. Therefore, in patients with a Class I or Class II occlusal relationship, the posterior speaking space is greater than the anterior speaking space. In terms of dental reconstruction, these patients can usually accept variance in their vertical dimension of occlusion as long as it remains within the vertical dimension of speech (Fig. 1-17). Because the speaking space of patients with a Class III occlusal relationship is approximately the same anteriorly and posteriorly, such patients cannot tolerate as much variation of their vertical dimension of occlusion because it would interfere with their speaking space.[29,30]

Proportion and idealism

The term *idealism* serves to study and replicate ideal tooth forms before creating variation and character-

ization. The term *proportion* implies geometry and arithmetic — associating beauty with numerical values conforms to the concept that beauty is fundamentally exact.[10] Throughout the ages artists have tried to standardize the proportions of the human body into rules or canons. Early on, beauty was equated with a harmony of proportions,[31] because certain proportions appeal to our emotions whereas others leave us indifferent. This preoccupation with mathematical formulas as the basis of art means that, up to a point, beauty can be rationally defined and taught to the student.[1–3]

Idealism and proportion are tools, not goals; they are merely a useful guide within which the artist's imagination has free play.[31] Lombardi[6] pointed to the importance of the proportion between width and length in the dimensions of individual teeth and between the respective size of the anterior teeth. In esthetic dentistry, proportion and idealism serve to determine *(1)* the optimum size of the maxillary central incisors and *(2)* the optimum relationship between the dimensions of the maxillary central incisor, lateral incisor, and canine (Figs. 1-18–1-23). These two elements are further discussed in chapter 3.

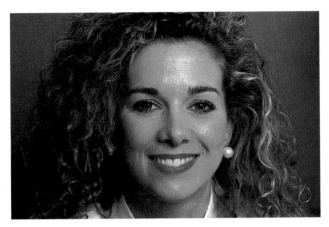

Fig. 1-18 Central incisors are dominant in this pleasing natural smile. An esthetic dental composition needs a dominant element, which should be the central incisors. Lack of dominance of the central incisors is a most common deficiency with anterior crowns.

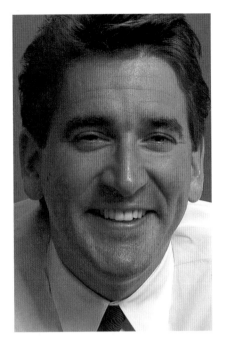

Fig. 1-19 A dynamic youthful smile is associated with dominant, prominent central incisors, and a convex smile line.

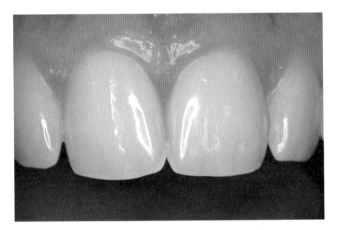

Fig. 1-20 Pleasing proportions of the central incisors are expressed in a width-to-length ratio of approximately 75% to 80%. Pleasing central incisors of pleasing proportions are an essential aspect of a successful esthetic rehabilitation.

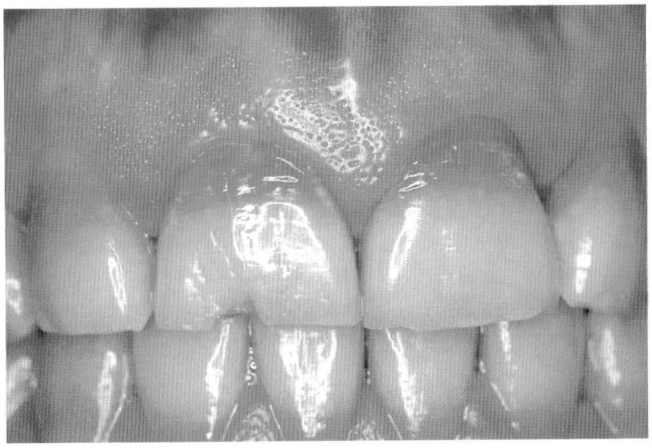

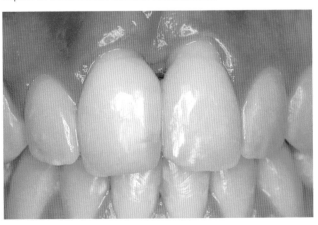

Fig. 1-21 Short square or short tapered incisors are displeasing because their width-to-length ratio exceeds 85%. This can be corrected by incisal elongation with porcelain laminate veneers or crowns, as long as this does not result in excessive incisal display, or with surgical elongation followed by restorations of the appropriate length.

Fig. 1-22 Long narrow incisors are displeasing because their width-to-length ratio is below 65%. This can be corrected either by shortening the clinical crown with a full crown, as long as there is sufficient incisal display remaining, or with a root coverage procedure. If these are not feasible, restorations should impart an illusion of shorter and wider teeth.

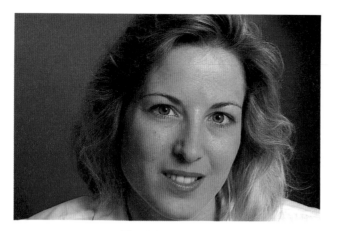 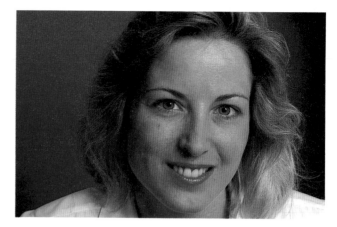

Fig. 1-23a and b Dominant central incisors. The four maxillary incisors are restored with porcelain foil crowns. The dominance of the central incisors over the lateral incisors may be accentuated slightly more than necessary as long as the central incisor is proportionate and maintains a pleasing width-to-length ratio.

Symmetry and diversity

Symmetry refers to the regularity or balance of tooth arrangement and serves to define how much regularity is required and how much asymmetry is allowed in the dental composition. As observers we desire to see objects in a stable position because the eye is conditioned by expectations based on past experience. We unconsciously expect to perceive a reasonable amount of facial symmetry, which is reinforced by the smile. This perception of order in the face relies on parallel lines, symmetry, and recurring ratios. Confusion and tension are produced with obvious or unusual facial asymmetries, such as that which occurs with Bell's palsy.

Patients' preferences

Brisman[32] demonstrated that many patients prefer equilibrated smile arrangements with either alike teeth on a straight incisal plane (horizontal symmetry) or normal-sized teeth on a mildly convex incisal plane (radiating symmetry[33]). This comes from a desire of acceptability in our society,[34] which associates youth and success with regularity and aging and disorder with irregularity and misalignment.

The patient's perception of his or her own dentofacial appearance is subject to cultural variations. Some dental irregularities are acceptable to lay groups according to European surveys,[35,36] whereas in North America many adolescents are already sensitive to overbite, overjet, and dental crowding and their influence on facial features.[37–39] This image of the ideal smile[8] is constantly reinforced in all facets of media and advertising.

Given these circumstances, there is a need for good dentist-patient communication and education about artificial and natural-looking dentitions. The clinician must initially determine the patient's desires. According to Miller, the "media smile" is characterized by white and aligned teeth with an absence of gingival and incisal embrasures and long contact areas.[8] These patients characteristically seek to have a noticeable smile. Patients who prefer a pleasing natural appearance still seek the benefits of a youthful smile but consent to various degrees of dental irregularities. The dentist should involve and solicit the patient's input as early as possible in the treatment[40,41] to determine in which of these two categories the patient belongs. The active participation of the patient is crucial in the final acceptance of the treatment.[5,42]

Pleasing natural symmetry

An esthetic composition involves an arrangement of elements conceived around a unifying principle (unity in variety) but with sufficient diversity to create interest (diversity in unity). Unity is the prime requisite for giving a composition order and purpose with proportion and symmetry.[43]

Symmetry is almost synonymous with unity,[43] but subtle diversity is needed because excessive regularity is monotonous. Harmonious facial features are more symmetrical close to the facial midline and more asymmetrical away from the facial midline. For a pleasing smile, this means: the closer to the dental midline, the more symmetrical the smile must be; the further away from the dental midline, the more asymmetrical the smile may be. Therefore, in a natural pleasing smile, pleasing tooth symmetry is found close to the

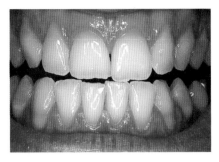
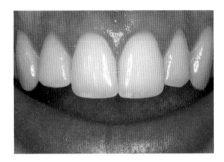
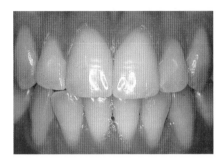

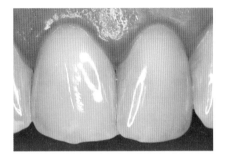
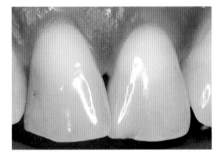

Fig. 1-24a–c   In these three esthetically pleasing dentitions, the central incisors are mostly symmetrical with subtle minor asymmetries. The lateral incisors are definitely asymmetrical in form and position, and the canines are asymmetrical mostly in position. Usually, the smile is symmetrical close to the midline and asymmetrical away from it: pleasing symmetry is observed at the central incisors and pleasing asymmetry at the lateral incisors and canines.

Fig. 1-25a and b   Subtle patterns of asymmetry are commonly found on the central incisors: the dental midline may be slightly oblique, one of the two central incisors may be either slightly rotated or assume a more facial position, or the distal aspect of the incisal edges and the distal incisal corners may be bilaterally asymmetrical.

midline and pleasing irregularity away from the midline. This rule combines order and spontaneity: the "T" between the facial midline and the pupillary line must not be antagonized with pronounced asymmetry close to the midline, but at the same time, dentofacial features do not need to be totally symmetrical to impart beauty. This is because lateral asymmetries are more pleasing to the eye than median asymmetries. A very tilted dental midline or a slanted incisal plane are displeasing. The patient or the observer may not precisely discriminate the problem, but confusion and uneasiness ensue.

The goal in a natural smile is to achieve a pleasing balance between idealism and diversity[43] because in a subtle way natural dentitions are always asymmetrical (Figs. 1-24, and 1-25).

Natural variations

Dental midline

A perfectly vertical dental midline reinforces the perception of order and organization but also imparts some artificiality.[46] Miller et al found that the dental midline coincided with the median line of the face in 70.4% of the population.[47] This is consistent with the "dentogenic" concept, which states that an eccentric midline, if not too exaggerated, is acceptable and lends to the illusion of the natural dentition.[46]

Maxillary central incisors

These teeth must be kept symmetrical within reasonable limits. Minor asymmetries are allowed, because bilateral asymmetry between maxillary central incisors was found not to exceed 0.3 to 0.4 mm in mesiodistal width.[48,49] The shape and outlines of the central incisors studied were strictly identical in only 14% of the subjects, were similar in 23% (one or two dimensions not exceeding 0.2 mm), and were dissimilar (differences in all three dimensions, one of which was more than 0.2 mm) in 63% of subjects.[49]

Maxillary lateral incisors

Maxillary lateral incisors display more variations in shape than central incisors and are often bilaterally asymmetrical in the same mouth. Variations in the mesiodistal diameter of lateral incisors are wide (3.98 mm average) and of greater magnitude than in central incisors (2.98 mm average).[50–53] This explains why extreme variations in shape are frequently observed within the same mouth. In addition, the gingival margins of lateral incisors are not aligned and displayed evenly during a smile. For this reason, gingival correction between the lateral incisors is indicated only with obvious and displeasing asymmetry. Within the same mouth, lateral incisors differ bilaterally in basic shape, abrasion, axis, rotation, and length. The diversity of the dental reconstruction, therefore, should rely on asymmetry of the lateral incisors.

Maxillary canines

The clinical crown length of both canines is similar, but their wear patterns may be different. A difference in their vertical alignment is a frequent finding. The gingival margins and cusp tip of the canines are usually not aligned on the same horizontal level because of asymmetry or cant of the maxilla. As a result, the canine tips are not displayed evenly during a smile and the incisal embrasure progression from central incisor to canine is bilaterally asymmetrical. There seems to be no valid reason to align the canines on the same horizontal level unless the patient requests perfect alignment; therefore, full surgical correction of the gingival plane is rarely indicated to realign the canines unless it is used to compensate for the cant of the maxilla. Another common finding is the difference in buccolingual inclination of the canines, which results in bilateral asymmetry of the incisal embrasures and of the buccal corridors. Therefore, an important role of the canines is to control the effective width of the smile by occluding part of the buccal corridors.

Perspective and illusion

The term *perspective* is used in dentistry to express (1) how the perception of the shape of an individual tooth may be altered and (2) how the elements of an esthetic composition may affect one another.

Altering the perception of an individual tooth

Widening and narrowing

The illusion of larger or narrower teeth in the same space is created by varying the outline or silhouette form, which in turns affects light reflection. Pincus[54] described the silhouette form of the tooth as the portion that reflects light straight forward. Therefore, by narrowing or enlarging the silhouette form, the illusion of a smaller or larger tooth is created by deflecting more or less light to the side. The eye is susceptible to trickery of lines and curves, and procedures for altering shape have been well docu-

---

Rules of Symmetry/Asymmetry for Maxillary Anterior Teeth

Symmetry	Asymmetry
• The dental midline is straight.	• The dental midline may be slightly oblique in relation to the facial midline.
• The smile line follows the convexity of the lower lip.	• The incisal edges of the central incisors may be slightly misaligned if their gingival margins are not level.
• The central incisors are symmetrical.	
• The gingival margins of the central incisors are symmetrical.	• Teeth should not be aligned in all three planes of space to suggest alignment; they should diverge in at least one plane.
• Incisal embrasures gradually deepen from the central incisor to the canine.[44]	• A central incisor may slightly overlap the other or occupy a more facial position or may be slightly rotated facially.[45]
• The incisal plane is either convex, sinuous, or a combination of both.	• A central incisor may be more mesially inclined than the other.[45]
• Mesial tooth inclinations are more pleasing than distal inclinations.[13]	• The distal incisal angle of the central incisors may be bilaterally asymmetrical.[45]
	• Lateral incisors may differ bilaterally in shape, inclination, abrasion, and rotation; their gingival margins do not need to be level.
	• The labiolingual inclination of the canines may be slightly asymmetrical.

mented.[54–56] Eissman[56] pointed out that, separately, these changes are moderately effective and that for a meaningful effect they should be used in combination. Some effects are also more effective in one direction than another. For example, central incisors that appear too narrow are not easily altered by displacing the line angles laterally. This is because the line angles may already be close enough to the proximal contacts and because it is difficult to obtain a pleasing natural aspect with a flattened central incisor. When central incisors appear slightly too wide, displacing their line angles and increasing the convexity of their facial aspect effectively suggests a narrower silhouette because there is comparably more leeway to displace line angles medially and to emphasize the median ridge if necessary (Fig. 1-26).

Altering Maxillary Incisors

Widening

- Displace line angles laterally
- Flatten facial outline
- Highlight texture and gloss with horizontal lines and ridges
- Decrease facial embrasures
- Displace proximal contacts labially
  Applications include:
- To correct crowding (limited result)
- To increase narrow pontic space
- To improve tooth proportions
- To correct elongated clinical crowns after periodontal or implant surgery

Narrowing

- Displace line angles medially
- Increase the convexity of the facial outline
- Highlight texture and gloss with vertical lines and ridges
- Displace proximal contacts lingually
- Increase the facial embrasures
- Shadow the proximal aspects with extrinsic staining
  Applications include:
- To close diastema
- To reduce large pontic space
- To control tooth proportions

Shortening

- Emphasize the prominence of the cervical convexity
- Displace the cervical convexity coronally
- Accentuate the downward tilt of the incisal third
- Highlight texture and gloss with horizontal lines and ridges
- Emphasize the cementoenamel junction
  Applications include:
- Asymmetry of the maxillary central incisors
- Long pontics
- To control proportions
- To correct elongated clinical crowns after periodontal or implant surgery

Lengthening

- Flatten the cervical convexity
- Displace the cervical convexity apically
- Highlight texture and gloss of the line angles and create vertical ridges
- Lighten the cervical aspect
  Applications include:
- Asymmetry of the maxillary central incisors
- To correct a short maxillary central incisor that cannot be lengthened surgically

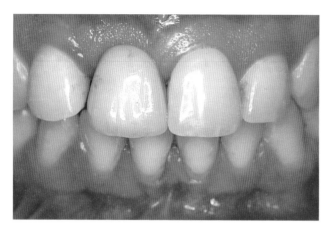

Fig. 1-26 An implant crown replaces the maxillary central incisor. This patient wished to close the original diastema, which required that the crown be made significantly wider than the adjacent central incisor. The distal line angle had to be displaced toward the center of the tooth to narrow its silhouette and suggest the illusion of a narrower crown. (In collaboration with A. Mendez, DDS.)

Shortening and lengthening

The illusion of shorter or longer teeth is produced by varying the outline or silhouette form, which in turn affects light reflection. The cervical portion of the incisor curves toward the gingival aspect and reflects light upward, whereas the incisal third curves lingually and reflects light downward.[54] By shortening or lengthening the silhouette form, the illusion of a shorter or longer tooth is created by deflecting more or less light vertically.

As explained earlier, several effects must be used in combination to produce a meaningful illusion. These techniques have limited applications in lengthening a central incisor that appears to be too short because there is little latitude in a short tooth to displace lines and prominences and maintain pleasing anatomy and tooth proportions. Surgical repositioning of the gingival margin provides better esthetic results.

Widening and Shortening

A challenge in creating illusions of tooth shapes is the restoration of the periodontally involved dentition after the teeth have been lengthened. If restored as such, the principles of pleasing proportions are violated because the central incisors are too long and not dominant enough, even if the lateral incisors are narrowed mesiodistally. Tooth-to-tooth proportions are thus also violated. There are two possible solutions according to the length of the patient's lip:

1. *Short lip*. The patient can tolerate a shortening of the clinical crowns by as much as 3 to 4 mm so that harmonious proportions may be reestablished and still maintain tooth visibility during speech. The control of at least a whole arch is necessary, and most frequently all abutments need endodontic therapy.[57,58] The vertical dimension of occlusion is often preserved because the anterior teeth are frequently found to have supraerupted and need to be shortened to some degree.

2. *Long lip*. Shortening of the clinical crown on a patient with a long lip may compromise tooth exposure and result in an aged appearance. Only some cosmetic recontouring and leveling are permitted with a long lip.

Several effects must be used in combination to suggest pleasing intrinsic proportions of the central incisors, dominance of the central incisors, and expansion of the whole arch in order to avoid a narrow smile effect with long teeth. All the elements outlined to shorten and widen a maxillary central incisor must be emphasized to the fullest (Fig. 1-27).

Prosthetic Options for Periodontally Involved Teeth that Cannot be Shortened

- Widen the central incisors
- Narrow the lateral incisors mesiodistally as much as possible
- Overlap the central incisors over the lateral incisors
- Rotate the mesial surfaces of the lateral incisors to suggest wider central incisors
- Rotate the distal surfaces of lateral incisors and canines facially
- Straighten or tilt the long axis of the canines distally
- Increase the depth and width of the mesial embrasure of the canines

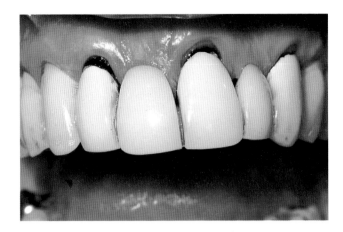

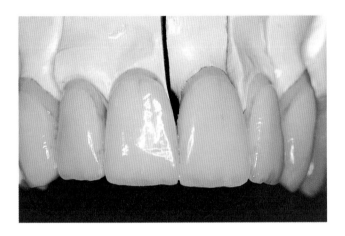

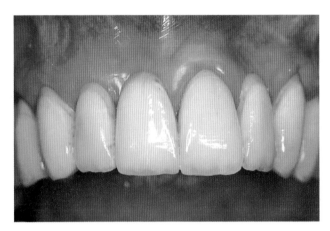

Fig. 1-27a–c   This patient initially had minimal tooth display in relation to the upper lip, thus the incisal edge could not be relocated apically to improve tooth proportion after periodontal surgery. A combination of several measures was necessary to suggest the illusion of wider and shorter teeth. The central incisors are restored by: *(1)* flattening their facial aspect and displacing the line angles to the lateral aspects to suggest width; *(2)* accentuating the root effect of the central incisors to displace their cervical convexity coronally; *(3)* narrowing the lateral incisors as much as possible in order to emphasize the dominance of the central incisors.

Altering perception between teeth

Tooth length and position are perceived by comparison or contrast with the adjacent teeth. Altering individual tooth shape may cause an altered perception of adjacent teeth. Therefore, anterior teeth are interpreted in perspective of one another. The cardinal rule is: everything is relative to something else.

Perspective by contrast

A maxillary incisor may be perceived longer than it really is if the two adjacent teeth are made shorter. Conversely, it may be perceived shorter than it really is if the two adjacent teeth are made longer. This effect is useful with lateral incisors to create a perspective by contrast; if the maxillary central incisor needs to be lengthened to improve its proportion and to accentuate its dominance, the lateral incisor may be shortened to suggest contrast (Fig. 1-28). Alternatively, if the lateral incisor appears too short and misaligned, it is converted into a small canine so that most of its crown is kept shorter, but only the incisal tip reaches the incisal plane to suggest some length (Fig. 1-29).

Parallel perspective

If the axis of a maxillary canine crown is too facial as dictated by root position or preparation axis, this contrast may be reduced by bringing the labial outline of the first premolar facially (Fig. 1-30). Similarly, if the axis of the maxillary first premolar is too facial (as dictated by an implant position, for example), the distal portion of the canine could be rotated outward to suggest alignment with the first premolar (Fig. 1-31).

Shading perspective

In natural dentition, the four maxillary incisors usually have the same shade, whereas the canines appear darker. This is difficult to replicate prosthetically because four maxillary incisor crowns of identical shade may appear artificial. The patient may also object to the abrupt color change between the lateral incisors and the canines. It is preferable to create a smooth transition with a progressive shade saturation from the central incisor to the canine. This also emphasizes the dominance of the maxillary central incisors because their value is higher than the lateral incisors and it generates pleasing diversity and individuality between the crowns[45] (Fig. 1-32).

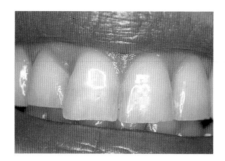
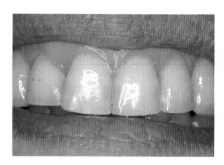

Fig. 1-28a and b Perspective by contrast: the right lateral incisor is too short, and the patient wished to avoid any restoration if possible. Reshaping and shortening the distal incisal aspect of the adjacent central incisor gives the illusion of a longer lateral incisor in a new perspective.

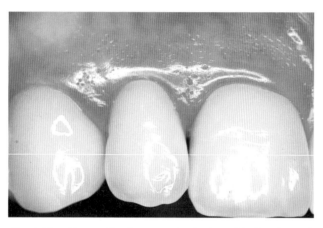

Fig. 1-29 Perspective by contrast: the lateral incisor is much shorter than the central incisor and the canine, but it could appear too narrow and long if it were aligned with the other teeth. This pointed canine shape recaptures some of the desired alignment while maintaining a balanced shape of the lateral incisor.

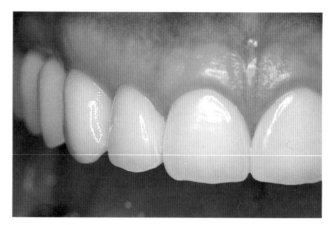

Fig. 1-30 Parallel perspective: with a wide pontic space, the illusion of a narrow lateral incisor was suggested by displacing the line angles toward the center of the tooth. In addition, the canine had to be restored slightly to the facial aspect because of restrictions imposed by the preparation; therefore, the first premolar pontic was displaced facially to reduce the prominence of the canine and suggest an illusion of alignment.

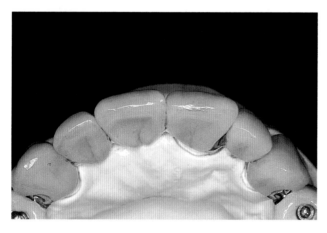
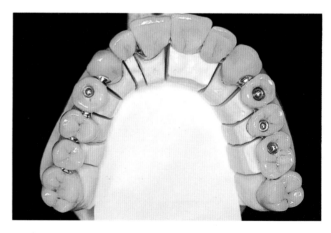

Fig. 1-31a and b Parallel perspective: implant position and screw emergence dictated a facial position of the premolars. To minimize the esthetic liability caused by facially inclined premolars, the canines were rotated so that their distal aspects could be more prominent and suggest a correct alignment of the first premolars.

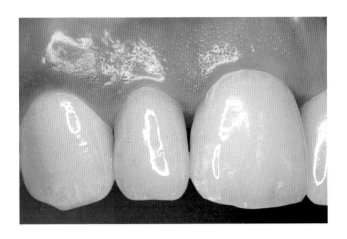

Fig. 1-32 Shading perspective: the central incisors are restored with a lighter shade than the lateral incisors to highlight the prominence of the central incisors. In addition, this softens the natural contrast between the normally darker shade of canines and of the lighter lateral incisors, which could be objectionable to some patients.

References

1. Loomis A. *Drawing the Head and Hands*. New York: Viking, 1956.

2. Parramon JM. *Le Grand Livre de la Peinture à l'Aquarelle*. Paris: Editions Bordas, 1984.

3. Perard V. *Anatomy and Geometry*. New York: Bonanza Books, Crown, 1989.

4. *Webster's Ninth New Collegiate Dictionary*. Springfield, Mass.: Merriam-Webster, 1985.

5. Goldstein RE. *Change Your Smile*. Chicago: Quintessence, 1984.

6. Lombardi RE. The principles of visual perception and their clinical application to denture esthetics. *J Prosthet Dent* 1973; 29:358.

7. Roach RR, Muia PJ. Communication between dentist and technician: An esthetic checklist. In: Preston JD (ed). *Perspectives in Dental Ceramics. Proceedings of the Fourth International Symposium on Ceramics*. Chicago: Quintessence, 1988: 445.

8. Miller L. Porcelain crowns and porcelain laminates: Problems and solutions. Presented at the International Ceramic Symposium, New Orleans, May 31, 1991.

9. Shavell H. Mastering the art of esthetic dentistry. Louisiana State University School of Dentistry, New Orleans, May, 1988.

10. Rufenacht CR. *Fundamentals of Esthetics*. Chicago: Quintessence, 1990.

11. Vig RG, Brundo GC. The kinetics of anterior tooth display. *J Prosthet Dent* 1978;39:502.

12. Lammie GA, Posselt U. Progressive changes in the dentition of adults. *J Periodontol* 1965;36:443.

13. Kessler JC. Maximizing the esthetic potential of ceramo-metal restorations. The American Academy of Crown and Bridge Prosthodontics. Fourtieth Annual Scientific Seminar. Chicago, February 15, 1991.

14. Allen P. Use of mucogingival surgical procedures to enhance esthetics. *Dent Clin North Am* 1988;32:307.

15. Golub J. Entire smile pivotal to teeth design. *Clin Dent* 1988;33.

16. Frush JP, Fisher RD. The dynesthetic interpretation of the dentogenic concept. *J Prosthet Dent* 1958;8:558.

17. Kokich V. Esthetics and anterior tooth positioning: An orthodontic perspective. American Academy of Esthetic Dentistry, 16th Annual Meeting, August 8, 1991; Santa Barbara, Ca.

18. Burstone CJ. The integumental profile. *Am J Orthod* 1958;44:1.

19. Subtelny JD. A longitudinal study of soft tissue facial structures and their profile characteristics, defined in relation to underlying structures. *Am J Orthod* 1959;45:481.

20. Tweed CH. The diagnostic facial triangle in the control of treatment objectives. *Am J Orthod* 1991;55:651.

21. Peck S, Peck H. A concept of facial esthetics. *Angle Orthod* 1970;40:284.

22. Pound E. Applying harmony in selecting and arranging teeth. *Dent Clin North Am* March 1962:241.

23. Maritato FR, Douglas JR. A positive guide to anterior tooth placement. *J Prosthet Dent* 1964;14:848.

24. Pound E. *Personalized Denture Procedures. Dentist's Manual*. Anaheim: Denar, 1973.

25. Dawson PE. Determining the determinants of occlusion. *Int J Periodont Rest Dent* 1983;3(6):9.

26. Augsburger RH. Occlusal plane relation to facial type. *J Prosthet Dent* 1953;3:755.

27. *Glossary of Prosthodontic Terms*, ed 5. St Louis: CV Mosby, 1987.

28. Spear F. Facially generated treatment planning: A restorative viewpoint. American Academy of Esthetic Dentistry, 16th Annual Meeting, Santa Barbara, Calif., August 8, 1991.

29. Pound E. Let "S" be your guide. *J Prosthet Dent* 1977;38:482.

30. Pound E. Applying the vertical dimension of speech to restorative procedures. In: Lefkowitz W (ed). *Proceedings of the Second International Prosthodontic Congress*. St Louis: Mosby, 1979.

31. Richer P. *Artistic Anatomy*. New York: Watson-Guptill, 1971.

32. Brisman AS. Esthetics: A comparison of dentists' and patients' concepts. *J Am Dent Assoc* 1980;100:345.

33. Hambidge J. Dynamic symmetry. *Sci Am* 1921;4:23.

34. Albino JE, Tedesco LA, Conny DJ. Patients' perceptions of dento-facial esthetics: Shared concerns in orthodontics and prosthodontics. *J Prosthet Dent* 1984;52:9.

35. Shaw WC, Lewis HG, Robertson NRE. Perception of malocclusion. *Br Dent J* 1975;March:211.

36. Andersen BP, Boersma H, Van der Linden FPG, Moore AW. Perceptions of dentofacial morphology by laypersons and general dentists. *J Am Dent Assoc* 1979;98:209.

37. Graber LW, Luckner WG. Dental esthetic self-evaluation and satisfaction. *Am J Orthod* 1980;77:163.

38. Albino JE, Cunnat JJ, Fox RN, Lewis EA, Slakter MJ, Tedesco LA. Variables discriminating individuals who seek orthodontic treatment. *J Dent Res* 1981;60:1661.

39. Tedesco LA, Albino JE, Cunnat JJ, Green LJ, Lewis EA, Slakter MJ. A dental-facial attractiveness scale. Part I. Reliability and validity. *Am J Orthod* 1983;83:38.

40. Hirsch B, Levin B, Tiber N. Effect of dentist authoritarianism on patient evaluation of dentures. *J Prosthet Dent* 1973;30:745.

41. Hirsch B, Levin B, Tiber N. Effect of patient involvement and esthetic preference on denture acceptance. *J Prosthet Dent* 1972;28:127.

42. Brigante RF. Patient-assisted esthetics. *J Prosthet Dent* 1981; 46:18.

43. Parramon JM. *Comment Peindre une Nature Morte*. Paris: Bordas, 1980.

44. Greenberg JR. Shaping anterior teeth for natural esthetics. *Esthet Dent Update* 1992;3:86.

45. Geller W. Dental Ceramics and Esthetics. Chicago, February 15, 1991.

46. Frush JP, Fisher RD. The dynesthetic interpretation of the dentogenic concept. *J Prosthet Dent* 1958;8:558.

47. Miller EL, Bodden WR, Jamison HC. A study of the relationship of the dental midline to the facial median line. *J Prosthet Dent* 1979;41:657.

48. Garn SM, Lewis AB, Walenga AJ. Maximum-confidence value for the human mesiodistal crown dimension of human teeth. *Arch Oral Biol* 1968;13:841.

49. Mavroskoufis F, Ritchie GM. Variation in size and form between left- and right maxillary central incisor teeth. *J Prosthet Dent* 1980;43:254.

50. Bjorndal AM, Henderson WG, Skidmore AE, Kellner FH. Anatomic measurements of human teeth extracted from males between the ages of 17 and 21 years. *Oral Surg Oral Med Oral Pathol* 1974;38:791.

51. Woelfel JB. *Dental Anatomy: Its Relevance to Dentistry*, ed 4. Philadelphia: Lea & Febiger, 1990.

52. Sanin C, Savara BS. An analysis of permanent mesiodistal crown size. *Am J Orthod* 1971;59:488.

53. Ballard ML. Asymmetry in tooth size: A factor in the etiology, diagnosis and treatment of malocclusion. *Angle Orthod* 1944; 14:67.

54. Pincus CL. Color and esthetics. In: *Dental Porcelain: The State of the Art—1977*. Los Angeles: University of Southern California, School of Dentistry, 1977:303.

55. Goldstein RE. *Esthetics in Dentistry*. Philadelphia: Lippincott, 1976.

56. Eissman H. Visual perception and tooth contour. In: *Dental Porcelain: The State of the Art—1977*. Los Angeles: University of Southern California, School of Dentistry, 1977:297.

57. Bori J. Cours C.E.S. Prothèse Scellée. University Paris V, 1976–1979.

58. Perelmuter S, Trichet D. Facteurs influencant la forme de contour des infrastructures céramo-métalliques. *Cahiers de Proth* 1981;36:141.

Chapter 2

Diagnosis and Treatment Planning of Esthetic Problems

Gerard Chiche, Vincent G Kokich, and Richard Caudill

With advances in metal ceramic technology, implant therapy, and all-ceramic systems, numerous techniques are currently available for the fixed prosthetic restoration of the anterior dentition. Goldstein[1] stressed that communication and patient education are essential in order to match the dentist's and patient's definitions of success. The most successful esthetic results are frequently team efforts involving other specialists but always involve close personal communication with the patient.[1,2] Disappointment with the outcome of prosthodontic care is often the result of poor communication and poor understanding of the limitations of treatment by the patient.[1-3] Improving communication calls for increased sophistication in the dental examination[1,4] in the form of thorough esthetic diagnostic and treatment planning, detailed patient self-examination, and computer-assisted patient evaluation. Many esthetic problems may be solved with surgery, orthodontics, or prosthodontics alone, but others often require a multidisciplinary approach.[5]

Orthodontic considerations

Because alignment of anterior teeth is an important aspect of dental esthetics, orthodontics has traditionally been intimately involved in esthetic dentistry. Alignment, however, is not the only esthetic aspect that may be modified by orthodontics. Now that orthodontists are treating a wider age range of patients with underlying restorative requirements, the role of orthodontics in esthetic dentistry has broadened. The ability to intrude, extrude, and move teeth mesially, distally, labially, and lingually, in conjunction with re-

storative dentistry, has expanded the esthetic possibilities. The astute diagnostician must first recognize these possibilities and plan the appropriate treatment accordingly to achieve the ultimate esthetic result. The following discussion will provide an orthodontic perspective of the four esthetic aspects of tooth position that may be influenced by orthodontic treatment: vertical position, mediolateral position, crown length, and crown width.

Vertical tooth position

When assessing the esthetic appearance of anterior teeth, the vertical position of the maxillary incisors is important. Of course, all assessments such as this are relative. We must therefore assess the position of the maxillary incisors relative to other facial landmarks. From an orthodontic perspective, two major landmarks are critical to the analysis. The first is the level of the lip when the patient is smiling, and the second is the interpupillary line. When a patient smiles, the upper lip should expose the entire crown of the maxillary central incisors in addition to about 1 mm of the maxillary labial gingiva. This would be considered esthetically ideal. Exposed gingiva of 2 to 3 mm is also esthetically acceptable. Second, the incisal edges as well as the posterior maxillary occlusal plane should be parallel with the interpupillary line. Excessive display of maxillary gingiva upon smiling or an oblique occlusal or incisal plane may be unesthetic. Orthodontics can improve both of these conditions. The clinician, however, must correctly diagnose the problem, because several options for treatment are possible.

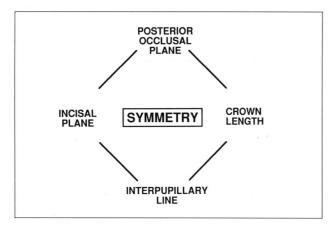

Fig. 2-1 Four factors help the orthodontist create the proper orientation of the incisal and posterior occlusal planes relative to the patient's interpupillary line.

Interpupillary line

If the incisal plane of the maxillary anterior teeth does not coincide with the interpupillary line, orthodontic planning depends on the interrelationship of four factors: incisal plane, posterior occlusal plane, interpupillary line, and crown length (Fig. 2-1).

If neither the incisal plane nor the posterior occlusal plane are parallel with the interpupillary line but they are symmetrical, asymmetrical skeletal growth has occurred and is usually the result of unilateral condylar hyperplasia or hypoplasia. This in turn results in unilateral supraeruption of maxillary teeth. When viewing such a patient anteriorly, the right and left posterior facial heights, represented by the lengths of the mandibular rami, will differ. This problem cannot be corrected merely with orthodontics. To reorient the maxillary occlusal plane, maxillary surgery must be performed to intrude the maxilla unilaterally to level the occlusal plane (Fig. 2-2). The interpupillary line is used as a guide during surgical positioning of the maxilla.

Not all incisal plane problems are treated surgically. When the incisal plane and posterior occlusal plane are not coincident, it is important initially to determine if the posterior occlusal plane is coincident with the interpupillary line. If so, the skeleton is probably symmetrical, and the problem is due only to the position of the maxillary anterior teeth.

The next critical assessment is the relative crown lengths of the maxillary central and lateral incisors. If the lengths of the contralateral incisors are similar, the underlying incisal plane problem is caused by over- or undereruption of the incisors. This problem is corrected easily with orthodontic treatment. Using the posterior occlusal plane as anchorage and a refer-

ence, the incisors may be extruded or intruded to make the incisal plane symmetrical with the posterior occlusal plane and interpupillary line (Fig. 2-3).

In some situations, restorative dentistry is also required. When the incisal plane and posterior occlusal planes are asymmetrical with one another, but the posterior occlusal plane is coincident with the interpupillary line, the asymmetry is not skeletal but is confined to the maxillary anterior teeth. In this situation, when the crown lengths of the right and left central and lateral incisors are compared, there is a significant difference in the lengths of the teeth. This unesthetic oblique incisal plane is caused by a combination of asymmetrical wear of the incisors and uneven eruption of the anterior teeth. Treatment requires a combination of orthodontics to level the gingival margins and restorative dentistry to re-create symmetrical lengths of the right and left central and lateral incisors. In this latter situation, the orthodontist and restorative dentist must communicate during diagnosis and treatment phases to provide the most esthetic result (Fig. 2-4).

Upper lip line

When a patient smiles, the upper lip should expose the entire crown of the central incisors. However, some patients show excessive amounts of gingiva when they smile, which may be unesthetic. The correct diagnosis and treatment are based on an evaluation of the interrelationship between four factors: incisal plane, posterior occlusal plane, gingival margins, and crown length (Fig. 2-5).

The first step in establishing the diagnosis is to evaluate the level of the gingival margins relative to the upper lip when the patient smiles. If the patient shows excessive gingiva, it should first be determined if the entire anatomic crown of the tooth is uncovered. In some patients, the excess gingiva can be removed surgically to expose more clinical crown length.

If the entire anatomic crown lengths of the central incisors are visible, the next assessment should compare the incisal plane and posterior occlusal plane. First, if these two planes are at the same level, and the patient displays excess gingiva, the cause of the problem is vertical maxillary hyperplasia. This is an overgrowth of the maxilla in a vertical direction. This unesthetic situation cannot be corrected with orthodontics only. The solution for this problem requires orthognathic surgery to remove a wedge of bone from the maxilla and reposition the entire maxilla and maxillary anterior teeth superiorly to reduce the display of gingiva.

Second, if the incisal and occlusal planes are at different levels and the posterior occlusal plane is

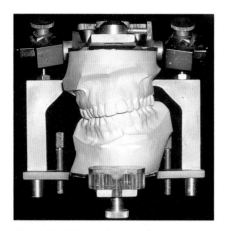

Fig. 2-2 Mounted casts of a patient with a skeletal asymmetry. The incisal plane did not coincide with the interpupillary line, and the incisal and posterior occlusal planes were coincident. This skeletal asymmetry was due to overgrowth of the mandibular ramus on the right side and will have to be corrected surgically by reorienting the maxillary occlusal plane and shortening the right mandibular ramus.

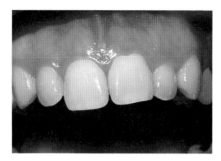 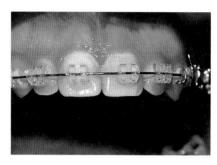

Fig. 2-3a and b In this patient, the incisal plane did not coincide with the interpupillary line or the posterior occlusal plane. This problem was corrected by orthodontically extruding the left incisors to level the incisal plane.

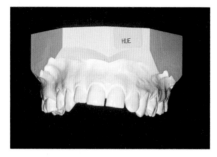 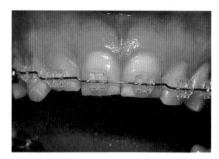

Fig. 2-4a and b Here the incisal plane did not coincide with the interpupillary line or with the posterior occlusal plane. Orthodontics was required to level the gingival margins, and restorative dentistry will be indicated to reestablish proper crown length.

positioned properly, the problem is supraeruption of the maxillary incisors. This requires intrusion of the incisors to produce leveling of the incisal and occlusal planes, as well as movement of the gingival margin superiorly as the tooth is intruded in order to reduce gingival display. The orthodontic mechanics involved in this type of movement can be accomplished intraorally with an intrusive force to the incisors, or extraorally using a headgear to move the maxillary incisors superiorly (Fig. 2-6).

If the problem is not corrected at an early age, overeruption and the resulting deep overbite may cause excessive wear of the incisal edges with increasing age. Subsequent treatment of these patients often requires orthodontics in conjunction with restorative dentistry. In these latter situations, patients usually display excess gingiva upon smiling and have a discrepancy in the levels of the incisal and occlusal planes. In addition, the maxillary incisors are short because of years of abrasion. If the posterior occlusal plane is at the proper vertical level, then intrusion is required to move the gingival margin superiorly, followed by restoration to reestablish proper crown length (Fig. 2-7).

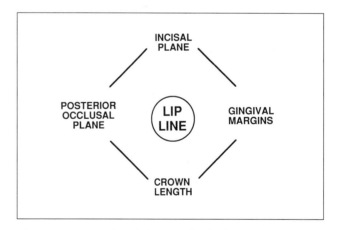

Fig. 2-5 Four factors help the orthodontist make the proper decisions regarding vertical positioning of the maxillary incisors relative to the lip line.

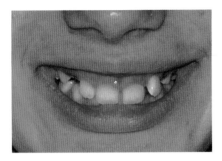

Fig. 2-6 This young patient showed excess gingiva upon smiling because the supraeruption of the maxillary incisors produced a step between the incisal and posterior occlusal planes. This discrepancy will require intrusion of the maxillary incisors to eliminate the excess gingival display.

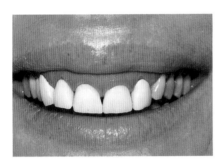 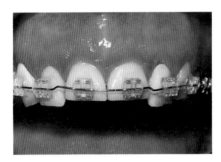 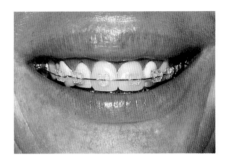

Fig. 2-7a–c This patient showed excess gingiva upon smiling. The central incisors had supraerupted, and their crown lengths were shorter than the lateral incisors. First, the central incisors were intruded to level their gingival margins relative to the upper lip. Then the incisal edges were restored with provisional crowns to re-create the correct crown length pending the final restorations.

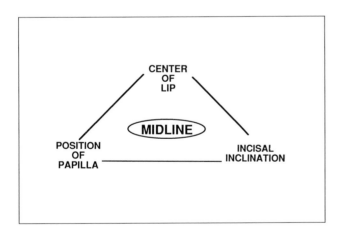

Fig. 2-8 Three factors help the orthodontist determine the proper treatment for midline discrepancies.

Mediolateral position

The mediolateral position of the maxillary central incisors is an important aspect of esthetics. In some situations, the maxillary dental midline will deviate to one side. When correcting these situations, it is important to distinguish between a true midline deviation and improperly inclined incisors. The treatment for these two situations differs, and the clinician must evaluate the relationship between three factors: the center of the upper lip, the position of the papilla, and the inclination of the central incisors (Fig. 2-8).

The maxillary midline must be related to a specific facial landmark. The most reliable one is the center of the philtrum because very few asymmetries (except cleft lip deformities) will occur in the upper lip. The nose is not adequate as reference because often the tip of the nose will deviate laterally. It is also important not to use the contact point between the maxillary central incisors as a reference. The true reference for the maxillary anterior teeth is the interproximal papilla between the central incisors.

If the tip of the papilla deviates from the center of the philtrum of the upper lip, a true maxillary dental midline problem exists. This is usually the result of a

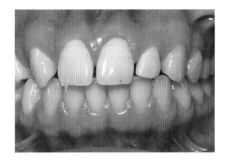

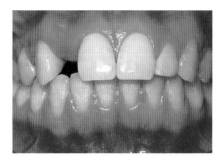

Fig. 2-9a and b The maxillary dental midline deviated to the right because of congenital absence of the maxillary right lateral incisor. This problem was corrected by orthodontically moving the maxillary incisors to the left, reorienting the maxillary dental midline, and creating space for an implant or a pontic.

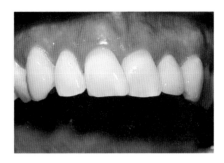

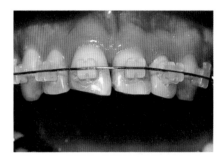

Fig. 2-10a and b Although this patient's dental midline apparently deviated to the left, the papilla between the central incisors was centered in the middle of the face. This deceptive midline deviation was caused by tipping of the right central incisor to the left and abnormal wear of the distoincisal edge. This required orthodontic tipping of the root of the right central incisor mesially. The discrepancy in the incisal edges will then have to be corrected by restoring the abraded portions of the central incisors.

missing tooth on the side toward which the midline is deviated. The maxillary midline is seldom deviated in a completely dentulous maxillary arch. If a tooth is missing near the anterior portion of the arch, the midline deviates more.

If the missing tooth is located more posteriorly, the midline deviates less. This type of midline deviation is easily corrected orthodontically. In order to move the dental midline back into the center of the upper lip, either extracting a similar tooth on the opposite side of the arch or opening space for the missing tooth is required. The decision between these two alternatives depends on the arch length and facial profile (Fig. 2-9).

Some apparent maxillary anterior midline deviations may be misinterpreted. It is important to assess the position of the papilla relative to the philtrum. If the papilla and philtrum coincide but the contact point between the central incisors is deviated, the problem may be oblique inclination of the incisors. Orthodontic treatment involves tipping the incisors to improve their inclination and to relocate the contact point beneath the papilla and philtrum. As the inclination of the incisors is corrected, the restorative dentist may need to reshape or restore the incisal edges to re-create proper crown form (Fig. 2-10).

Crown length

The relative crown lengths of the maxillary incisors are important in the esthetic appearance of the anterior teeth, and this relationship is often overlooked by orthodontists. Assessment of crown length discrepancies is important in order to determine proper treatment because several options exist for correcting crown length discrepancies. The correct diagnosis and treatment are based on an evaluation of the interrelationship between four factors: lip level, sulcular depth, amount of incisal wear, and relative crown length of contralateral incisors (Fig. 2-11).

The typical crown length problem encountered by the orthodontist is a discrepancy between the lengths of two central incisors. The first assessment to be made is the esthetic importance of this discrepancy, which involves evaluating the level of the upper lip when the patient smiles. If the patient does not have a high lip line, discrepancies between the lengths of the central incisors are not esthetically important. If a discrepancy in crown lengths is apparent during smiling, then it should be corrected during orthodontic treatment.

In some patients, both the clinical and anatomic crown lengths of the central incisors differ. The typical cause of disproportionate anterior crown lengths in adult patients is asymmetric wear of the central inci-

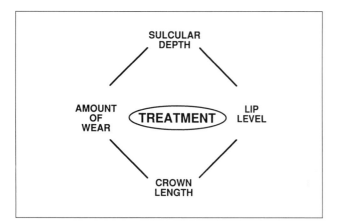

Fig. 2-11 Four factors help the orthodontist determine the proper treatment of maxillary incisor crown length discrepancies.

sors due to tooth malposition. Because worn incisors have much thicker incisal edges, assessing the incisal edges of the central incisors from an occlusal view will yield the amount of wear. Typically when an incisor abrades, it continues to erupt, and as it abrades more, it will erupt more, resulting in a shorter tooth. To determine the appropriate treatment, the relative crown lengths of the central and lateral incisors must be evaluated. If the shortest central incisor is still longer than the lateral incisors, extrusion and reduction of the incisal edge of the longer central incisor will correct the discrepancy. If the shorter central incisor is the same length or shorter than the lateral incisors, however, it should be intruded. Intrusion of the shorter central incisor will move the gingival margin apically (Fig. 2-12).

Crown width

An important but often overlooked aspect of maxillary anterior esthetics is crown width. Orthodontists often treat patients with disproportionate widths of anterior

teeth. The most common discrepancies exist in patients with peg-shaped lateral incisors. Usually the root length of the malformed lateral incisor is adequate, but the narrow crown is caused by lack of width at the incisal edge. In most situations, the cervical width of the malformed lateral incisor is within normal limits. If insufficient space exists to restore these teeth, an orthodontist can open interproximal space to permit restoration of proper crown width. A helpful step in coordinating this interdisciplinary treatment is to construct a diagnostic wax-up prior to orthodontic treatment. This will permit visualization of the final result and allow for input from both the restorative dentist and orthodontist during the planning stage of treatment (see Fig. 2-21).

Periodontal considerations

The clinician's concept of what constitutes an ideal smile must be balanced with the patient's wishes. Periodontal diagnosis should be aimed at an esthetic treatment that preserves but does not compromise health,[6,7] adequate periodontal support, and speech.

Esthetic restorations for a previously unrestored dentition

An existing reversible gingivitis or mild periodontitis should be corrected by proper home care procedures, scaling, polishing, and root planing. Patients with moderate-to-severe periodontitis in the esthetic zone may require tooth extractions with edentulous ridge preservation, or regenerative procedures to salvage teeth or create esthetic pontic areas for the final restoration.

Traditional surgical pocket elimination around teeth with extensive osseous loss may create a healthy situation yet leave the patient with teeth that are of exaggerated length and without interproximal papillae. Crowning may be required to close open em-

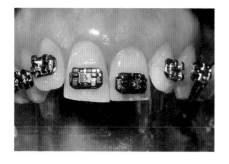
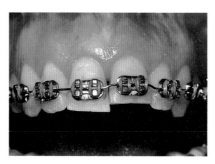

Fig. 2-12a and b This patient had a crown length discrepancy between the central incisors caused by excessive wear of the left central incisor and gradual supraeruption of this tooth relative to the adjacent teeth. The left central incisor was intruded orthodontically to level the gingival margins so that the discrepancy in the incisal edges could be restored to establish identical crown lengths of the central incisors.

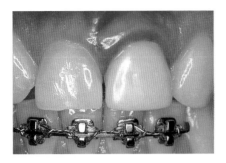

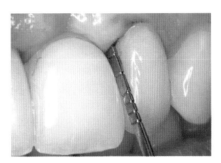

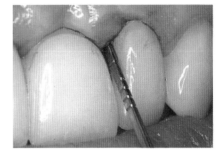

Fig. 2-13 The tissue around this existing crown is inflamed. The problem is either caused by overcontouring, poor marginal adaptation, hypersensitivity to a nickel alloy, or violation of biologic width.

Fig. 2-14a and b Violation of biologic width by a deep crown margin may be suspected in the presence of inflammation when the patient exhibits adequate plaque control and cervical contour and marginal adaptation are deemed satisfactory. This restoration was fabricated with a gold-platinum alloy. Before anesthesia the probing depth was 2.5 mm, and after anesthesia the probe could be pushed to the bone crest with only an additional 0.5 mm. This probably indicates that the required dimensions of 1 mm of connective tissue and 1 mm of junctional epithelium have been violated by the crown margin in the proximal aspect.

brasures or to shorten any surgically lengthened teeth according to the lip length.

Restorations for a previously restored dentition

If a patient presents with preexisting crown restorations and gingival inflammation (Fig. 2-13), the inflammation could be caused by one or several simultaneous factors as summarized by Spear and Townsend.[8] The most common factor is gingivitis from plaque, and in such cases both restored and adjacent nonrestored teeth exhibit equivalent degrees of gingival inflammation. Gingival inflammation can also be caused by noncleansable gingival pockets due to deficient crowns with open or overhanging margins,[9,10] or with bulbous emergence profiles.[11] This can usually be detected radiographically or clinically with an explorer.

Patients who perform adequate plaque control yet show inflamed gingival tissues localized around existing crowns may be subject to allergy or "inadequate biologic width." Allergy to nickel-containing alloys is rare but has been reported around crowns fabricated with nickel-containing alloys.[12] Previous studies reported that approximately 10% of women in the United States and Europe display hypersensitivity to nickel,[13,14] usually in the form of skin allergic responses to jewelry containing nickel.

If gingival inflammation persists, it is probably due to inadequate "biologic width,"[15,16] which results from the placement of a deep crown margin compromising the apical-coronal width of the connective tissue attachment to the tooth, which averages 1.07 mm.[17] Similarly, when the interproximal margins of crowns approximate the level of crestal bone on radiographs,

they may be suspected of violating the biologic width.[18] Siverton and Burgett[19] demonstrated that the most coronal aspect of the connective tissue attachment on the facial line angles of teeth with periodontal attachment loss can be accurately assessed by routine periodontal probing without anesthesia. After anesthesia, determination of adequate biologic width on the radicular aspect can then be made by sounding the bone level with a periodontal probe. With healthy gingival tissues, this probe reading should be approximately 1 to 2 mm greater than the preoperative reading. The patient is not anesthetized first because the periodontal probe tip barely penetrates the junctional epithelium (which is approximately 1 mm in width). No penetration into connective tissue occurs unless the gingival tissue is inflamed.[20,21] In crown preparations, when the bone level is sounded in relation to the finish line of the tooth preparation, there should be at least 2 mm between the finish line and the bone crest. A 2-mm difference means that although the biologic width is being respected, the finish line is located at the base of the crevice; a greater distance is preferred to ensure that the finish line is located just within the crevice, well within the reach of plaque-control devices (Fig. 2-14).

Impingement on biologic width may not manifest for several months after tooth preparation. This impingement, in the form of unresolved interproximal inflammation,[16] may be especially evident where anterior teeth are prepared to the same level circumferentially, because interproximal bone levels follow the contour of the cementoenamel junction[22,23] and are, especially in the anterior region, considerably more coronal than on the facial and lingual aspects.[24]

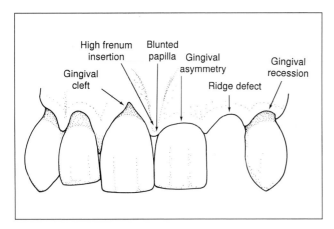

Fig. 2-15 These noninflammatory periodontal defects require plastic periodontal surgery.

Correction of noninflammatory periodontal defects (Fig. 2-15)

Inadequate attached keratinized gingiva

Maynard and Wilson[25] advocated providing "approximately 5 mm of keratinized tissue, composed of 2 mm of free gingiva and 3 mm of attached gingiva" where restorative procedures will enter the gingival crevice. They also believed that if a periodontal probe could be seen through thin marginal gingiva, the ability of that tissue, even if keratinized, to support intracrevicular restorative procedures would be doubtful. Stetler and Bissada[26] reported that teeth with subgingival restorations and narrow zones of keratinized gingiva (less than 2 mm) showed statistically significantly higher gingival inflammatory scores than teeth having submarginal restorations with wide zones of keratinized gingiva and similar plaque indices; teeth without subgingival restorations showed no statistically different inflammation scores between narrow and wide zones of keratinized gingiva. The amount of keratinized gingiva can be clinically evaluated by "rolling up" the mucosal tissue apical to the mucogingival junction using the side of a periodontal probe held horizontally. Subtracting the probing depth from that measurement determines the amount of attached keratinized gingiva. If an insufficient amount is present initially, it can be increased by one or more augmentation techniques.

Prominent frena

The maxillary anterior frenum is usually associated with a nonkeratinized epithelium and often contrasts with the pinker adjacent keratinized gingiva. Some investigators have found it to contain muscle fibers,[27]

while others found no muscle fibers in the frenum proper.[28] The presence of the frenum has been implicated by some clinicians in orthodontic relapse, causing reopening of a diastema between the maxillary central incisors.[29] When the frenum approximates the marginal gingiva, it may retract the gingival margin or the interproximal papilla when the lip is manipulated.[30] Besides this indication, the frenum is not usually resected (frenectomy) or relocated (frenotomy) unless: (1) the position of the gingival margin is changed by progressive recession or surgery; (2) toothbrush trauma to the frenum is caused by its proximity to the gingival margin; (3) orthodontic relapse is probable because of the frenum's presence; or (4) the frenum itself creates an unsightly appearance because of an unusually high lip line.

Localized gingival recessions

Localized gingival recessions may be caused by traumatic tooth-cleaning techniques, especially when teeth are prominent in the dental arch[31,32] and the overlying soft tissue is thin. Localized gingival recessions such as gingival clefts may be attributed to: local irritants such as plaque and calculus, especially in the presence of excessive occlusal forces[33]; severe orthodontic tipping of teeth[34]; trauma from occlusion[35]; temporary crowns[36]; periodontal surgery[37–39]; mechanical traumatic factors such as fingernail-biting habits[40]; and the extraction of adjacent teeth.[41] Surgical correction of gingival recession is often required together with restorative therapy, but total correction may be difficult or impossible depending on the level of interproximal bone and soft tissues.

Miller[42] classified gingival tissue recessions and predicted the outcome of corrective surgery based on his classification. In Class I defects where marginal tissue recession does not extend to the mucogingival junction and there is no loss of interproximal periodontium, full coverage of the exposed root can be anticipated postsurgically. Total root coverage can also be anticipated for Class II recessions, which are different only in that they extend to or beyond the mucogingival junction. Partial root coverage can be expected in Class III recessions where interproximal tissue loss poses problems for new attachment. Due to the severity of interdental bone or soft tissue loss and/or tooth malpositioning in the Class IV situation, root coverage cannot be expected.

Deficient pontic areas

Because the pontic/gingival interface is important for proper esthetics in visible anterior regions, alveolar ridge deformities present special challenges during fixed prosthetic reconstruction. These deformities origi-

Table 2-1 Classification Systems for Edentulous Ridge Deformities

	Apicocoronal	Buccolingual	Combination
Seibert[45]	Class II	Class I	Class III
Allen, et al[46]	Type A	Type B	Type C

nate from developmental defects, traumatic injury, surgical trauma, and advanced periodontal disease. Where teeth have been extracted, and especially where facial alveolar bone has been destroyed by periodontitis, there is a narrowing of the faciolingual dimension of the edentulous ridge,[43] later followed by apically progressing bone loss.[44]

Seibert[45] originally presented a system for classifying various edentulous ridge deformities: Class I—buccolingual loss of ridge contour; Class II—apicocoronal loss of ridge contour; and Class III—combined loss of ridge contour in both apicocoronal and buccolingual dimensions. This classification system was further modified by Allen et al[46] to describe the depth of the defect relative to the adjacent (intact) gingiva as: mild (less than 3 mm); moderate (3 to 6 mm); and severe (greater than 6 mm). They also referred to edentulous ridge defects using an easy-to-remember format: type A—apicocoronal loss of ridge contour; type B—buccolingual defects; and type C—combined type A and B deformities. Table 2-1 compares the classification systems of Seibert and Allen et al.

Gingival asymmetries

Gingival asymmetries are common findings in the esthetic zone. Symmetry between the maxillary central incisors is more critical than bilateral symmetry between the central incisors, lateral incisors, and canines. For natural pleasing results, esthetic surgical alignment of the gingival margins mostly involves the central and lateral incisors and, to a lesser extent, the canines. Holding a straight edge in front of the patient, parallel to the interpupillary line,[47] will aid in detecting asymmetries in maxillary anterior gingival margins. Whether or not asymmetries can be surgically corrected depends on whether crown lengthening or root-coverage procedures are feasible without compromising bone support; also, severe root angulation can preclude an esthetic result after gingiva is repositioned at the desired level.

Any periodontal pockets must first be resolved, and the likelihood of exposing the cementoenamel junction must be assessed. This is essential if bonded laminates versus full crowns are to be fabricated, or if the tooth to be lengthened is intact and does not need crowning or veneering.

Gingival asymmetries may also be treated with orthodontic eruption or intrusion. When teeth are extruded slowly, the attachment apparatus and overlying gingiva will follow the cementoenamel junction, assuming the periodontium is healthy.[48] On the other hand, if the clinical crown needs to be elongated while the gingival level remains stationary, sequential fiberotomies should be performed while the tooth is being forcefully erupted.[49] With multiple gingival margin discrepancies, conventional orthodontics may be initially undertaken to properly align roots and cementoenamel junctions, followed with surgical elongations as needed. Proper tooth diameter is an important consideration when crowns are to be lengthened, because root form at the final gingival margin must remain consistent with proper emergence profiles in the final restoration.

Excessive gingival display (the "gummy smile")

The "gummy smile" is often encountered in patients who have short lip lines and/or where more than 3 mm of gingiva in the maxillary anterior region is displayed during a relaxed smile. Proper treatment planning is based on the location of the cementoenamel junction, the potential for root exposure, and an appraisal of the existing tooth length and incisal edge position.[50] Proper incisal position must first be evaluated in relation to the lips, then an average tooth length of pleasing proportion should be visualized from this incisal edge. The decision between reduction with gingivectomy, flap surgery, orthodontic intrusion, or orthognathic surgery is made according to the severity of the gummy smile (Figs. 2-16 and 2-17).

Restorative dentistry considerations

Bleaching, composite resin bonding, cosmetic contouring, and porcelain laminate veneers used singly or in various combinations provide conservative solutions or economic alternatives for numerous esthetic problems that would conventionally have required extensive crown preparations.[51–54] Various treatment alternatives are available,[54] but making the right decision is perplexing at times because the indications of the procedures overlap. According to Weinstein,[2] the treatment decision is based on: (1) the esthetic and functional needs of the patient; (2) the motives and expectations of the patient; (3) the integrity of the remaining tooth structure; (4) the esthetic potential of the restoration; (5) the occlusal relations and the intensity of the occlusion, and (6) the durability, invasiveness, and cost of the procedure.

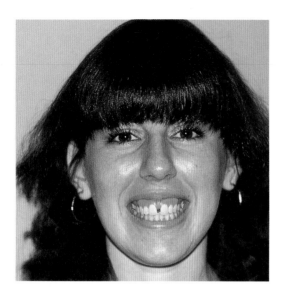 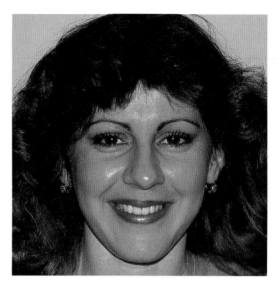

Fig. 2-16a and b   Excessive display of gingival tissue in the smile position. Extensive surgical elongation is not advised in this situation because it would have to be extended to the posterior teeth, would likely expose the cementoenamel junctions excessively, and would result in elongated teeth difficult to restore with full crowns. Fig. 2-16b: Correction after orthognathic surgery. (Surgical treatment performed by Dr JN Kent.)

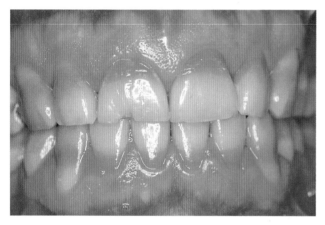 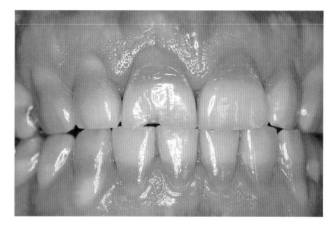

Fig. 2-17a and b   Moderate gummy smile corrected with surgical elongation of the incisors before porcelain laminate veneer treatment. The central incisors were short and square and required elongation to improve their proportions. Because the incisal display was already adequate, only surgical elongation could significantly improve the intrinsic proportion of the incisors. The favorable location of the cementoenamel junction allowed for up to 2 mm of elongation without exposing root structure.

Direct composite resin bonding

The main advantages of direct composite resin bonding are to obtain an immediate esthetic result and patient satisfaction in one-to-two office visits, conservatively and at a relatively low cost.[55–59] The entire procedure is controlled by the dentist and yields good results if he or she is skilled. Strength and wear resistance are moderate, and repeated chipping or discoloration can occur. Longevity is fair to good, and coverage of certain discolorations is difficult. Good ability with shade and contour is essential for medium and large restorations.

Porcelain laminate veneers

This minimally invasive procedure results in limited pulp and periodontal involvement because tooth preparation is mostly confined to the enamel and relies on supragingival margins. The anterior guidance is usually preserved, and tissue compatibility, color stability, and translucency are good. The esthetic results depend on the artistic ability of the technician and are very satisfactory with proper indications[60–65] (Figs. 2-18–2-22).

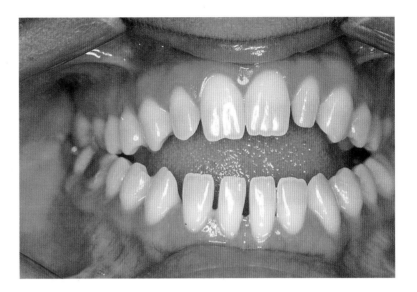

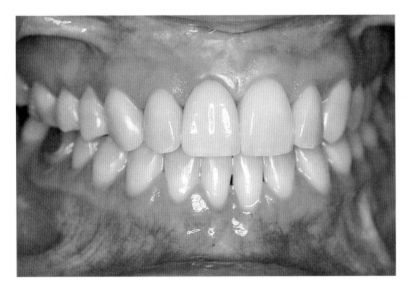

Fig. 2-18a–c This patient underwent orthognathic surgery, orthodontics, and porcelain veneers. Midface hypoplasia and mandibular prognathism resulted in this anterior open bite. Surgery consisted of a segmental maxillary Le Fort I osteotomy, vertical ramus osteotomy, and bilateral malar implants. Setting the canines in Class I occlusion resulted in diastemas between the maxillary incisors that had to be corrected with four porcelain laminate veneers. The original narrow aspect of the central incisors was modified to a wider outline of improved proportion. Widening of the central incisors required that the lateral incisors be rotated to emphasize the dominance of the central incisors. (Surgery: Dr Dale J Missiek; orthodontics: Dr David R Hoffman.)

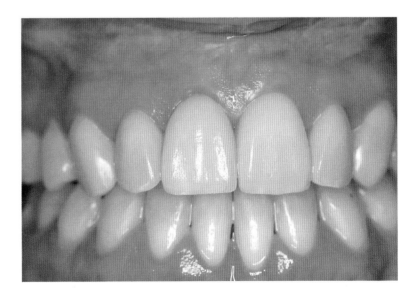

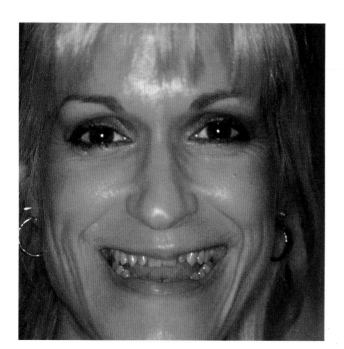 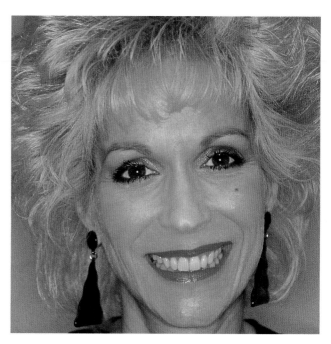

Fig. 2-19a and b Before and after treatment. Even though the central incisors were widened to improve their dominance over the lateral incisors, they are in good harmony with the face.

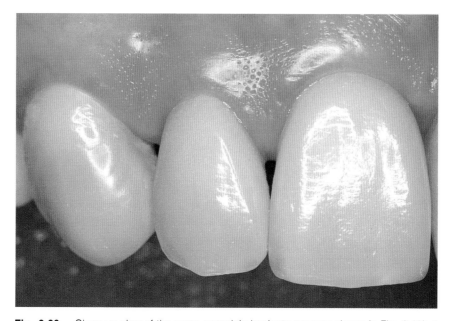

Fig. 2-20 Close-up view of the same porcelain laminate veneers shown in Fig. 2-19b 4 years postoperatively. The integrity of the cervical margins is well maintained because of their supragingival location and bonding to cervical enamel, preventing microleakage. If the margins had been located on cementum, the prognosis would probably have been more guarded because of the possibility of microleakage.

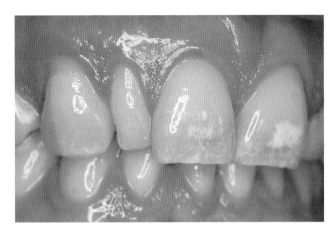
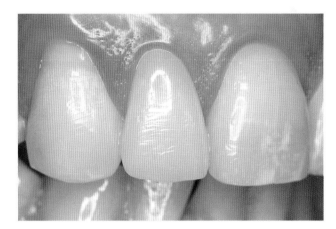

Fig. 2-21a and b This patient underwent treatment with orthodontics and porcelain laminate veneering (Opal porcelain, 3M Dental Products, St Paul, MN). The peg-shaped maxillary lateral incisor had to be corrected first by opening the interproximal space between the lateral incisor and the adjacent teeth orthodontically. This allowed for restoration of proper crown width with a porcelain laminate veneer. (Orthodontic treatment: Dr J Sheridan.)

Fig. 2-22a–c Combination treatment of orthodontics and porcelain laminate veneers (Opal porcelain, 3M Dental, St Paul, MN). When closing diastemas, it is preferable to emphasize dominance of the central incisors by widening their distal aspect as long as their outline remains proportionate. The lateral incisor had to be distalized orthodontically to widen the central incisor with the laminate veneer. The lateral incisor was widened distally with the veneer until it contacted the mesial aspect of the canine.

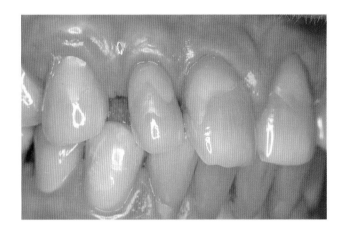

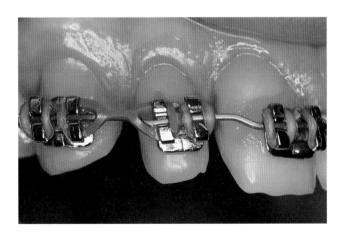
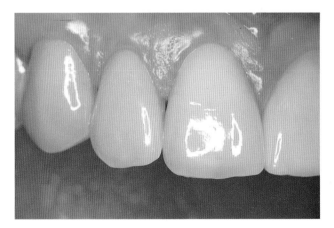

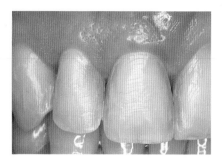
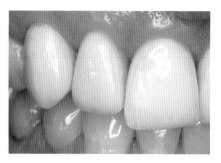

Fig. 2-23a and b   Adequate tooth reduction is essential for proper esthetic rendition with porcelain laminate veneers. Proper shade must be incorporated into the porcelain to lessen the influence of the background. This requires a veneer thickness of approximately 0.8 mm. Because the enamel thickness of a maxillary central incisor is on the average 0.8 mm in the incisal third, tooth reduction may have to be confined within 0.6 to 0.7 mm, requiring slight overcontouring of the porcelain veneers. In this patient, the anterior teeth were in linguoversion and did not require reduction at the incisal third. These porcelain veneers were used to increase the display and prominence of the anterior teeth.

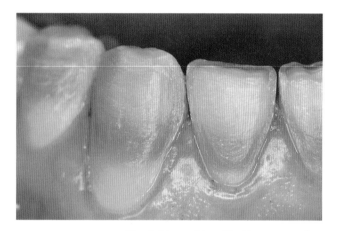
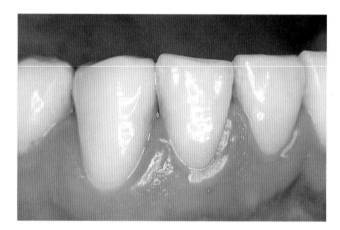

Fig. 2-24a and b   Masking tetracycline stains with porcelain veneers is difficult and may result in an opaque and monochromatic result. The preparation may have to be extended into the dentin for maximum veneer thickness, and the die relief must be increased for additional cement thickness and increased masking ability.

The longevity potential, mechanical strength, and wear resistance are excellent due to the reliability of the composite resin bond to etched ceramic and etched enamel.[66–70] Porcelain laminate veneers are contraindicated with severely fractured teeth or deep composite resin restorations, and parafunctional activity may cause chipping or fracture over a period of time[71] unless an occlusal guard is prescribed.[64] Crossbite or edge-to-edge relationships require careful planning,[72] and management of protrusive and lateral excursions, because most failures may be traced to improperly adjusted occlusion.[73]

Tooth preparation for porcelain laminate veneers is exacting (Fig. 2-23). It requires that at least 50% of enamel be available for etching and that an intact enamel periphery be maintained.[74] Cervical margins should preferably be located in enamel, but if cervical margins are bonded to dentin or cementum, the long-term prognosis of porcelain veneers may be uncertain because of the possibility of leakage at the margin[69–70]; the patient should be informed that this is not an ideal indication for the procedure.[68–70] Adequate masking of severely tetracycline-stained teeth is difficult and requires excellent laboratory support and good communication between the dentist and ceramist. It may result in opaque and monochromatic veneers unless the preparation is extended deeper into dentin[75] (Fig. 2-24).

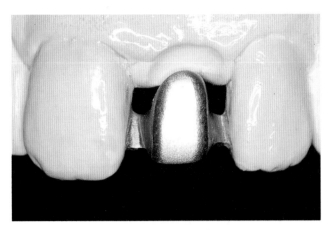
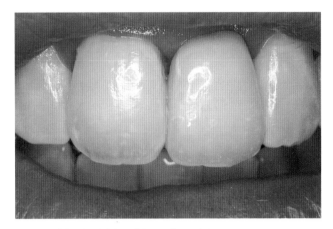

Fig. 2-25a and b A resin-bonded fixed partial denture (Maryland bridge) has a favorable prognosis with proper indications. The abutments must exhibit no mobility, no more than one tooth should be replaced, and no additional abutments should be used besides the two proximal teeth. It is essential that maximum etched-enamel surface be available for resin cement bonding. This mandates proximal extensions as allowed by the esthetic requirements, surgical elongation at the cervical lingual aspect if necessary, definite proximal grooves or lingual pinholes, and extension of the preparation close to the incisal edge.

Full-coverage crowns

Metal ceramic crowns

Mechanical strength, durability, simplicity, and excellent esthetic potential are traditionally associated with metal ceramic restorations. While tooth preparation may not be as exacting as with all-ceramic crowns, insufficient tooth reduction invariably results in opacity and overcontouring. To achieve a proper shade, tooth reduction may have to be invasive and result in pulp trauma or dictate elective endodontic therapy.

All-ceramic crowns

All-ceramic crowns have maximum esthetic potential because of the absence of a metal coping.[76] Existing ceramic systems differ significantly in terms of technique sensitivity, flexural strength, and translucency. For maximum predictability, all-ceramic crowns are presently best suited for maxillary incisors with proper indication; in addition, their mechanical properties may be enhanced with resin luting cements. They have potential for fracture and breakage in patients with parafunction or deep vertical overbite. Tooth reduction is slightly more conservative than with metal ceramic restorations, but it must be precise and crown thickness requirements are exacting.

Etched-metal resin-bonded prosthesis (Maryland bridge)

The main advantage of this type of prosthesis is its conservative nature.[77] The performance of an etched-metal retainer relies on proper patient selection, retainer design, and adequate bonding of the resin cement to enamel and to the metal casting[78–80] (Fig. 2-25). Inadequate tooth preparation, poor metal treatment, or misuse of the cement properties could result in debonding of the restoration; the reported failure rate ranges from 13% to 34%.[81–86]

Sufficient etchable enamel should be available for adhesion to metal, and since the area available for bonding is often small in the anterior region, surgical elongation of the lingual aspect of the abutments may be required 13% of the time.[87] Deep cingulum rests may also have to be added to the abutment preparation.[88] Replacement of a single missing incisor as an alternative to implant therapy, or splinting of mobile teeth when there is no missing tooth,[78] are the most predictable indications of etched-metal resin-bonded prostheses. No more than one tooth should be replaced.[81]

Abutments must not have large carious lesions or large restorations and must exhibit no mobility. The difficulty of tooth preparation varies according to the location and depth of the occlusal contacts, and clearance may be required at the expense of the opposing dentition.[78] Adequate proximal extensions, retention grooves, and connector dimensions may be restricted by the shape of the abutments and by the esthetic imperatives. Esthetic results may be affected when abutment shape (eg, tapered teeth) imposes limitations on pontic and embrasure form, or when the width of the abutments and the pontic cannot be harmonized.

Preoperative Analysis

Laminate Veneers

- Tooth alignment: rotation; lingual or labial version
- Extent of previous restorations and carious lesions
- Extent and distribution of enamel, incisal wear
- Gingival recession and root exposure
- Occlusal relations, heavy function, or parafunction
- Crown length and extent of lengthening of the incisal aspect
- Thickness of the incisal edge
- Curvature of the facial and proximal surfaces
- Severity of discoloration

Full Veneer Crowns for Anterior Teeth

- Tooth length
- Tooth thickness
- Tooth taper and extent of gingival recession
- Pulp status: pulp size, deep restorations, previous crowning
- Occlusal relations: heavy function, bruxism, location of occlusal contacts, horizontal and vertical overlap, crowding of mandibular dentition

Resin-Bonded Prostheses

- Crown length
- Surface area of etchable enamel
- Composite resin restoration or incipient decay
- Abutment mobility
- Occlusal relations: crowding of opposing teeth and protrusive relations, horizontal and vertical overlap
- Incisogingival dimensions for adequate connectors
- Mesiodistal taper of the abutments and volume of the interdental papillae
- Pontic size and need for reshaping of the abutments

Anterior Implant Crowns and Bridges

- Availability of bone and location of the anatomical structures
- Dimensions of the alveolar ridge and location of cortical bone
- Mesiodistal interdental and interradicular spaces
- Proximity and direction of adjacent roots
- Ridge trajectory and depth of apical bone undercuts
- Soft tissue and bone height in relation to adjacent teeth
- Height of the interdental papillae
- Occlusal relations with mounted diagnostic casts

Implant crowns

The predictability of osseointegrated implants has been extensively documented[89–93] and has influenced all areas of fixed prosthodontics because replacement of missing teeth is no longer equated with automatic tooth reduction of the adjacent teeth and construction of a fixed partial denture. In addition, to preserve the existing bone height and reduce the number of surgical procedures, implants may be placed immediately after atraumatic tooth extraction if implant stability can be achieved.[94,95] As a rule, dental implants are contraindicated with bruxism and parafunctional activity. The mesiodistal dimension of the edentulous space and the interradicular distance must be sufficient to accommodate the body of the implant without risk of encroaching on the interdental papillae and the adjacent roots. The buccolingual thickness of the alveolar ridge must be sufficient, otherwise it requires a ridge augmentation procedure with bone grafting.

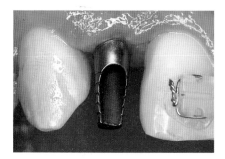
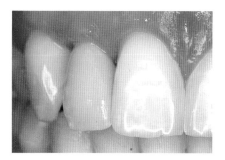
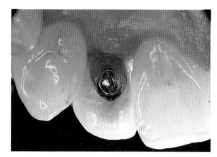

Fig. 2-26a–c   When the implant location is inclined facially, a prepared titanium abutment or a preangled abutment screwed in the implant body is required. The metal ceramic crown is either temporarily cemented over these abutments or may be screw-retained for maximum retrievability with an accessory transverse screw with little or no cement. (Integral Implant, Calcitek Inc. Carlsbad, CA.)

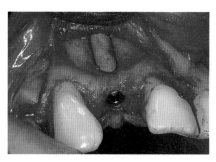
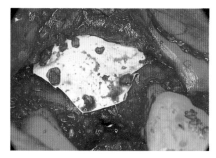

Fig. 2-27a and b   When the alveolar ridge is inclined facially and the implant requires a straight axis for restorative purposes, the implant preparation must be performed in conjunction with grafting of a demineralized freeze-dried bone allograft and placement of a poly-tetrafluoroethylene barrier for guided bone regeneration. The implant is stabilized with anchorage in the nasal cortical plate. (Surgery: Dr John N Kent.)

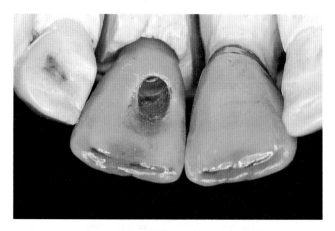
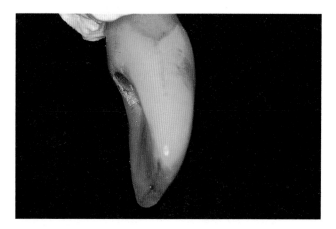

Fig. 2-28a and b   Ideally, implant location in the anterior region should be such that the screw emerges through the cingulum area and the cervical aspect of the crown is restored without overcontouring in proper continuity with the implant. This relationship is jeopardized when the implant axis is labial to the incisal edge position or when the screw emergence is just lingual to the incisal edge and could weaken it. The facial convexity of the crown may also result in an incisal edge that interferes with the path of insertion of the screw. (In collaboration with Dr D Palmisano.)

Success requires a well-coordinated team to achieve satisfactory prosthetic results.[96-98] Implant placement and axis must be precise to facilitate fabrication of the optimal prosthesis, but anatomy and inclination of the residual ridge are also important factors. Implants that incline toward the facial aspect are a frequent problem in the anterior maxilla because the alveolar process resorbs at the expense of its facial aspect[97] (Fig. 2-26). Ideally, crestal bone resorption in height and thickness should be minimum, and with unfavorable situations ridge grafting should be considered whenever possible to achieve a straighter implant inclination consistent with the expected crown anatomy[94,99] (Fig. 2-27). This is because facially angled fixtures increase the complexity of the restorative process and compromise retrievability to some degree,[100,101] and because lingual placement of fixtures may dictate a ridge-lapped crown, restrict access for cleaning, and cause abnormal loading of the implant. Prosthetically, the objective is to achieve properly contoured and retrievable restorations with the emergence of the abutment screw through the cingulum aspect whenever possible (Fig. 2-28).

References

1. Goldstein RE. *Change Your Smile*. Chicago: Quintessence, 1984.

2. Weinstein AR. Anterior composite resins and veneers: Treatment planning, preparation and finishing. *J Am Dent Assoc* (special issue) 1988;38.

3. Nicholson JW, Highton R, Malone WFP. Esthetic bonding. In: Malone WFP, Kohl DL (eds). *Tylman's Theory and Practice of Fixed Prosthodontics*. St Louis: Ishiyaku, 1989;195.

4. Lackey AD. Examining your smile. *Dent Clin North Am* 1989; 33:133.

5. Goldstein RE, Goldstein CE. Is your case really finished? *J Clin Orthod* 1988;22:702.

6. Löe H, Listgarten M, Terranova V. The gingiva: Structure and function. In: Genco R, Goldman H, Cohen DW (eds). *Contemporary Periodontics*. St Louis: Mosby, 1990:3–32.

7. Caton J. Periodontal diagnosis and diagnostic aids. In: *Proceedings of the World Workshop in Clinical Periodontics*. Chicago: American Academy of Periodontology, 1989: I–II.

8. Spear F, Townsend C. Esthetics: A multidisciplinary approach. Presented at the American Academy of Periodontology, 77th Annual Meeting, October 2, 1991, Vancouver, BC.

9. Waerhaug J. Tissue reactions around artificial crowns. *J Periodontol* 1953;24:172–185.

10. Lang P, Kiel RA, Anderhalden K. Clinical and microbiological effects of subgingival restorations with overhanging or clinically perfect margins. *J Clin Periodontol* 1983;10:563–578.

11. Perel ML. Axial crown contours. *J Prosthet Dent* 1971;25: 642–649.

12. Lamster IB, Kalfus DI, Steigerwald PJ, Chasens AI. Rapid loss of alveolar bone associated with nonprecious alloy crowns in two patients with nickel hypersensitivity. *J Periodontol* 1987; 58:486–492.

13. Peltonen L. Nickel sensitivity in the general population. *Contact Dermatitis* 1979;5:27.

14. Prystowsky SD, Allen AM, Smith RW, et al. Allergic contact hypersensitivity to nickel, neomycin, ethylenediamine and benzocaine: Relationships between age, sex, history of exposure and reactivity to standard patch tests and use tests in a general population. *Arch Dermatol* 1979;115:959.

15. Ingber FJS, Rose LF, Coslet JG. The "biologic width"—a concept in periodontics and restorative dentistry. *Alpha Omegan* 1977;10:62–65.

16. Tal H, Soldinger M, Dreiangel A, Pitaru S. Responses to periodontal injury in the dog: Removal of gingival attachment and supracrestal placement of amalgam restorations. *Int J Periodont Rest Dent* 1988;8(3):45–55.

17. Gargiulo AW, Wentz FM, Orban B. Dimensions and relations of the dento-gingival junction in humans. *J Periodontol* 1961; 32:261.

18. Nevins M, Skurow HM. The intracrevicular restorative margin, the biologic width, and the maintenance of the gingival margin. *Int J Periodont Rest Dent* 1984;4(3):31–49.

19. Siverton JF, Burgett FG. Probing of pockets related to the attachment level. *J Periodontol* 1976;47:281–286.

20. Listgarten MA, Mao R, Robinson PG. Periodontal probing and the relationship of the probe tip to the periodontal tissues. *J Periodontol* 1976;47:511–513.

21. Fowler C, Garrett S, Crigger M, Egelberg J. Histologic probe penetration in treated and untreated periodontal tissues. *J Clin Periodontol* 1982;9:373–385.

22. Ritchey B, Orban B. The crests of the interdental alveolar septa. *J Periodontol* 1953;24:75–87.

23. O'Connor TW, Biggs NL. Interproximal bony contours. *J Periodontol* 1964;35:326–330.

24. Weisgold AS. Contours of the full crown restoration. *Alpha Omegan* 1977;10:77.

25. Maynard JG Jr, Wilson RDK. Physiologic dimensions of the periodontium significant to the restorative dentist. *J Periodontol* 1979;50:170.

26. Stetler KJ, Bissada NF. Significance of the width of keratinized gingiva on the periodontal status of teeth with submarginal restorations. *J Periondontol* 1987;58:697–700.

27. Ross RO, Brown FH, Houston GD. Histologic survey of the frena of the oral cavity. *Quintessence Int* 1990;21:233–237.

28. Henry SW, Levin MP, Tsaknis PJ. Histologic features of the superior labial frenum. *J Periodontol* 1976;47:25–28.

29. Edwards JG. The diastema, the frenum, the frenectomy: A clinical study. *Am J Orthodont* 1977;71:489–508.

30. Kopczyk RA, Saxe SR. Clinical signs of gingival inadequacy: The tension test. *J Dent Child* 1974;41:352–355.

31. O'Leary TJ, Drake RB, Crump PP, Allen M. The incidence of recession in young males: A further study. *J Periodontol* 1972;42:264–267.

32. Gorman WJ. Prevalence and etiology of gingival recession. *J Periodontol* 1967;38:316.

33. Novaes AB, Ruben MP, Kon S, Goldman HM, Novaes AB. The development of the periodontal cleft. A clinical and histopathologic study. *J Periodontol* 1975;46:701–709.

34. Batenhorst KF, Bowers GM, Williams JE Jr. Tissue changes resulting from facial tipping and extension of incisors in monkeys. *J Periodontol* 1974;45:660–668.

35. Stillman P. Early clinical evidence of disease in the gingiva and pericementum. *J Dent Res* 1921;3:25.

36. Donaldson D. The etiology of gingival recession associated with temporary crowns. *J Periodontol* 1974;45:468.

37. Knowles JW, Burgett FG, Nissle RR, et al. Results of periodontal treatment related to pocket depth and attachment level. *J Periodontol* 1979;50:225–233.

38. Pihlstrom BL, Ortiz-Campos C, McHugh RB. A randomized four-year study of periodontal therapy. *J Periodontol* 1981;52:227–242.

39. Ramfjord SP, Caffesse RG, Morrison EC, et al. Four modalities of periodontal treatment compared over 5 years. *J Clin Periodontol* 1987;14:445–452.

40. Moskow B, Bressman E. Localized gingival recession. Etiology and treatment. *Dent Radiogr Photo* 1965;38:3.

41. Lammie G, Posselt V. Progressive changes in the dentition of adults. *J Periodontol* 1965;36:443.

42. Miller PD. A classification of marginal tissue recession. *Int J Periodont Rest Dent* 1985;5(5):9–13.

43. Abrams H, Kopczyk RA, Kaplan AL. Incidence of anterior ridge deformities in partially edentulous patients. *J Prosthet Dent* 1987;57:191–194.

44. Atwood DA. Bone loss of edentulous ridges. *J Periodontol* 1979;(special issue):11–21.

45. Seibert JS. Reconstruction of deformed, partially edentulous ridges, using full thickness onlay grafts. Part I. Technique and wound healing. *Compend Contin Educ Dent* 1983;4:437.

46. Allen EP, Gainza CS, Farthing GG, Newbold DA. Improved technique for localized ridge augmentation. A report of 21 cases. *J Periodontol* 1985;56:195–199.

47. Roach RR, Muia PJ. Communication between dentist and technician: An esthetic checklist. In: Preston JD (ed). *Perspectives in Dental Ceramics. Proceedings of the Fourth International Symposium on Ceramics.* Chicago: Quintessence, 1988:445.

48. Ingber JS. Forced eruption. Part I. A method of treating isolated one- and two-wall infrabony osseous defects. Rationale and case report. *J Periodontol* 1974;45:199–206.

49. Kozlovsky A, Tal H, Lieberman M. Forced eruption combined with a gingival fiberotomy. A technique for clinical crown lengthening. *J Clin Periodontol* 1988;15:534–538.

50. Allen EP. Use of mucogingival surgical procedures to enhance esthetics. *Dent Clin North Am* 1988;32:307.

51. Goldstein RE. *Esthetics in Dentistry.* Philadelphia: Lippincott, 1976.

52. Jordan RE, Boksman L, Comfortes I. *Esthetic Composite Bonding.* St Louis: Mosby, 1986.

53. Feinman RA, Goldstein RE, Garber DA. *Bleaching Teeth.* Chicago: Quintessence, 1987.

54. Goldstein RE. Diagnostic dilemma: To bond, laminate, or crown. *Int J Periodont Rest Dent* 1987;7(5):9.

55. Feigenbaum NL, Mopper WKA. *A Complete Guide to Bonding.* East Windsor, NJ: M.E.D. Communications, 1984.

56. Heymann HO. The artistry of conservative esthetic dentistry. *J Am Dent Assoc* 1987;(special issue):14.

57. Sockwell CL, Heymann HO, Brunson WD. Tooth colored restorations and additional conservative and esthetic treatments. In: Sturdevant CM (ed). *The Art and Science of Operative Dentistry.* St Louis: Mosby, 1985:267.

58. Christensen GJ. Veneering of teeth: State of the art. *Dent Clin North Am* 1985;29:373.

59. Christensen GJ. Comparison of veneer types. *CRA Newsletter* 1986;10:4.

60. Faunce FR, Myers DR. Laminate veneer restoration of permanent incisors. *J Am Dent Assoc* 1976;93:790.

61. Horn HR. Porcelain laminate veneers bonded to etched enamel. *Dent Clin North Am* 1983;27:671.

62. Calamia JR. Etched porcelain facial veneers: A new treatment modality based on scientific and clinical evidence. *NY Dent J* 1983;53:255.

63. Nixon RL. *The Chairside Manual for Porcelain Bonding.* Wilmington, Del: BA Videographics, 1987.

64. Friedman MJ. Multiple potential of etched porcelain laminate veneers. *J Am Dent Assoc* 1987;December (special issue):83.

65. Garber DA, Goldstein RE, Feinman RA. *Porcelain Laminate Veneers.* Chicago: Quintessence, 1988.

66. Calamia JR, Simonsen RJ. Effects of coupling agents on bond strength of etched porcelain. *J Dent Res* 1984;63:162.

67. Calamia JR, Calamia S, Lemler J, Hamburg M, and Scherer W. Clinical evaluation of etched porcelain laminate veneers: Results at six months–three years [abstract 1110]. *J Dent Res* 1987;66 (special issue):245.

68. Tjan AHL, Dunn JR, Sanderson IR. Microleakage patterns of porcelain and castable ceramic laminate veneers. *J Prosthet Dent* 1989;61:276.

69. Lacy AM, Wada C, Weiming D, Watanabe L. In vitro microleakage at the gingival margin of porcelain and resin veneers. *J Prosthet Dent* 1992;67:7.

70. Sorensen JA, Strutz JM, Avera D, Materdomini D. Marginal fidelity and microleakage of porcelain veneers made by two techniques. *J Prosthet Dent* 1992;67:16.

71. Nixon RL. Porcelain veneers: An esthetic therapeutic alternative. In: Rufenacht CR (ed). *Fundamentals of Esthetics.* Chicago: Quintessence, 1990.

72. Calamia JR. Materials and techniques for etched porcelain facial veneers. *Alpha Omega* 1988;81:48.

73. Porcelain veneers. *The Adept Report* Santa Rosa, Calif: Adept Institute, 1990;1:17.

74. Friedman MJ. Augmenting restorative dentistry with porcelain veneers. *J Am Dent Assoc* 1991;122:29.

75. Nixon R. Masking severely tetracycline-stained teeth with porcelain veneers. *Pract Perio Aesth* 1991;2:14.

76. McLean JW. *The Science and Art of Dental Ceramics,* monographs I and II (1974) III and IV (1976). Louisiana State University School of Dentistry.

77. Rochette A. Attachment of a splint to enamel of lower anterior teeth. *J Prosthet Dent* 1973;30:418.

78. Simonsen R, Thompson V, Barrack G. *Etched Cast Restorations: Clinical and Laboratory Techniques.* Chicago: Quintessence, 1983.

79. Thompson VP, Grolman KM, Liao R. Bonding of adhesive resins to various nonprecious alloys. *J Dent Res* 1985;64:314.

80. Council on Dental Materials, Instruments and Equipment. Etched-metal resin-bonded prostheses. *J Am Dent Assoc* 1987;115:95.

81. Chang HK, Zidan O, Lee IK, Gomez-Marin O. Resin-bonded fixed partial dentures: A recall study. *J Prosthet Dent* 1991;65:778.

82. Al-Shammery AR, Ibraheem HS. Acid etch bridge: 36 cases reported in 38 months follow-up [abstract 1545]. *J Dent Res* 1988;62:306.

83. Priest GF, Donatelli HF. A four-year clinical evaluation of resin-bonded fixed partial dentures. *J Prosthet Dent* 1988;59:542.

84. Creugers NH, Snoek PA, Vant'Hof MA, et al. Clinical performance of resin-bonded bridges: A five year prospective study. III. Failure characteristics and survival after rebonding. *J Oral Rehabil* 1990;17:179.

85. Crispin BJ. A longitudinal clinical study of bonded fixed partial dentures: The first 5 years. *J Prosthet Dent* 1991; 66:336.

86. Olin PS, Hill EME, Donahue JL. Clinical evaluation of resin-bonded bridges: A retrospective study. *Quintessence Int* 1991;22:873.

87. Hansson O, Moberg LE. Clinical evaluation of resin-bonded prostheses. *Int J Prosthodont* 1992;5:533.

88. Lacy AM. Improved retention for bonded cast metal rests: A case report. *Quintessence Int* 1991;22:439.

89. Brånemark P-I, Hansson BO, Adell R, et al. Osseointegrated implants in the treatment of the edentulous jaw. Experience from a 10-year period. *Scand J Plast Reconstr Surg* 1977;16 (suppl).

90. Adell R, Lekholm U, Rockler B, Brånemark P-I. A 15-year study of osseointegrated implants in the treatment of the edentulous jaw. *Int J Oral Surg* 1981;10:387.

91. Zarb G, Symington J. Osseointegrated dental implants. Preliminary report on a replication study. *J Prosthet Dent* 1983; 50:271.

92. Brånemark P-I, Zarb G, Albrektsson T (eds). *Tissue-Integrated Prostheses: Osseointegration in Clinical Dentistry*. Chicago: Quintessence, 1985.

93. Laney W, Tolman DE, Keller EE, Desjardin RP, Van Roekel NB, Brånemark P-I. Dental implants and osseointegration. *Mayo Clin Proc* 1986;61:91.

94. Lazzara RJ. Immediate implant placement into extraction sites: Surgical and restorative advantages. *Int J Periodont Rest Dent* 1989;9:333.

95. Krauser J, Boner C, Boner N. Immediate implantation after extraction of a horizontally fractured maxillary lateral incisor. *Pract Perio Aesth* 1991;3:33.

96. Blustein R, Jackson R, Rotskoff K, Coy R, Godan D. Use of splint material in the placement of implants. *Int J Oral Maxillofac Implants* 1986;1:47.

97. Schwartz MS, Stauts B. Fixture placement. *CDA J* 1987; November:45.

98. Engleman MJ, Sorensen JA, Moy P. Optimum placement of osseointegrated implants. *J Prosthet Dent* 1988;59:467.

99. Bahat O. The anatomic abutment strategic implant placement in the maxilla. Presented at the American Academy of Esthetic Dentistry, 17th Annual Meeting, Santa Fe, NM, August 8, 1992.

100. Lewis SG, Avera S, Engleman M, Beumer J. The restoration of improperly inclined osseointegrated implants. *Int J Oral Maxillofac Implants* 1989;4:147.

101. Chiche GJ, Weaver C, Pinault A, Elliott R. Auxiliary substructure for screw-retained prostheses. *Int J Prosth Odont* 1989;2:407.

Chapter 3

Replacement of Deficient Crowns

Gerard Chiche and Alain Pinault

Maxillary anterior crowns often need to be replaced after several years of service for esthetic or functional reasons. With the growing esthetic awareness of patients and the available ceramic technology, this type of retreatment is becoming common in the dental office.

Esthetic analysis

A methodical analysis is required for retreatment that harmonizes the smile with the face and fulfills the patient's self-image. It must be conducted in a logical progression from the incisal edge of the deficient crowns toward their gingival aspect, so that tooth structure is evaluated before gingival tissue. This is because the assessment of the proper incisal edge position and crown length determines whether the gingival position will eventually need to be modified to achieve a pleasing tooth shape.

Analysis of Deficient Crowns

- Incisal plane
- Incisal length
- Incisal profile
- Tooth proportion
- Tooth-to-tooth proportion
- Gingival outline

Incisal plane

Morphology

In natural dentition, three pleasing patterns are typically encountered in the young to middle-aged patient and result in a progressive widening of the incisal embrasures from the central incisors to the canines (Abrams Rule 1).[1] The incisal edges of the anterior teeth follow either a mild convexity, a "gull wing," or a combination of a convexity on one side of the arch and a "gull wing" on the other side. A flat incisal plane represents an acceptable pattern in the older age group only. Displeasing patterns include a flat plane in the young to middle-aged patient; a concave or reverse smile line; or, an excessive convexity.[2]

With deficient crowns, a straight incisal plane is a most common mistake and typically results in a lack of progression of the incisal embrasures from the central incisors to the canines. This also means that either the central incisors are too short or that the lateral incisors are too long, or possibly both. The systematic goal of the clinician is to restore an acceptable convexity in the incisal plane[3] (Figs. 3-1–3-6). Accessorily, the convexity of the incisal plane may be restored to distract attention from displeasing facial features.[4] Riley[5] recommends compensating a pointed chin with a flatter smile curve, or conversely balancing a square face with a relatively accentuated smile curve.

Inclination

The inclination of the incisal plane is best evaluated by facing the patient to evaluate its orientation in the face. The direction of the dental midline and of the gingival plane from one canine to the other is also useful in the

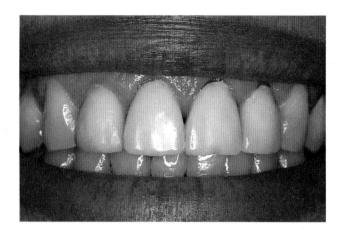

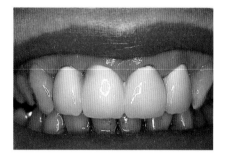

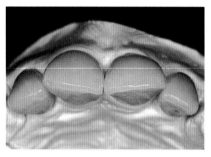

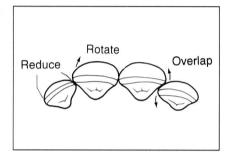

Fig. 3-1 This incisal plane is flat with no progression of incisal embrasures. Correction to an esthetically pleasing plane will involve either lengthening the central incisors, shortening the lateral incisors, or possibly a combination of both.

Fig. 3-2 This patient wanted these crowns as aligned as possible. Correcting crowding with crowns may result in narrower central incisors with loss of their dominance and lateral incisors that are slightly too wide. Also note the straight smile line.

Fig. 3-3 The new central incisor crowns are overlapped over the lateral incisors to restore their dominance. This pattern was modeled on a photograph of the patient with her natural teeth.

Fig. 3-4 Representation of the correction in composition.

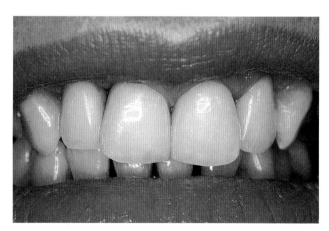

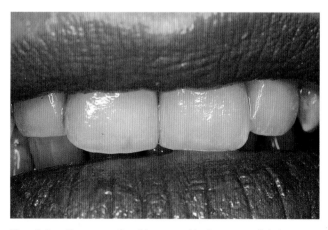

Fig. 3-5 Cemented crowns. The incisal plane has a convex pattern on one side and a "gull wing" configuration on the other side. The central incisors are also a lighter shade than the lateral incisors to emphasize their prominence.

Fig. 3-6 The convexity of the central incisors was slightly accentuated so that the incisal third could be in proper harmony with the lower lip.

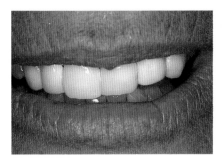

Fig. 3-7a This patient shows severe incisal plane discrepancy in relation to the upper lip line and the interpupillary line.

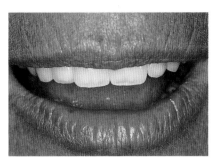

Fig. 3-7b Correction of the incisal plane with an anterior fixed partial denture in harmony with the lip line and the interpupillary line. The visibility of the incisal edges was reduced to a more acceptable display.

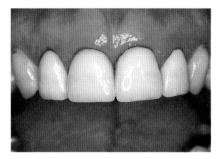

Fig. 3-8 Inclined incisal plane. The dental midline is perpendicular to the incisal plane. A lack of communication between the dentist and the technician probably caused the aligned crowns on the articulator to assume a different inclination in the mouth.

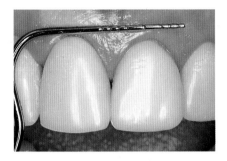

Fig. 3-9a When the maxilla is moderately tilted and the gingival plane follows its inclination, partial correction of the incisal plane is required before completing the crown restorations. Flap surgery will realign the gingival plane of the central incisors parallel to the interpupillary line and is usually sufficient to reestablish symmetry of the gingival plane before crown reconstruction.

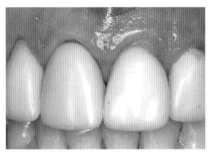

Fig. 3-9b Postoperative healing 3 months before definitive tooth preparations.

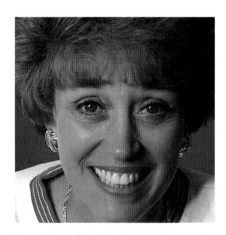

Fig. 3-9c Completed metal ceramic crowns cemented on the four maxillary incisors. Note the inclination of the maxilla in relation to the interpupillary line. The crowns are in good harmony with the face because alignment of the gingival plane with the interpupillary line was restored at the midline before reconstruction. As a rule, lateral asymmetry in the smile is not esthetically objectionable if there is symmetry at the midline.

final appraisal. The incisal plane is generally either parallel to the pupillary line or slightly to moderately canted. Severe cants are infrequent but do exist. With deficient crowns, a canted incisal plane frequently exists, with the dental midline perpendicular to it. This results from the incorrect orientation of the working cast in the articulator, which leads to a different inclination of the incisal plane of the crowns in the mouth as compared on the articulator (Figs. 3-7 and 3-8).

A slightly canted incisal plane requires either minor incisal reshaping of the incisal edges or no correction at all. A moderately canted incisal plane either requires a partial or a full correction of the gingival plane before prosthetic reconstruction. In the partial correction of a moderate cant, the key to success is to ensure that the gingival margins of the central incisors are parallel with the pupillary line. A moderately canted plane can be made esthetically pleasing even with misalignment of the canines as long as the gingival margins of the maxillary central incisors are horizontal and the central incisors are restored aligned with the interpupillary line. If the orientation of the gingival

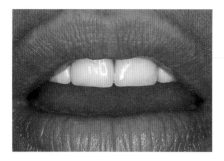

Fig. 3-10a Analysis of crown length with the lips at rest. A display of 4 mm is common for young female patients or individuals with a short lip.

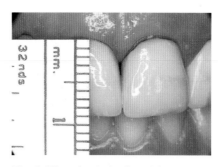

Fig. 3-10b Analysis of tooth length may also be based on statistical averages of the anatomic crown length. The average length of a maxillary central incisor varies between average values of 10.4 and 11.2 mm. This crown measures 9 mm and may need to be lengthened if its proportion needs to be improved or if there is insufficient incisal visibility.

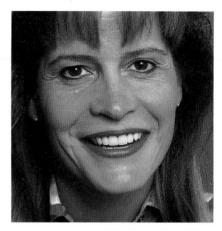

Fig. 3-10c The patient's desired visibility of his or her smile is an important determinant of incisal length. Proper communication with the patient is essential so that proper tooth length is established with these anterior crowns.

plane follows the cant of the maxilla and appears oblique in relation to the interpupillary line, a unilateral surgical elongation of the central incisor on the lower aspect is indicated. A partial realignment of the incisal plane is often all that is desired by the patient, but the patient must be informed that the progression of incisal embrasures resulting from realignment of the incisal plane will be much steeper on the side of the higher canine (Fig. 3-9).

When the patient desires a full correction of the smile in order to suggest a perfect alignment, or if the maxilla is severely canted, a more aggressive treatment is indicated and requires consultations with the orthodontist and the oral and maxillofacial surgeon (see chapter 2). From a sole restorative treatment standpoint, one alternative of treatment consists in first realigning the gingival plane through surgical elongation of its lower aspect (if this does not compromise bone support) and through root coverage procedures on its higher aspect. The incisal plane is then correspondingly realigned with full crown restorations.[6]

Incisal length

Determinants

The incisal edge of the central incisor is the cornerstone from which the smile is built, because once it is set, it serves to determine proper tooth proportion and gingival level. Elongation of the incisal aspect is often indicated to correct incisal wear, insufficient

Table 3-1 Average Maxillary Incisor Display (mm) with Lips at Rest[8]

Sex		Lip Length		Age	
Men	Women	Short	Long	Young	Middle-aged
1.91	3.40	3.65	0.59	3.37	1.26

tooth display, or displeasing tooth or crown proportion. Shortening the incisal edge may be required to compensate for unesthetic elongation after periodontal surgery, to correct excessive tooth display, or to correct a displeasing tooth or crown proportion. The desire to project a noticeable or prominent smile also depends significantly on the patient's self-image and how much of a youthful, dynamic appearance is desired.[7]

The primary determinants of incisal length are: the age and sex of the patient; the length and curvature of the upper lip; and the patient's preference (Fig. 3-10 and Table 3-1).

The accessory determinants of incisal length are the posterior plane of occlusion[2] and average anatomic crown length values for the maxillary central incisor,[9–12] which range from 10.4 to 11.2 mm (Fig. 3-10b). There is some subjectivity in incisal edge determination, therefore additional diagnostic tests are often required during treatment, with the patient's input, for actual visualization of the final incisal edge

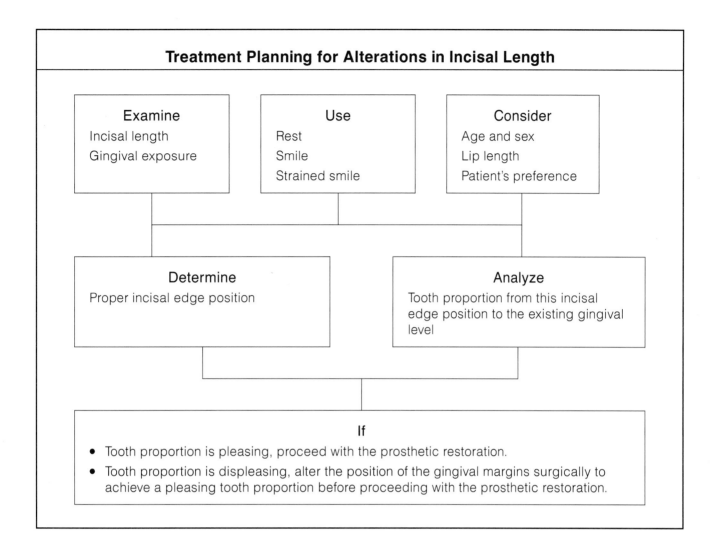

Treatment Planning for Alterations in Incisal Length

Examine	Use	Consider
Incisal length	Rest	Age and sex
Gingival exposure	Smile	Lip length
	Strained smile	Patient's preference

Determine

Proper incisal edge position

Analyze

Tooth proportion from this incisal edge position to the existing gingival level

If

- Tooth proportion is pleasing, proceed with the prosthetic restoration.
- Tooth proportion is displeasing, alter the position of the gingival margins surgically to achieve a pleasing tooth proportion before proceeding with the prosthetic restoration.

position. These additional tests include computer imaging to communicate with the patient and the dental technician, direct addition of composite resin at the desired length, diagnostic waxing, provisional restorations, and trial denture tooth set-up.

Incisal length modification

It is easier to modify tooth length prosthetically with a crown or a porcelain veneer than to surgically alter gingival position. When incisal length needs to be altered, many issues face the clinician: If a short tooth needs to be lengthened, can it be done at the incisal level only with a crown or a veneer? If significant tooth elongation is desired, what is the maximum tooth length allowed by the lips and face? If a long tooth needs to be shortened, can it be done at the incisal level only with a crown or a veneer? If significant reduction in length is planned, what is the minimum tooth length allowed by the lips and face? Decisions are based on an assessment and a preview of the proper incisal edge position and of the desired crown length. This in turn determines whether the existing gingival position is adequate, or whether it must be altered surgically to achieve a maxillary central incisor of pleasing proportions in the final result (Figs. 3-11 and 3-12).

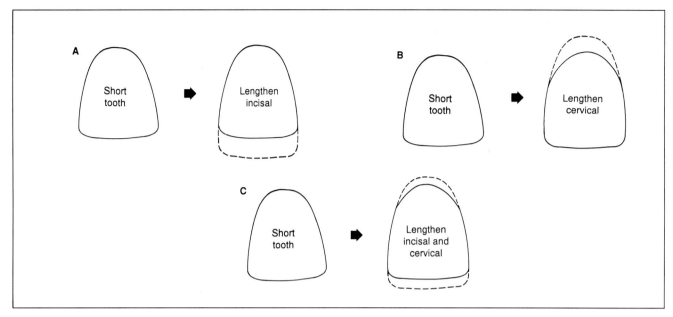

Fig. 3-11 Modifying proportions of a short maxillary incisor according to the lip dictates: **A,** If there is insufficient incisal display, the tooth may be elongated incisally; **B,** If there already is sufficient display, the tooth may only be elongated surgically; **C,** A combination of incisal and cervical elongation may also be indicated.

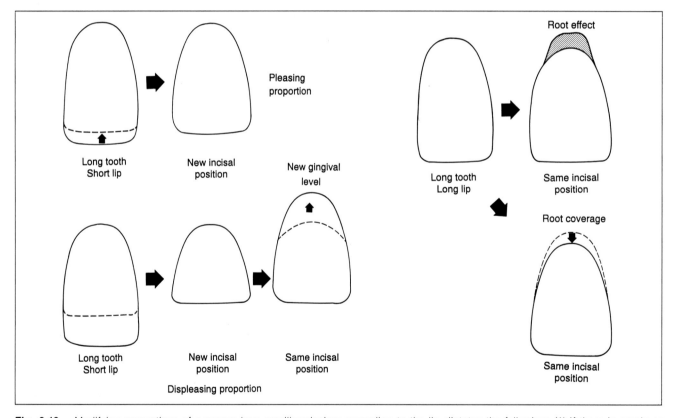

Fig. 3-12 Modifying proportions of a narrow long maxillary incisor according to the lip dictates the following: *(1)* If there is ample or excessive incisal display because of a short or concave upper lip, the tooth may be shortened incisally to achieve a pleasing proportion; *(2)* If there is excessive incisal display because of faulty restorations in combination with a short or concave upper lip, the tooth may be shortened incisally to achieve a pleasing proportion. However, with an adequate incisal edge position and display, the tooth proportion may be inadequate and require cervical elongation; *(3)* If there is normal incisal display and the upper lip is long, the long tooth may not be shortened incisally, or there will be insufficient tooth exposure, resulting in an aged appearance. A root effect with displacement of the cervical convexity coronally may give the illusion of a shorter tooth, or, in selected situations, root coverage procedures may be indicated to reduce the length of the clinical crown.

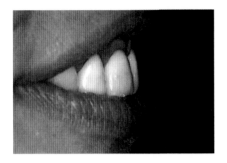

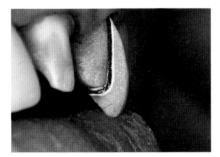

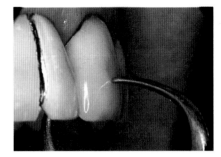

Fig. 3-13a During "f" or "v" sounds, the incisal third of the crown should make contact with the mucous part of the lip. This contact with the cutaneous portion of the lip suggests overcontour of the incisal third.

Fig. 3-13b Overcontouring of the incisal third is usually caused by insufficient tooth reduction at the incisal aspect of the preparation.

Fig. 3-13c Overcontouring of the incisal third may also be diagnosed by measuring the crown labiolingual thickness at the junction between the middle third and the incisal third. Overcontouring is suspected when the crown thickness exceeds 3.5 mm.

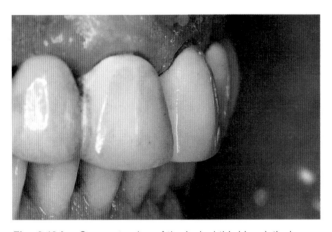

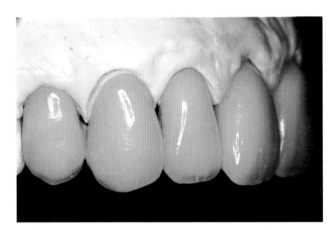

Fig. 3-13d Overcontouring of the incisal third is relatively easy to diagnose by direct profile observation or analysis of the study cast. The excessive thickness of the incisal edge is also an obvious clue to abnormal contour.

Fig. 3-14 Correct facial convexity of the central incisors. It is essential that the tooth preparation allow for proper curvature of the labial aspect of the crown as long as anterior guidance allows it.

Incisal profile

The pleasing aspect of the natural maxillary central incisor lies in its pronounced facial curvature, in part because it creates varied reflection patterns. This convexity is most evident in a direct profile observation where a straight incisal profile (or an overcontoured incisal edge) is probably the most common defect encountered in poorly contoured crowns[13] (Fig. 3-13) because it leads to a monochromatic bright appearance. Overcontouring the incisal third of anterior crowns does not seem to lead to significant occlusal or functional disturbance. This is probably because the incisal edge of the crown was relocated outward in relation to the original natural tooth and caused the envelope of function to be opened.

The challenge in correcting the incisal profile is to push back the incisal edge to its original esthetic appearance and still preserve a comfortable and unrestricted anterior guidance (Fig. 3-14). If the incisal edge of the deficient crown is too bulky, the incisal third may simply be reduced and pushed back in the new crown with the same original anterior guidance. Gross overcontouring of the incisal third may be detected by measuring the buccolingual thickness of the crown at the junction of the middle and incisal third. The average thickness of a natural maxillary central incisor ranges in this zone from 2.5 mm for a thin tooth to 3.3 mm for a thick tooth. Overcontouring may be suspected when crown thickness exceeds 3.5 mm (Fig. 3-13c).

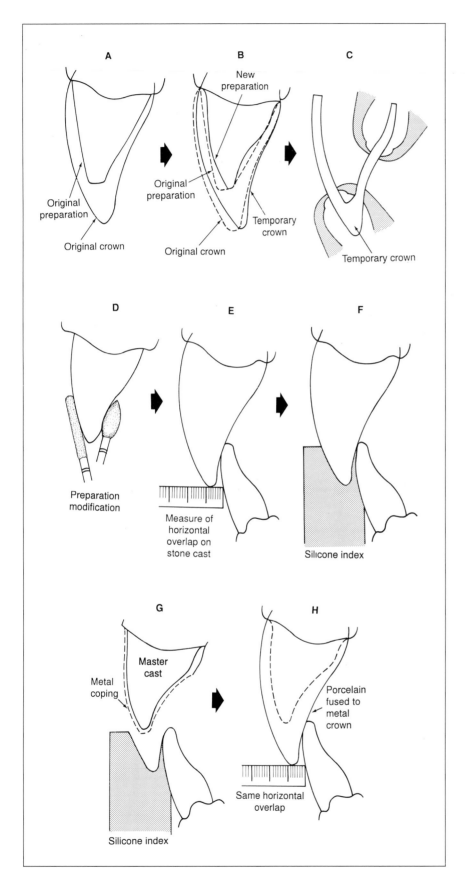

Fig. 3-15   Sequence of Retreatment

A and B, The first step after removal of the deficient crowns in the absence of references is to arbitrarily reprepare the incisal third until the incisal edge thickness is approximately 0.5 mm. Adequate lingual clearance must be maintained. Provisional restorations that satisfy esthetic and occlusal requirements are fabricated and serve as reference.

C and D, The thickness of the provisional restorations with the temporary cement in place is measured at a subsequent appointment and may dictate additional reduction to achieve adequate thickness for the restorations.

E and F, When the preparations and the provisional restorations are deemed satisfactory, impressions of the provisional restorations and of the opposing arch are made and the casts are articulated into centric occlusion. The horizontal overlap is monitored with a ruler and a silicone index.

G and H, The silicone index serves to verify that the waxed framework is properly constructed with adequate support for the porcelain, and location of the interproximal connectors. The ruler serves to precisely compare the horizontal overlap between provisional and final restorations.

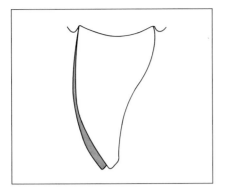

Fig. 3-16 To correct overcontouring of deficient crowns, a normal facial convexity must be restored by relocating the incisal third slightly toward the lingual aspect and reducing the labiolingual thickness of the tooth to a normal anatomic dimension.

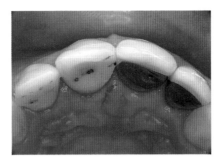

Fig. 3-17 The straight facial profile of the original metal ceramic crowns was corrected with new provisional restorations. The incisal third is pushed 0.5 mm lingually in relation to the original crown to restore an anatomic curvature to the central incisor. This must be accomplished carefully by harmonizing the anterior guidance in the provisional restoration with the existing guidance. The two metal ceramic crowns are then removed and replaced with two provisional restorations that incorporate the new incisal edge position and the original guidance.

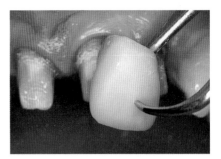

Fig. 3-18 After the provisional crowns and the tooth preparations are completed, the provisional crown thickness must be measured, at a subsequent appointment, at the junction of the incisal third and middle third with the temporary cement still in place. This allows the clinician to determine whether the tooth preparation was sufficiently reduced. For a metal ceramic crown, a minimum thickness of 1.5 mm is necessary in this area.

If relocating the incisal third of the crown more lingually results in a different anterior guidance, function must first be monitored with provisional restorations to ensure that the patient adapts to the new incisal position and that there is no discomfort, tooth mobility, or pain. Reproducing a pleasing normal curvature in the facial aspect of the maxillary incisor is theoretically ideal, but it may at times prove difficult to achieve if: the patient cannot tolerate alterations in anterior guidance; crowding of the lower incisors prevents any significant modification of maxillary edge position, or the clinical crown is thin labiolingually, thus limiting further tooth reduction.

The incisal edge position of the preparation dictates the amount of curvature that can be developed in the final crown. When removing deficient crowns, there is no reference available for proper position of the incisal edge of the preparation. Therefore, when the incisal third of the new crown has to be relocated lingually in relation to the deficient crown, the new tooth preparation must be methodically executed; in the lingual aspect, the clearance is kept minimal (0.6 to 0.8 mm) but is not accentuated because the clinician may eventually restore a thin tooth and must make provision for adequate reduction on the facial aspect by keeping a minimum workable clearance in the lingual aspect. On the facial aspect, the incisal third is arbitrarily reprepared until the incisal aspect of the tooth preparation is 0.5 mm and the tooth preparation is completed. This sequence ensures that the

---

Analysis of Overcontoured Incisal Profile
• Direct visual observation
• Relation to the lower lip in the "F" or "V" position
• Assessment of the thickness of the incisal edge
• Buccolingual thickness measurement
• Insufficient tooth reduction

incisal edge position is sufficiently modified to create a more convex facial contour but, as stated above, there must be greater reliance on provisional restorations when significant esthetic and functional alterations are planned (Figs. 3-15–3-18).

Tooth proportion

Once the incisal edge position is determined, the outline and proportion of the central incisor can be evaluated (Fig. 3-19). Tooth proportion is computed by dividing the width of the clinical crown by its length.[14,15] As a rule, pleasing width-to-length ratios

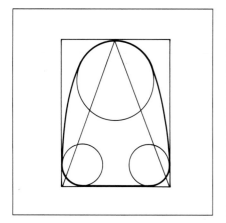

Fig. 3-19 Intrinsic proportions of a central incisor. The outline of a maxillary central incisor is a combination of a circle, a rectangle, and a triangle. In a pleasing proportionate outline, there is no obvious imbalance between these three elements.

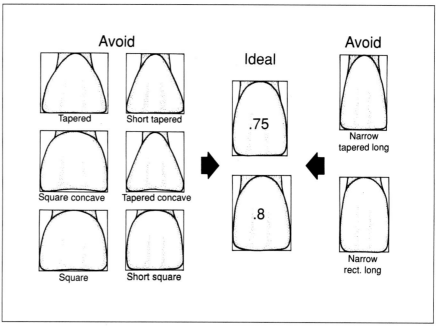

Fig. 3-20 A proportionately balanced central incisor has an intrinsic proportion (width: length ratio) of approximately 0.75 to 0.8. Numerous pleasing outlines may be produced with this ratio. It is important to avoid short tapered square or narrow long central incisors, which have displeasing proportions.

for maxillary central incisors are between 75% to 80%. Below 65%, the central incisor may appear too narrow, as could occur with implant crowns or after periodontal surgery. Above 85%, the incisor may appear too short and square, as occurs with attrition or with altered passive eruption (Fig. 3-20). Selecting a pleasing proportion for the central incisor involves determining its ideal shape in relation to the face. The question for the clinician is: what are the determinants of an ideal tooth proportion?

Proportion determined by statistical average

The mesiodistal diameter of the maxillary central incisor was measured in numerous studies[10–12,16–24] and ranges from a low average of 8.37 mm to a high average of 9.3 mm. The average crown length on extracted teeth[10–12] ranges from 10.4 mm to 11.2 mm. Therefore, the average width-to-length ratio extends from a low value of 0.74 to a high value of 0.89. The proportion suggested by Wheeler for carving techniques is 0.8 (8.5 mm/10.5 mm)[30] and is consistent with the averages of 0.8, 0.8, and 0.76 respectively found by Shillingburg et al (8.5 mm/10.4 mm),[10] Bjorndal et al (9.0 mm/11.2 mm),[11] and Woelfel (8.6 mm/ 11.2 mm).[12]

Proportion determined by face form

In 1887 Hall[31] proposed the "typal form concept," classifying natural teeth into ovoid, tapering, and square categories. Berry's[32] "biometric ratio" method advocated that the outline form of the inverted maxillary central incisor closely approximate the outline form of the face. He also postulated with House and Loop[33] that the mesiodistal width of the tooth was 1/16 of the bizygomatic width. In 1914 Williams[34] introduced under the "typal form method" his concept of harmony of tooth form with face form, which was almost universally accepted as the standard determinant of tooth form through the following 40 years.[34–38]

This geometric theory was challenged when Frush and Fisher introduced in 1956 the Dentogenic theory, where tooth selection is governed primarily by sex, personality, and age (SPA).[39–44] In spite of the SPA theory and the ambiguity and subjectivity inherent in any face form classification,[44,45] the geometric theory remains most dentists' method of choice for selecting anterior artificial teeth. Scientifically, however, the validity of correlating tooth form with facial form or size is widely refuted by biometric and standardized photographic research.[21,45–48] Therefore, face form is not a precise determinant of tooth form.

Proportion determined by dentist and patient preference

Woodhead[23] demonstrated that several molds of maxillary central incisors were narrower mesiodistally than any extracted tooth he measured and further concluded that very few denture molds were available for teeth larger than the average width of 9.0 mm. McArthur[49,50] studied casts from completed orthodontic patients and computed an average difference of 0.51 mm between the maxillary central incisor and typical denture molds. Kern[51] studied 509 skulls with good dentition and analyzed the relation between the bizygomatic measurements and the width of the maxillary central incisors and only found the biometric ratio of 1/16 on 31% of skulls, whereas 60% of skulls revealed ratios of 1/14 and 1/15. This means that the "biometric ratio" method would select a too-narrow mold 60% of the time. Brisman[52] evaluated the preferences of patients, dentists, and dental students and found preference on drawings of central incisors for the 0.75 or 0.80 width-to-length ratio. On photographs, however, patients still favored the 0.8 ratio whereas dentists and dental students selected longer and narrower teeth with a ratio of 0.66. This means that clinicians may be somewhat conditioned by denture tooth selection and narrow central incisors, as Woodhead and McArthur had suspected.

Proportion determined by anatomic characteristics

Isolated studies find some relation between the size of the maxillary central incisor and various anatomic features.[21,51,53,54] However, the evidence remains too thin to strictly correlate the shape of the maxillary central incisor with a facial landmark.

Ideal dimensions of the maxillary central incisor cannot scientifically be generated from face form or any privileged proportion. Instead, subjective criteria prevail: esthetically pleasing proportions are expressed with a width-to-length ratio ranging between 0.75 to 0.8. Despite wide variations in personal interpretation and perception, the clinician must refine a sense of proportion based on observation of pleasing natural dentition. Restrictions may be imposed by tooth position, arch width, and gingival outline; however, narrow and elongated or short and wide central incisors must always be avoided in esthetic reconstruction.

Proportions in Dental Composition

- Maxillary central incisor of pleasing proportions
- Dominance of the maxillary central incisors
- Pleasing proportion between maxillary central and lateral incisors
  Relative priorities include:
- Pleasing proportion between maxillary lateral incisors and canines
- Same recurring proportion between maxillary central and lateral incisors and between maxillary lateral incisors and canines

---

Optimum tooth-to-tooth relationship

The optimum relationship between central incisors, lateral incisors, and canines is governed by rules borrowing from dominance and rhythm (repeated ratio). With deficient crowns, the question is: what is the ideal arrangement between the anterior teeth, and does it follow precise rules?

Dominance and rhythm

Frush and Fisher[41] and Lombardi[14] emphasized the need for maxillary central incisors to be of sufficient size to dominate the smile, because any composition is based on dominance of a major element. Lombardi also stressed the importance of order in the composition, with the same recurring ratio from the central incisor to the first premolar. Levin[27] felt that the most harmonious recurrent tooth-to-tooth ratio was found in the "golden proportion." This implies that the maxillary central incisor should be approximately 60% wider than the lateral incisor and that the lateral incisor should be approximately 60% wider than the mesial aspect of the canine. In this summation series, each term is composed of the sum of the two preceding terms. One consequence is that when a canine is in golden proportion to a lateral incisor, the distal aspect of the canine must not be visible from the facial aspect. Ricketts[26] also determined rules of dentofacial harmony based on the golden proportion and on recurring proportions for the features of an attractive face.

Ideal central incisor-to-lateral incisor ratio

The golden proportion between the mesiodistal diameter of the maxillary lateral incisor and central incisor dictates I2/I1 = 0.618. Instead, mesiodistal measurements of natural teeth[11,12,20,22,28] reveal an average I2/I1 ratio ranging from 0.75 to 0.79. Only when the lateral incisor is rotated in the arch and appears narrower would the I2/I1 ratio fall in the 0.60-to-0.70 range. Variations in mesiodistal diameter of lateral incisors are very wide (3.98 mm average) and greater than those of central incisors (2.98 mm average) so that the only conclusion drawn from natural teeth studies is that ideal proportions between the maxillary incisors may vary within a wide range as long as definite dominance of the central incisors is established (Figs. 3-21–3-27).

A common mistake in esthetic restorations is to restore maxillary incisors out of proportion with another: the lateral incisors are often slightly oversized at the expense of the central incisors. The goal of the clinician is to shift the dominance from the lateral incisor to the central incisor. When in doubt, the central incisors should be slightly oversized because their line angles may be readjusted later to give the illusion of a narrower tooth.

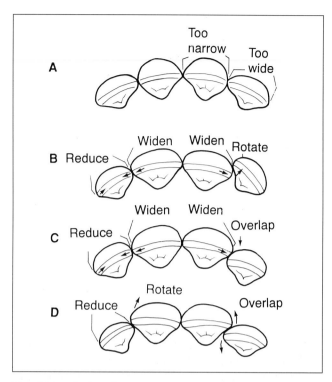

Fig. 3-21 Options for reharmonizing tooth-to-tooth proportions in a smile of normal width: **A,** Deficient crowns with deficient tooth-to-tooth proportions are shown; **B,** Widening the central incisors results in width reduction and/or rotation of the lateral incisors; **C,** Widening the central incisors results in width reduction and/or overlapping the central incisors over the lateral incisors (Geller modification); **D,** Widening the central incisors results in rotation of the central incisors for additional width, reduction, and/or overlapping the central incisors over the lateral incisors.

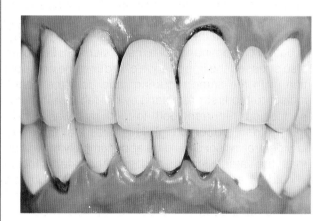

Fig. 3-22a Root decay will require surgical elongation of the maxillary anterior teeth so that the crown margins will extend into sound tooth structure. The central incisors are already narrow and long and will be further elongated by surgery. The incisal edge position cannot be modified in this situation because the patient has a long lip and there is already minimal incisal display.

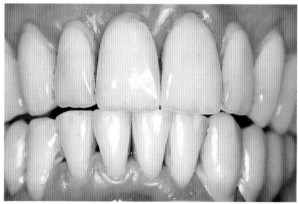

Fig. 3-22b The final restoration gives an illusion of shorter teeth: the facial aspect of the central incisors is flattened, the line angles are displaced laterally to suggest width, and the root effects are prominent with a definite cementoenamel junction to displace the cervical convexity coronally and suggest shorter teeth. The lateral incisors are as narrow as possible to suggest dominance of the central incisors by contrast. All these illusions must be incorporated simultaneously to be effective.

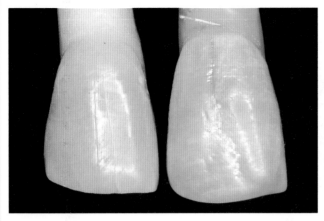

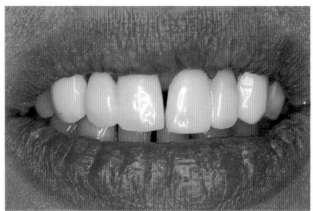

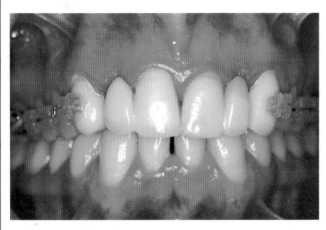

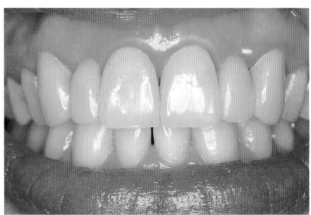

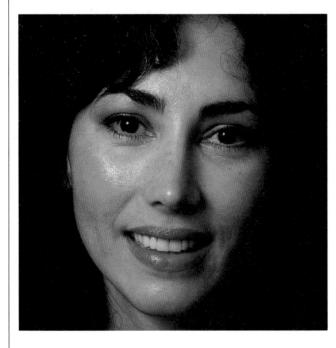

Fig. 3-23a Narrow central incisors lack intrinsic proportion and dominance over the lateral incisors. It is essential to avoid this type of geometry in the final esthetic result.

Fig. 3-23b This patient presents with acrylic resin restorations that incorporate long narrow central incisors. Because the lateral incisors are narrow, widening the central incisors would either result in overlapping over the lateral incisors or in having to expand the whole smile.

Fig. 3-23c Orthodontic movement of the canines distally was the option of choice because the smile appeared too narrow in relation to the face. Orthodontic correction provided for an additional space of 1 to 1.5 mm bilaterally. (Orthodontic treatment: Dr G Dongieux.)

Fig. 3-23d Final reconstruction with two three-unit fixed partial dentures. The facial aspect of the central incisors was slightly flattened to suggest additional width, and the canine tips were distalized to widen the effective width of the smile.

Fig. 3-23e Final appearance of the anterior restorations.

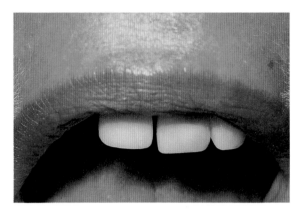

a

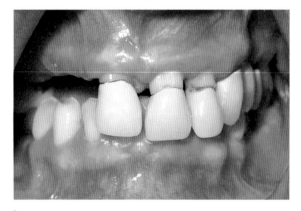

b

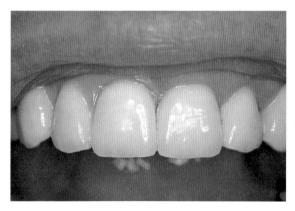

c

Fig. 3-24a–c Figure a and b: Narrow long crowns after periodontal surgery. The incisors are also elongated because of supraeruption, the vertical overlap is excessive, and there is ample incisal display. The lip is short and concave and can accommodate less incisal exposure. Fig. c: The final rehabilitation after extraction of the right central incisor consists of a removable partial denture with a precision attachment between the central incisors. The denture teeth are customized metal ceramic restorations. The anterior teeth have been shortened to more acceptable proportions, and there is still adequate tooth display due to the short lip.

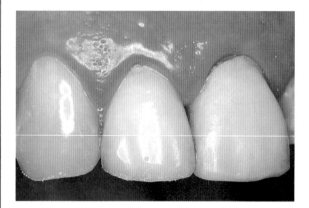

Fig. 3-25a The three most common mistakes with deficient anterior crowns are: a flat facial aspect of the central incisor; too wide lateral incisor and/or too narrow central incisor; and a straight incisal plane.

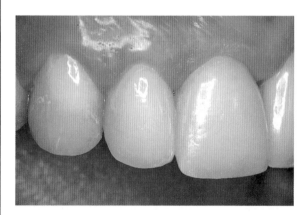

Fig. 3-25b Final correction. The objective was to shift the dominance from the lateral incisors to the central incisors. If the central incisors must be widened, they often must also be elongated for optimal intrinsic proportions.

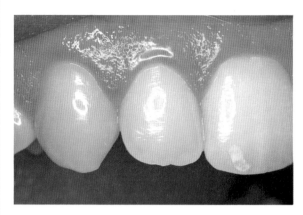

a

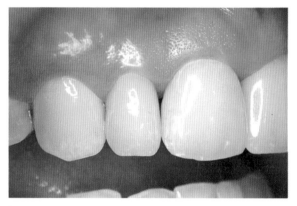

b

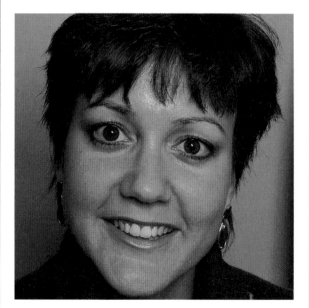

c

Fig. 3-26a Natural shade progression. The central and lateral incisors are significantly lighter than the canines. This abrupt color change between incisors and canines is frequently observed in natural dentition.

Fig. 3-26b and c Color progression in prosthetic restorations should be less abrupt than in natural dentition. When the lateral incisor shade is a combination between the canine and central incisor shade, there is a smooth transition that makes the darker canine less noticeable to the patient and also emphasizes the prominence of the central incisors. In this facial view, there is no abrupt color change from the central incisor crowns to the canines.

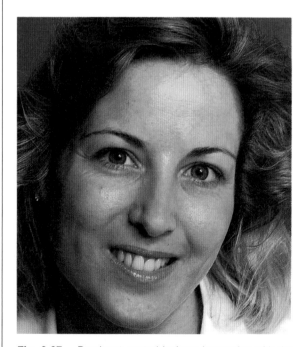

Fig. 3-27 Dominant central incisors harmonize with the face as long as their intrinsic proportion is pleasing. If the central incisors are judged slightly too wide, their line angles may be adjusted toward the center of the tooth to suggest a narrower tooth. If the central incisors appear too narrow, it is more difficult to suggest additional width by displacing the line angles laterally.

Gingival outline

The final evaluation of deficient crowns is made at the gingival level. Gingival contours may require alteration to: *(1)* eliminate residual periodontal defects; *(2)* improve symmetry between the maxillary central incisors; *(3)* enhance tooth proportion; *(4)* achieve a pleasing gingival outline; *(5)* reduce excessive gingival display; or *(6)* facilitate the restorative process.

Asymmetry

Asymmetry in length between the maxillary central incisors requires special attention because excessive asymmetry close to the dental and facial midline is unattractive. It often results from different patterns of wear or eruption between the central incisors, leading to uneven gingival margins. With medium to high lip lines, obvious cervical disharmony between the maxillary central incisors requires either surgical elongation, root coverage, or orthodontic correction. Gingival symmetry between the lateral incisors or between the canines is not mandatory; unilateral display of the free gingival margin of a lateral incisor or a canine in various smile positions is esthetically acceptable.

Tooth proportion

Tooth proportion may be significantly enhanced by relocating the gingival margin either apically or coronally, according to the desired effect. It is most commonly indicated for the maxillary incisors.

Gingival outline

Gingival margins normally follow two pleasing outlines. The sinuous pattern occurs when the gingival margin of the lateral incisor is coronal to the tangent drawn between the gingival margins of the central incisor and of the canine unilaterally. The straight pattern occurs when the gingival margins of the central incisors, lateral incisors, and canines are aligned along the same tangent unilaterally. These tangents may be bilaterally asymmetric in the same mouth. A combination pattern is also observed where a sinuous and a straight outline coexist on either side of the midline. A displeasing gingival outline occurs when the gingival margin of the lateral incisor is apical to the tangent drawn between the gingival margins of the central incisor and canine. If possible, surgical or orthodontic correction of this outline should be attempted before any crown restorations are planned (Figs. 3-28–3-32).

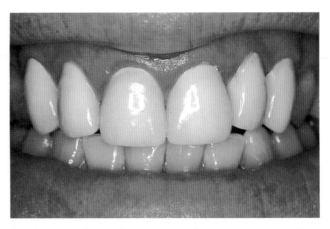

Fig. 3-28 A displeasing gingival outline causes the lateral incisors to extend beyond the level of gingival margins of the central incisor and the canine. A determination must be made whether the lateral incisor margins are too high or the central incisors are too low. In the latter situation, the central incisors would be diagnosed as having supraerupted and the lateral incisor margins as in correct position. Preprosthetic treatment will consist of either intrusion or surgical elongation of the central incisors.

Gingival exposure

Excessive gingival exposure is often encountered in patients with short lip lines and/or supraerupted maxillary anterior teeth. Proper diagnosis is essential[29] and is based on the location of the cementoenamel junction, the potential for root exposure, and an appraisal of the existing tooth length and incisal edge position. The decision between reduction with gingivectomy, flap surgery, orthodontic intrusion, or orthognathic surgery is made according to the severity of the "gummy smile."

Restorative procedures

Even though surgical elongation, root coverage, and ridge augmentation procedures may not fulfill the original expectations of the clinician, with good indications the restorative process is always facilitated by plastic periodontal surgery, as long as gingival alterations proceed in the desired direction. It is difficult to restore two central incisors displaying excessive gingival asymmetry because a shorter crown appears darker and also because the levels of the cervical convexities between the two teeth do not match and result in uneven light reflection at the surface, making the asymmetry even more noticeable. On young patients with high lip lines, root exposure caused by marked gingival recession, or the placement of a root form in a pontic caused by an apical ridge defect are difficult restorative challenges better resolved with root coverage or ridge augmentation procedures preprosthetically. These defects are otherwise conspicuous in this age group when left uncorrected.

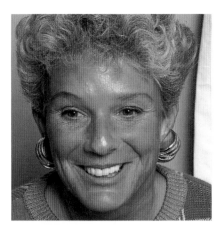

Fig. 3-29 In the initial esthetically deficient fixed partial denture there is ample tooth exposure.

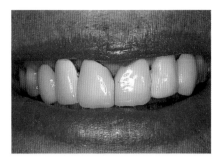

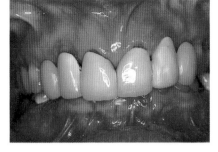

Fig. 3-30a and b The central incisors are too long (13 mm), the vertical overlap is excessive, and the anterior abutments exhibit Class 2 and 3 mobility. The gingival outline is abnormal and suggestive of supraeruption of the central incisors. The right lateral incisor needs root coverage, and the canine pontics need to be relocated at a level consistent with a pleasing gingival outline in relation to the incisors. The objectives of treatment are to shorten the incisors at the incisal edge and to relocate the central incisor crowns more apically, to reduce the vertical overbite and to achieve an esthetic gingival outline.

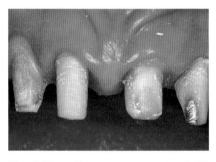

Fig. 3-31a Abutments were restored with post and core buildups and were provisionalized. The initial preparation is completed, and residual periodontal defects must be corrected surgically.

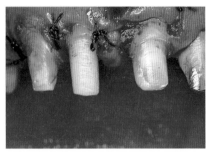

Fig. 3-31b Periodontal surgery consisted of apical repositioning of the gingival margins of the central incisors by 2 to 3 mm, root coverage of the right lateral incisor, and frenectomy. The deep mesial margin associated with the central incisor was not corrected in order to preserve the interdental papilla and because the patient was able to maintain that pocket and declined forced orthodontic eruption of the tooth.

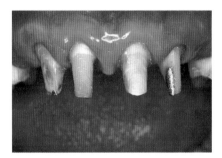

Fig. 3-31c Postsurgical appearance at 4 months with normal gingival outline.

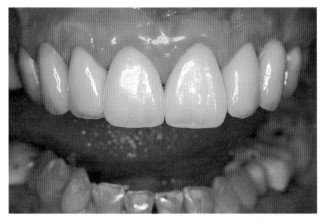

Fig. 3-31d Final esthetic rehabilitation with an eight-unit fixed partial denture.

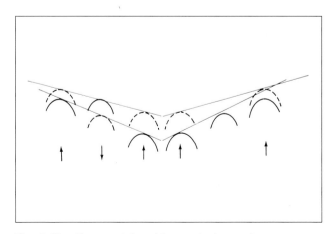

Fig. 3-32 Representation of the surgical procedure.

Replacement of deficient crowns

Before attempting any gingival correction it is preferable to replace deficient crowns with sound provisional restorations for the following reasons:

1. the shadow of a metal margin or dark root may give the false illusion of a shorter tooth and lead to an error in appreciation of tooth length.
2. gingival margins may recede after tooth preparation and scaling and result in a slight increase in crown length.
3. the level of gingival margins cannot be considered stable with deficient crowns, causing unequal degrees of gingival inflammation.[56] Correction of subgingival overhanging margins with sound provisional restorations as part of initial therapy is expected to result in significant changes in pocket depth and gingival architecture. Therefore, it is necessary to wait for 4 to 12 weeks[57] for stabilization of the gingival tissues before reevaluation and prescription of plastic periodontal surgery if necessary (Table 3-2).
4. the gingival outline may significantly change as it returns to health; scalloping is increased and marginal tissues regain their knife-edge configuration. Gingival asymmetry or irregularity that was not present initially may also result from this initial preparation and need to be corrected surgically. Therefore, before removing deficient crowns in the anterior region, the patient must be cautioned that plastic periodontal corrections may be eventually required, even though they do not seem to be indicated initially.

Table 3-2 Mean Pocket Depth (mm) after Elimination of Proximal Subgingival Overhangs*

	Test		Control	
	x	SD	x	SD
Preoperative	3.30 ± 1.15		3.53 ± 1.29	
4 weeks	2.40 ± 1.29		2.92 ± 0.99	
8 weeks	2.07 ± 0.98		2.63 ± 1.16	
12 weeks	1.71 ± 0.91		2.40 ± 1.13	

*Adapted from: Rodriguez-Ferrer HJ, Strahan JD, Newman HN. Effect on gingival health of removing overhanging margins of interproximal subgingival amalgam restorations. *J Clin Periodontol* 1980:7;457.

Endodontic considerations in prosthetic retreatment*

Assessing the status of the pulp

Pulp testing produces more accurate information after old crowns have been removed and replaced with temporary crowns. Temporary crowns can be easily removed for testing at a subsequent appointment without anesthesia, which is an appropriate time to evaluate their status. The results of all stimulation pulp tests are limited to information about vitality. A vital pulp implies only that neural elements are functioning. A vital pulp may be unhealthy or incapable of surviving additional irritation such as recrowning procedures, which is an essential consideration with retreatment of deficient crowns. There is no test that measures viability or health of the pulp, and therefore judgments must be made in many instances.

The guidelines for pulpal evaluation are as follows:
- Presence of pain. Lingering pain (30 seconds or longer) after thermal stimulation (hot or cold) is indicative of irreversible pulpitis. The process of removing existing crowns, preparation, and fabrication of temporary crowns can cause "stressed" pulps to become symptomatic. A patient may not be able to identify the offending tooth because the pulp lacks proprioceptive fibers. For an accurate diagnosis, the dentist can use thermal testing to reproduce symptoms of pain. Percussion or bite sensitivity indicates that the periodontal ligament is inflamed, with pulpal necrosis as the most common cause. Since the periodontal ligament contains proprioceptive fibers, identification of the offending tooth can be accomplished with the percussion test. It is critical to regularly question the patient about any episodes of lingering spontaneous pain, even mild pain, throughout the retreatment.

- Radiographic evaluation. Periapical radiographs should be evaluated for the presence of periodontal bone loss, periapical radiolucencies, and pulp cavity morphology.

- Vitality testing. Ideally, all teeth to be recrowned should be tested. In some instances, an air blast may quickly confirm vitality when the temporary crown is removed. Otherwise, electric testing or a cold test may be required, such as freon spray on a cotton pellet, which is especially effective. Endodontic therapy is advised if any tooth is nonresponsive or has a weaker response than neighboring teeth. The dentist may elect prophylactic endodon-

*Ron R Lemon, DDS, contributed this section.

tic therapy in instances with thin teeth and large pulps requiring significant reduction for esthetic purpose, where post build-ups are required for retention purpose, or where the prognosis of pulp viability is questionable. Special attention should be given to: presence of teeth within periodontal involvement; recurrent caries; calcification of the pulp cavity; "blushing" pulps; percussion sensitivity; large restorations; periapical radiolucency.

Assessing the endodontically treated tooth

Perhaps the least recognized relationship between restorative dentistry and the long-term endodontic success or failure is orthograde leakage. This leakage occurs at the tooth-restorative interface and can result in loss of the endodontic sealer within the canal, causing failure. Therefore, any endodontic filling material exposed to percolation (eg, caries and open margins, lost restorations) must be replaced.

Most Frequent Mistakes Found in Deficient Crowns

- The crowns are overcontoured or opaque because of underreduced preparations.
- The facial aspect of the central incisors is overcontoured.
- The central incisors are too narrow.
- The lateral incisors are too wide.
- The central incisors are asymmetrical at their gingival aspect.
- All four incisors are too aligned and narrow.
- The incisal plane is too straight.

Retreatment for Deficient Crowns

Objectives

- Determine the incisal edge position of the preparation
- Determine the incisal edge position of the central incisor
- Determine the facial curvature of the central incisor
- Determine pleasing proportions for the central incisor
- Establish pleasing symmetry at the midline
- Harmonize the proportions between the anterior teeth
- Harmonize the incisal and gingival planes with the face

Sequence

Phase 1

1. Remove the existing crowns, reprepare the abutments for proper reduction, and scale and root plane.
2. Determine the proper shape and incisal edge position of the central incisor in the provisional restoration and refine the incisal edge of the preparations.
3. Provide for dominance of the central incisors with respect to the lateral incisors; harmonize anterior guidance.

Phase 2

1. Reevaluate pulp status, gingival defects, anterior guidance, and tooth mobility.
2. Refer patient for endodontic and/or periodontal consultation and treatment as indicated.

Phase 3

1. Finalize crown build-ups, axial reduction, and margin placement on completion of endodontic therapy and periodontal healing.
2. Complete final restorations.

References

1. Greenberg JR. Shaping anterior teeth for natural esthetics. *Esthet Dent Update* 1992;3:86.

2. Spear F. Facially generated treatment planning: A restorative viewpoint. Presented at the American Academy of Esthetic Dentistry, 16th Annual Meeting, Santa Barbara, Calif., August 8, 1991.

3. Geller W. Dental Ceramics and Esthetics. Chicago, February 15, 1991.

4. Goldstein RE. *Change Your Smile*. Chicago: Quintessence, 1984.

5. Riley M. Creative approaches to total dento facial esthetics. Presented at the American Academy of Esthetic Dentistry, 17th Annual Meeting, Santa Fe, NM, August 8, 1992.

6. Shavell H. Mastering the art of esthetics. Presented at the New Orleans Dental Conference, New Orleans, September 1986.

7. Miller LL: Porcelain crowns and porcelain laminates. Problems and solutions. Quintessence International Symposium, 1991, New Orleans.

8. Vig RG, Brundo GC. The kinetics of anterior tooth display. *J Prosthet Dent* 1978;39:502.

9. Allen EP. Use of mucogingival surgical procedures to enhance esthetics. *Dent Clin North Am* 1988;32:307.

10. Shillingburg HT, Kaplan MJ, Grace CS. Tooth dimensions—a comparative study. *J South Calif Dent Assoc* 1972;40:830.

11. Bjorndal AM, Henderson WG, Skidmore AE, Kellner FH. Anatomic measurements of human teeth extracted from males between the ages of 17 and 21 years. *Oral Surg Oral Med Oral Pathol* 1974;38:791.

12. Woelfel JB. *Dental Anatomy: Its Relevance to Dentistry*, ed 4. Philadelphia: Lea & Febiger, 1990.

13. Dawson PE. Determining the determinants of occlusion. *Int J Periodont Rest Dent* 1983;3(6):9.

14. Lombardi RE. The principles of visual perception and their clinical application to denture esthetics. *J Prosthet Dent* 1973; 29:358.

15. Miller. The esthetic challenge. Les Journees Dentaires Quebec. 1990, Montreal.

16. Moores CFA, Thomsen SO, Jensen E, Yen PKJ. Mesiodistal crown diameters of the deciduous and permanent teeth in individuals. *J Dent Res* 1957;36:39.

17. Garn SM, Lewis AB, Kerewsky RS. Sex difference in tooth size. *J Dent Res* 1964;43:306.

18. Garn SM, Lewis AB, Swindler DR, Kerewsky RS. Genetic control of sexual dimorphism in tooth size. *J Dent Res* 1967; 46(supplement 5):963.

19. Goose DH. Preliminary study of tooth size in families. *J Dent Res* 1967;46(supplement 5):959.

20. Garn SM, Lewis AB, Walenga AJ. Maximum-confidence value for the human mesiodistal crown dimension of human teeth. *Arch Oral Biol* 1968;13:841.

21. Lavelle CLB. The relationship between stature, skull, dental arch and tooth dimensions in different racial groups. *Orthodontist* 1971;Spring:7.

22. Sanin C, Savara BS. An analysis of permanent mesiodistal crown size. *Am J Orthodont* 1971.

23. Woodhead MC. The mesiodistal diameter of permanent maxillary central incisor teeth and their prosthetic replacements. *J Dent* 1977;5:93.

24. Mavroskoufis F, Ritchie GM. Variation in size and form between left and right maxillary central incisor teeth. *J Prosthet Dent* 1980;43:254.

25. McArthur RD. Determining approximate size of maxillary artificial teeth when mandibular anterior teeth are present. Part I. Size relationship. *J Prosthet Dent* 1985;53:216.

26. Ricketts RM. The biologic significance of the divine proportion and Fibonacci series. *Am J Orthod* 1982;81:351.

27. Levin EI. Dental esthetics and the golden proportion. *J Prosthet Dent* 1978;40:244.

28. Ballard ML. Asymmetry in tooth size: A factor in the etiology, diagnosis and treatment of malocclusion. *Angle Orthod* 1944; 14:67.

29. Allen EP. Use of mucogingival surgical procedures to enhance esthetics. *Dent Clin North Am* 1988;32:307.

30. Ash MM. *Wheeler's Dental Anatomy, Physiology, and Occlusion*. Philadelphia: Saunders, 1984.

31. Hall WR. *Shapes and Sizes of Teeth From American System of Dentistry*. Philadelphia: Lea Bros, 1887:971.

32. Berry FH. Is the theory of temperament the foundation to the study of prosthetic art? *Dent Mag* 1905;61:405.

33. House MM, Loop JL. *Form and Color Harmony in the Dental Art*. Whittier, Calif.: M.M. House, 1939.

34. Williams JL. A new classification of human tooth forms with a special reference to a new system of artificial teeth. *Dent Cosmos* 1914;56:627.

35. Hughes GA. Facial types and tooth arrangement. *J Prosthet Dent* 1951;1:82.

36. Carson JW. Tooth form and face form, is it a "comedy of errors"? *J Prosthet Dent* 1951;1:96.

37. Young HA. Selecting the anterior tooth mold. *J Prosthet Dent* 1954;4:748.

38. Clapp GW. How the science of esthetic tooth-form selection was made easy. *J Prosthet Dent* 1955;5:596.

39. Frush JP, Fisher RD. Introduction to dentogenic restorations. *J Prosthet Dent* 1955;5:586.

40. Frush JP, Fisher RD. How dentogenics interpret the personality factor. *J Prosthet Dent* 1956;6:441.

41. Frush JP, Fisher RD. How dentogenic restorations interpret the sex factor. *J Prosthet Dent* 1956;6:160.

42. Frush JP, Fisher RD. The age factor in dentogenics. *J Prosthet Dent* 1957;7:5.

43. Frush JP, Fisher RD. The dynesthetic interpretation of the dentogenic concept. *J Prosthet Dent* 1958;8:558.

44. Frush JP, Fisher RD. Dentogenics: Its practical applications. *J Prosthet Dent* 1959;9:915.

45. Brodbelt RHW, Walker GF, Nelson D, Seluk LW. A comparison of face shape with tooth form. *J Prosthet Dent* 1984;52:588.

46. Bell RA. The geometric theory of selection of artificial teeth. Is it valid? *J Am Dent Assoc* 1978;97:637.

47. Mavroskoufis F, Ritchie GM. The face form as a guide for the selection of maxillary central incisors. *J Prosthet Dent* 1980; 43:501.

48. Seluk LW, Brodbelt RHW, Walker GF. A biometric comparison of face shape with denture tooth form. *J Oral Rehabil* 1987; 14:139.

49. McArthur RD. Are anterior replacement teeth too small? *J Prosthet Dent* 1987;57:462.

50. McArthur RD. Determination of approximate size of maxillary anterior denture teeth when mandibular anterior teeth are present. Part III. Relationship of maxillary to mandibular central incisor widths. *J Prosthet Dent* 1985;53:540.

51. Kern BE. Anthropometric parameters of tooth selection. *J Prosthet Dent* 1967;17:431.

52. Brisman AS. Esthetics: A comparison of dentists' and patients' concepts. *J Am Dent Assoc* 1980;100:345.

53. Cesario VA, Latta GH. Relationship between the mesiodistal width of the maxillary central incisor and the interpupillary distance. *J Prosthet Dent* 1984;52:641.

54. Singh S, Bhalla LR, Khanna VK. Relationship between width of maxillary central incisors and width of philtrum. *J Indian Dent Assoc* 1971;264.

55. Ballard ML. Asymmetry in tooth size: A factor in the etiology, diagnosis and treatment of malocclusion. *Angle Orthod* 1944; 14:67.

56. Shavell HM. Mastering the art of tissue management during provisionalization and biologic final impressions. *Int J Periodont Rest Dent* 1988;8(3):25.

57. Rodriguez-Ferrer HJ, Strahan JD, Newman HN. Effect on gingival health of removing overhanging margins of interproximal subgingival amalgam restorations. *J Clin Periodontol* 1980; 7:457.

Chapter 4

Metal Ceramic Crowns

Gerard Chiche and Alain Pinault

Metal ceramic and all-ceramic restorations have excellent esthetic potential when tooth preparation is correctly executed. Faulty tooth preparation may lead to overcontouring of the restoration, gingival inflammation, poor esthetics, or poor retention.

Anterior preparations for full veneer crowns

Tooth preparations are based on retention-resistance, preservation of the pulp, respect of the periodontium, occlusal function, and conservation of tooth structure.[1–4] Tooth reduction is dictated by three imperatives: *(1)* length of the preparation for adequate retention-resistance; *(2)* thickness of the ceramic veneer for proper esthetic rendition; and *(3)* occlusal clearance for occlusal function and anterior guidance (Fig. 4-1). Tooth preparation must be meticulous to reconcile these three antagonistic imperatives, especially in the anterior region where surface area is minimal. To identify factors that may compromise an ideal tooth preparation for a maxillary incisor, a detailed tooth analysis prior to preparation should evaluate: tooth length, tooth thickness, taper of the clinical crown, pulp size and status, and occlusal relations—vertical and horizontal overlap, location of occlusal contact, and crowding of mandibular incisors (Figs. 4-2–4-6).

Retention

The tooth preparation must be of sufficient length[5] and surface area[6,7] with an ideal 6° convergence angle[8] between the proximal walls and between the cingulum portion of the lingual wall and one half to two thirds of the facial wall. This ensures that the crown has only one path of insertion and that the luting cement is placed under as much compression as possible during function.[1–4]

Ideally, the clinician's objective is to achieve a convergence angle of 6° because retention values at 10° are only about half of those at 5°[8] and also because there is no significant difference in retention between 10° and 16° tapers.[9] Clinically, however, convergence angles of 15° to 23° are the rule rather than the exception[10–13] because a small taper free of undercuts is difficult to achieve.[11] Therefore, from a practical standpoint, the optimal degree of convergence of the axial walls should fall within a 6°-to-10° range.

Retention-resistance may be compromised with a short preparation, and with anterior tooth preparations it is frequently a challenge to create a lingual axial wall of sufficient length for retention and resistance.[14] This is because a uniform reduction of tooth structure often results in an overtapered preparation[15] or because the cingulum is not prominent or is abraded. In addition, deep lingual-occlusal contacts may compromise the length of the lingual axial wall of the preparation. If primary retention factors are insufficient, secondary factors should be incorporated.[4] Even though the small size of anterior teeth restricts the effectiveness of additional retention-resistance features, which in addition may weaken surrounding tooth structure, several solutions are available (Figs. 4-7 and 4-8):

- Increase parallelism between all axial walls; total taper in the 0°-to-3° range provides for the maxi-

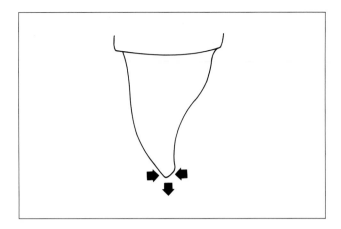

Fig. 4-1   The incisal edge position of the preparation depends on three antagonistic factors that dictate incisal position in three directions. Incisal edge location must be precise to reconcile esthetics, occlusion, and retention.

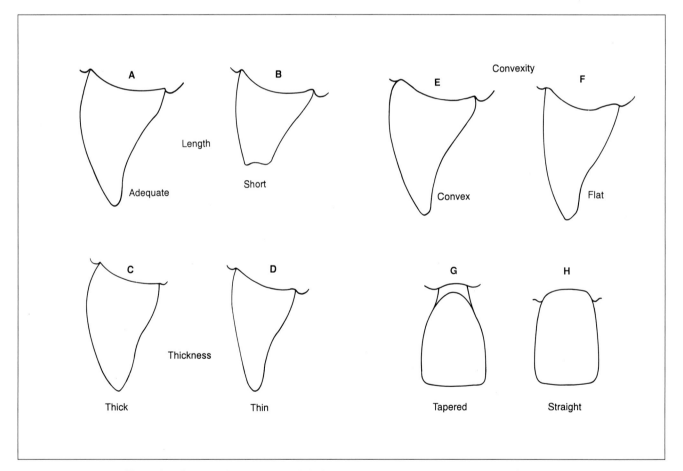

Fig. 4-2   Preoperative tooth analysis before tooth preparation is made consists of evaluation of length, labiolingual thickness, and convexity and taper.

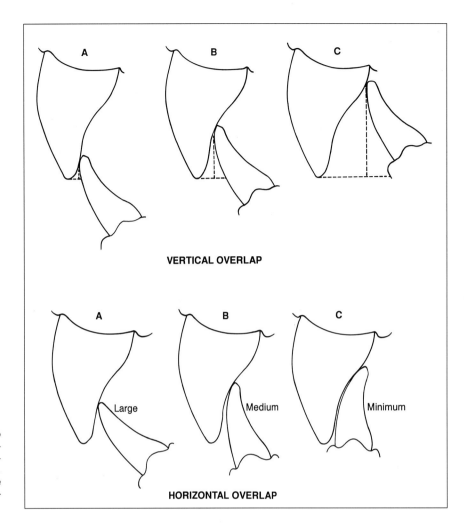

Fig. 4-3 Preoperative tooth analysis also includes evaluation of vertical overlap, horizontal overlap, and pulp size. These factors, together with those described in Fig. 4-2, determine the degree of difficulty of the tooth preparation and whether elective endodontic therapy may be required.

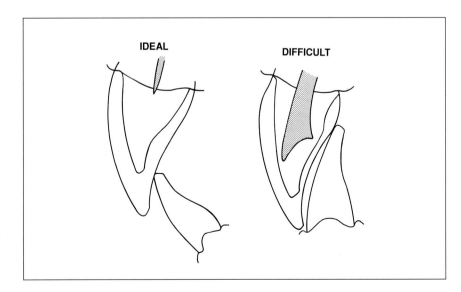

Fig. 4-4 A thick tooth of minimum convexity and taper, with a retracted pulp and with a large horizontal overlap and shallow vertical overlap, presents little difficulty at tooth preparation. A thin tooth with a severe convexity and taper, a large pulp, and small horizontal overlap and deep vertical overlap involves difficult preparation and possible elective endodontic therapy.

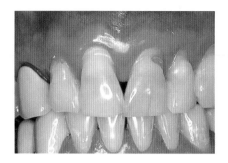

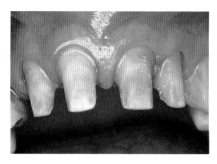

Fig. 4-5a Tapered teeth with cervical recession are difficult to prepare for optimum metal ceramic thickness. The patient must be warned before preparation of the possibility that teeth may be devitalized as needed to satisfy esthetic requirements.

Fig. 4-5b In the finished preparations the facial shoulder is 0.5 to 0.8 mm wide to minimize pulpal trauma.

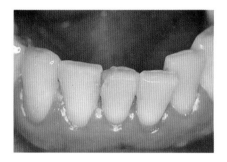

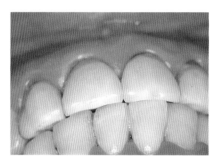

Fig. 4-6a and b Crowded opposing teeth may impose severe limitations when significant esthetic modifications in position or arrangement of the maxillary anterior teeth are planned. Unless crowding is corrected orthodontically, incisal edge position of the new crowns will not be significantly modified, and protrusive interferences will be difficult to eliminate.

mum retention[8] but is extremely difficult to achieve without creating undercuts.

- Prepare the lingual axial wall toward the center of the preparation and chamfer the edge of the lingual margin (ie, terraced design).[15]
- Prepare the lingual axial wall toward the center of the preparation and elongate it cervically with a thin tapered carbide bur (preparations for metal ceramic restorations only).
- When the occlusal contact is coronal to the cingulum, prepare the lingual axial wall so that most of the original height of the cingulum is preserved in the preparation.
- Sharpen the axiogingival line angles with a thin tapered carbide bur (for metal ceramic restoration preparations only).
- Prepare an axial groove if it can be of adequate length and does not weaken surrounding tooth structure (for metal ceramic restorations only).

Position of the incisal edge of the preparation

Stein[16] advocated "canting" the occlusal third of the preparation for proper positioning of the incisal table in relation to function and esthetics. A one-plane facial reduction may come dangerously close to the pulp[17] and may also result in an overtapered preparation or produce opaque showthrough or overcontouring of the incisal third of the restoration. To satisfy esthetic, occlusal, and retention requirements, the incisal edge of the preparation assumes a precise position. The clinician, therefore, must use a reference when preparing the incisal aspect of the preparation. Three situations are encountered (Figs. 4-9–4-19):

- *The facial convexity of the tooth to be prepared serves as a reference.* When the tooth preparation is developed from calibrated depth cuts, the incisal edge of the preparation will automatically assume a correct position[18] (Figs. 4-11–4-15).
- *The adjacent tooth serves as a reference for the incisal edge.* If the adjacent tooth does not need to be prepared, it serves as a convenient reference for the incisal edge of the preparation, which is simply aligned to it (Fig. 4-17). If the adjacent tooth needs to be prepared, preparations should be sequenced around this reference tooth, which as a rule should be prepared last (Figs. 4-9 and 4-10). The every-other-tooth[19] preparation technique or other variations are useful in this context.

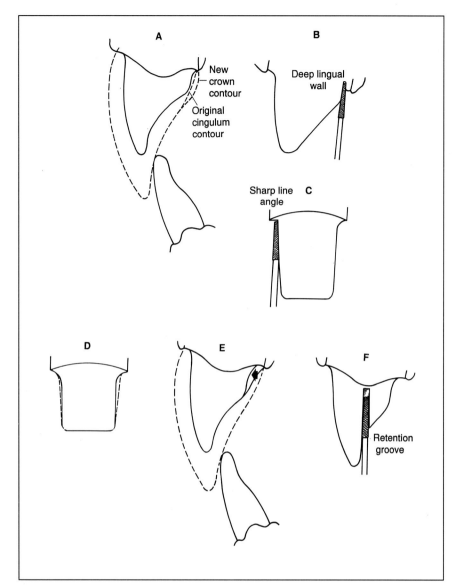

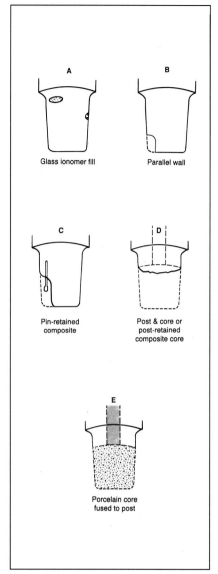

Fig. 4-7 To enhance retention of anterior preparations: **A,** The original height of the cingulum is maintained in the preparation when the centric contact is coronal to the cingulum. **B,** The short lingual wall is deepened apically with a thin carbide bur. Care should be taken not to make the lingual edge of the preparation fragile and to achieve a chamfer finish line in the lingual aspect (consider this option as a last resort). **C,** The internal line angles are sharpened with a thin carbide bur for additional length. **D,** The convergence of the axial walls is accentuated to a near-absolute parallelism. **E,** The lingual wall is further prepared toward the facial aspect until it is of adequate height. **F,** Retention grooves are prepared in the proximal aspects.

Fig. 4-8 Compensation of lost tooth structure for adequate retention of anterior preparations. (**E,** Design courtesy of de Cooman J, de Rouffignac M. Reconstitutions céramo-métalliques des dents dépulpées destinées à recevoir des coiffes sans alliages. lére partie. *RFPD* 1989;65:71.)

• *There is no reference available because of previous crowning.* In a retreatment situation, after crown removal, it is difficult to assess whether the abutments were adequately prepared or not because no reference is available. Repreparation is at first arbitrary, then provisional restorations are fabricated from the diagnostic wax-up, incorporating the prescribed corrections. Once the provisional restorations are deemed functional and esthetically pleasing, their facial thickness should be measured[15] and the preparations further refined to ensure adequate thickness for the ceramic crowns (Fig. 4-19).

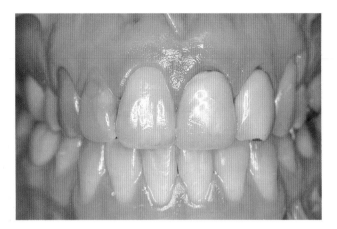

Fig. 4-9 This patient wanted to improve the esthetic appearance of the anterior teeth. The crown restorations will be removed first and the incisal edges aligned with the uncrowned central incisor serving as a reference.

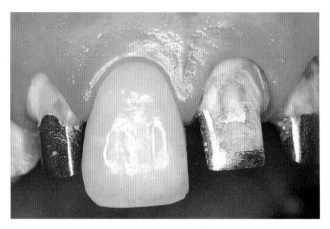

Fig. 4-10 The preparation sequence is organized so that the most intact central incisor is prepared last. The preparations and post and cores are reduced so that their incisal edge is aligned in reference to the unprepared tooth.

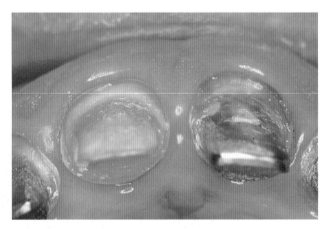

Fig. 4-11 Once the adjacent preparations are completed, the reference tooth is prepared using a half-preparation technique. With this sequence, the clinician ensures that the final crown restorations will incorporate the desired facial convexity.

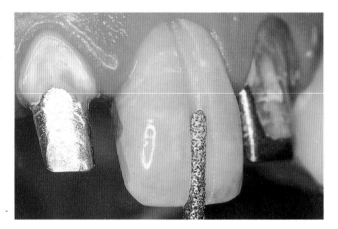

Fig. 4-12 The half-preparation technique involves cutting a depth groove to follow the facial aspect of the tooth with a round-ended diamond bur. Note the pronounced convexity of the facial aspect. At this stage the depth groove should extend to the gingival margin.

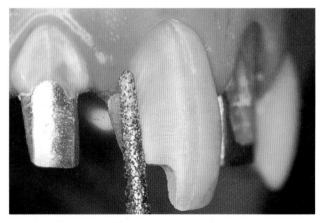

Fig. 4-13 A half-preparation is obtained by *(1)* cutting two facial depth grooves and connecting them, *(2)* reducing the incisal aspect by 2 mm, *(3)* extending a chamfer on the lingual aspect, and *(4)* providing occlusal clearance. The unprepared half of the tooth serves as a reference to ensure that the proper convexity is incorporated in the preparation. In this situation the tooth serves as its own reference.

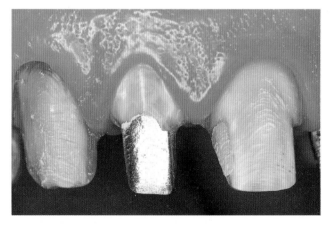

Fig. 4-14 The unprepared half is reduced by following the same previous sequence starting with two facial grooves, proceeding with the incisal reduction, and completing the lingual reduction. The subgingival depth of penetration is 0.5 mm.

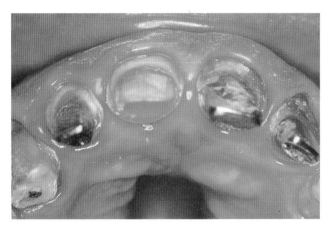

Fig. 4-15 The occlusal aspect of the completed preparations. The finish line consists of a 1.0- to 1.2-mm-wide facial shoulder and a 0.5-mm-wide lingual chamfer. A round-ended diamond bur is used to prepare both types of finish lines and provides a smooth transition between the shoulder and chamfer.

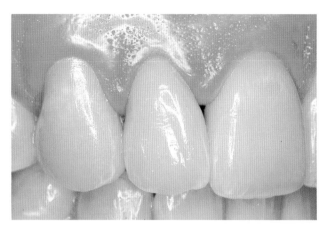

Fig. 4-16a For optimum esthetics, it is critical to reproduce in the final crowns the original facial convexity of the incisors.

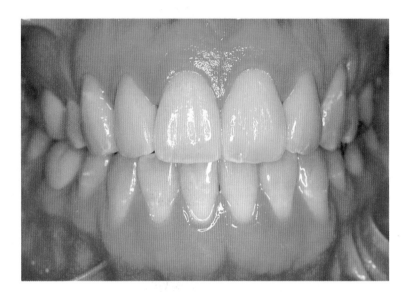

Fig. 4-16b Completed esthetic result with five metal ceramic crowns.

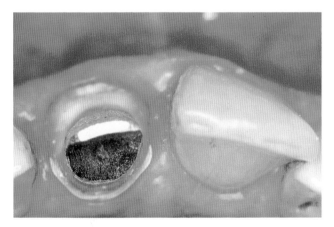

Fig. 4-17a The unprepared central incisor serves as reference for the position of the incisal edge of the prepared tooth so that the facial convexity of the crown is in harmony with the adjacent central incisor. The incisal edge of the cast post and core may have to be thinned to a sharp edge to provide for adequate lingual clearance.

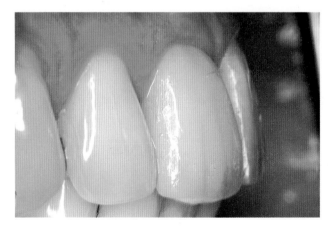

Fig. 4-17b Completed metal ceramic crown in harmony with the adjacent central incisor.

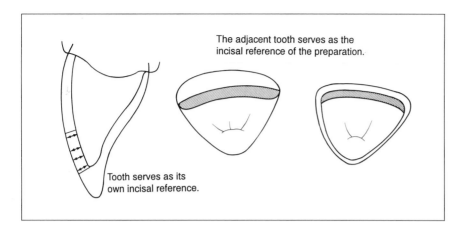

The adjacent tooth serves as the incisal reference of the preparation.

Tooth serves as its own incisal reference.

Fig. 4-18 Reference options for incisal edge position of the tooth preparation.

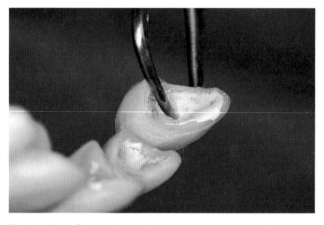

Fig. 4-19a Once old anterior crowns are removed, there is no reference for proper incisal edge location of the preparations, therefore tooth preparation is arbitrary. Measurement of the thickness of the provisional restorations at a subsequent appointment determines if the preparation was sufficiently reduced.

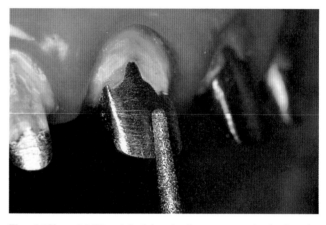

Fig. 4-19b Additional facial reduction was required after the provisional restoration was measured. For a metal ceramic crown, 1.5 to 1.8 mm of reduction should be provided at the junction of the incisal third and the middle third of the clinical crown according to the desired shade.

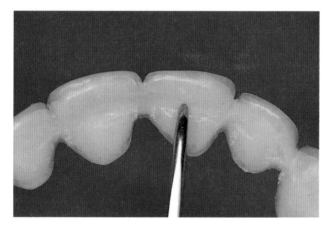

Fig. 4-19c Measurement of lingual thickness of the provisional restorations determines whether a lingual metal design is required along the protrusive path or whether the anterior guidance developed in the provisional restorations can be reproduced in porcelain fired over the metal coping.

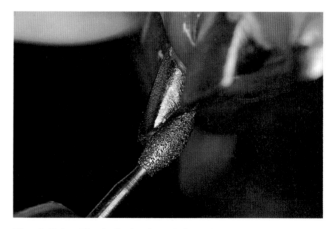

Fig. 4-19d The incisal edge of the preparation may have to assume a very precise position when both the labial and lingual aspects of the preparation are refined to conform to the thickness requirements imposed by the provisional restorations.

References for Incisal Edge of Preparation

Reference	Single Preparation	Multiple Preparations
Facial convexity of the natural tooth during preparation	→ Prepare with calibrated depth cuts	Prepare with calibrated depth cuts
Incisal edge of the intact adjacent tooth	→ Align the preparation to the adjacent tooth	Prepare the most intact central incisor last, after the incisal edges of the proximal teeth have been aligned to it
No reference from old crowns	→ Align the preparation to the adjacent tooth	Reprepare arbitrarily; create a new reference with provisional restorations; refine the preparations for optimum thickness

Precision of the preparation

Tooth preparation for anterior teeth must be exacting because of the comparatively limited surface area available for retention and resistance. The following guidelines are helpful:

- Use burs of known diameter.
- Plan a definite sequence of enamel removal with depth orientation cuts: the facial convexity of the tooth should be followed but not exaggerated because excessive labial reduction leads to insufficient clearance in the lingual aspect.[20]
- Identify and use references to properly position the incisal edge of the preparation.
- Establish shoulder depth at an early stage of the preparation so that reduction of the facial wall is established at the available subgingival diameter.[15]
- Measure the labial and lingual thicknesses of provisional restorations before making final impression to ensure that the preparation was sufficiently reduced.[15]

Armamentarium

Coarse or extra-coarse burs (ie, 100- to 150-μm grit) are recommended on the axial surfaces to increase the mechanical retention of the preparation.[21]

Armamentarium for Tooth Preparation

Facial Wall
Coarse or extra-coarse round-end tapered diamond bur

Lingual Wall
Coarse or extra-coarse round-end tapered diamond bur or torpedo diamond bur

Lingual Concavity
Pear-shaped diamond bur

Proximal Walls
Coarse or extra-coarse round-end tapered diamond bur or torpedo diamond bur or thin tapered tungsten carbide bur

Finish Lines
End-cutting diamond bur, rubber point, torpedo diamond bur, torpedo tungsten carbide bur

Preparations for metal ceramic crowns

Metal ceramic restorations owe their popularity to their esthetic potential, their strength and durability, their simplicity and versatility, and the ease of bridge construction. Primary and secondary soldering, interlocks, thin interproximal connections, thin lingual design, or screw-retained fixation are additional options provided with these restorations. Despite their relative simplicity of execution, insufficient reduction of the tooth preparation is a common problem that leads to overcontouring of the restoration or opacity and poor esthetics.

Finish lines

Various designs have been advocated for tooth preparations for anterior metal ceramic crowns, but from a survey of 51 dental schools conducted in the United States there is at present no consensus on the ideal finish line[22]: the flat shoulder is taught in 38% of institutions, the 45° beveled shoulder in 24%, the 135° shoulder in 15%, the chamfer in 10%, and the deep chamfer with bevel in 6%.

Shoulder with bevel

This design was advocated in the early development of metal ceramic restorations.[23] Because Rosner[24] demonstrated mathematically that the marginal opening of gold castings could be reduced by the use of a beveled finish line, this design remained popular with metal ceramic restorations for more than two decades. According to the same treatise, however, the bevel angle should be at least 45° to be effective, and only bevels in excess of 70° have major clinical effect on reducing leakage.[25] Furthermore, such a "long bevel"[26] would end at the base of the crevice and could not be accommodated in the shallow sulcus of an anterior tooth. Full-coverage castings constructed on beveled preparations may also display greater marginal discrepancies after cementation as compared with straight shoulders, possibly because hydrostatic pressure and filtration of the cement are increased as the crown is being seated on the beveled preparation.[27,28] The chamfer with bevel is a variation of the beveled shoulder advocated by Stein and Kuwata.[16]

Flat shoulder

The shoulder is easy to identify by the technician and allows for bulk of porcelain at the margin. It can be used equally in conjunction with a metal design or a porcelain butt margin. The axial line angle should be rounded because the stress concentration factor may be reduced up to 50% as compared with a sharp internal line angle.[29] Advantages associated with internally rounded shoulder preparations include ease of preparation, minimum potential for undercut, resistance to marginal distortion, and convenient transition to a lingual chamfer.[30]

The 135° sloping shoulder[31] provides for a more conservative preparation, especially on root structure, but it requires a feather-edge metal design or a metal collar. A porcelain butt margin is not recommended with the sloping shoulder.

Chamfer

This is the finish line of choice for most cast veneer restorations.[2] It can be conveniently prepared with torpedo-shaped burs,[32] and it has less potential for undercut than the shoulder preparation. It is also more conservative than the shoulder preparation and produces low stress[29] concentration on the cement. However, a shoulder is required for gold-based alloy restorations[33,34] because a chamfer does not provide sufficient rigidity against deformation of the thin facial metal margin of the crown during porcelain firing. Strating et al[35] and Weiss[36] reported on the other hand that this problem was not critical with nickel-chromium alloy restorations due to the superior mechanical properties of these alloys. A porcelain margin is not recommended with a chamfer finish because it would lack mechanical resistance and depth of translucency.

Margin design

A given crown design may be associated with several possible finish lines, but the present tendency is toward the reduction and the elimination of the metal collar facially or peripherally.

Metal collar

The labial metal collar is considered by some to be the ideal design in terms of marginal seal,[37] periodontal health, and rigidity during cementation. A wide facial metal collar (0.8 mm) offers sufficient rigidity against distortion caused by porcelain shrinkage in comparison with a feather-edge collar,[38] and it may be conveniently used with any of the finish lines described previously. The main disadvantage with metal collars is that they are difficult to conceal in a shallow crevice or with a thin or translucent gingival margin. In the case of gingival recession, the display of metal also becomes very conspicuous with a high lip line.

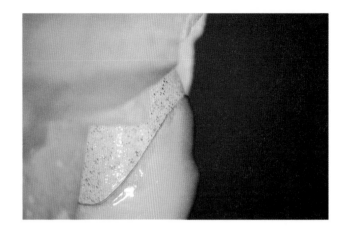

Fig. 4-20 Feather-edge metal design for a metal ceramic crown. This design is preferably used with a shoulder finish line with gold-based alloys to provide sufficient metal bulk at the internal line angle to resist deformation during porcelain firing. It is a difficult design to polish and it requires good dexterity to avoid overcontouring the cervical aspect or exposing the opaque. (Courtesy of Mr R Paschetta.)

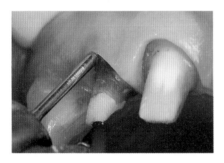

Fig. 4-21 A beveled end-cutting diamond bur is used to plane the edge of the facial shoulder. Its smooth bevel allows for finishing without laceration of the free gingival margin.

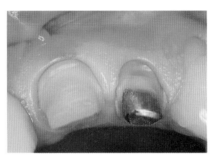

Fig. 4-22 Shoulder finish lines planed with a beveled end-cutting diamond bur and polished with a rubber point. No hand instrument was used to finish the shoulders.

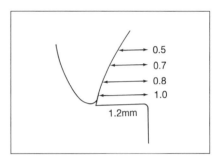

Fig. 4-23 When the facial shoulder width is narrow, the technician should suspect that the finish line is located on the cervical convexity of the tooth and that as the margin was prepared subgingivally, it became narrower. The clinician should properly communicate with the technician so that the crown is restored with a mild facial convexity.

Metal feather-edge

Reduction of the labial metal collar has been described as "triangular formation,"[39] "hairline collar,"[35] or "feather-edge" when metal, opaque layer, and porcelain simultaneously meet on the external edge of the tooth preparation. Even though it is theoretically attractive, this design is technique-sensitive and difficult to achieve without overcontouring the cervical aspect or exposing the opaque layer (Fig. 4-20). Finishing and polishing are difficult,[40] and microscopically the surface remains rough. Marginal adaptation after porcelain firing is subject to some distortion because as the metal collar thickness is decreased, the distortion caused by porcelain firing is increased.[38] The exact cause of this deformation is not known[41]: it is either caused by stress relaxation of the casting during its oxidation[41–43] or by the firing shrinkage of porcelain.[44–46] Shoulder preparations are recommended for the feather-edge metal design in order to provide rigidity of the metal in the cervical area. To limit

the potential for metal distortion prior to porcelain application, Campbell and Pelletier[43] recommend a separate thermal cycling of the metal at the oxidation temperature immediately following casting, either right before divestment or after divestment. Firing shrinkage of the porcelain produces significantly less distortion of the metal margin when thermal cycling and relaxation of casting stresses[47] precede grinding (cold working) of the castings.[43] As a precaution, the metal coping should be subjected to as little grinding and finishing before porcelain application.[40]

Porcelain margins

Esthetics of metal ceramic restorations have been significantly improved with the porcelain margin design because of the elimination of the facial metal collar, the improved depth in cervical translucency, and the possibility of light transmission through the root area. Furthermore, all conditions being equal, precious alloys seem to display greater plaque deposits than porcelain whether the porcelain is polished or rough,[48–49] because of low adhesive forces between dental plaque and ceramic surfaces.[50–52]

With adequate tooth preparation, porcelain margins are indicated with single-unit restorations and fixed partial denture retainers in the esthetic zone because of the improved depth of translucency at the cervical aspect. To provide optimum porcelain strength against tensile stresses at the margin, the ideal finish line should be a 0.8- to 1.2-mm-wide internally rounded shoulder, at a 90°-to-100° angle to the root surface, with a regular and smooth outline. Proper finishing techniques are essential to ensure the smoothest possible finish line and include various combinations of end-cutting burs,[2,53] rubber points,[54] or hand instruments[2,55,56] (Figs. 4-21–4-23).

A chamfer or sloping shoulder are contraindicated with porcelain margins because the porcelain margin would be too thin at the edge and be prone to chipping during clinical try-in. Additionally, it is difficult to achieve satisfactory marginal adaptation on the die as porcelain shrinkage proceeds towards its greatest bulk during firing (Fig. 4-24).

Various techniques of porcelain margin construction have been described using platinum matrix, refractory dies, separating varnish, wax, or resin binders.[57–63] Cooney et al[64] and West et al[65] demonstrated with conventional porcelain margin materials that rounded edges with rough and heterogenous surfaces were more likely to occur using direct lift-off techniques than with platinum matrix substrates.

For the direct lift-off method, it is therefore necessary to use shoulder porcelain materials instead of conventional porcelain because they fuse at a higher temperature (20° to 30°C higher than the regular body) and show greater resistance to pyroplastic flow compared with conventional porcelain materials.[40,66] They also allow the cervical margin to be completed separately in three firings prior to body porcelain build-up and yield clinically acceptable results in terms of surface texture, homogeneity, and translucency at the margin[66,67] (Fig. 4-25).

Previous reports indicate that various binders used as vehicles for shoulder porcelain powders facilitate the adaptation of porcelain to the die margin.[68–70] Hinrichs et al[71] compared density and tensile strength values of porcelain margins fired with various binder techniques and reported that distilled water and sodium silicate binders exhibited superior strength over wax and composite resin binders. The metal design required for a porcelain margin was investigated by Belles et al,[72] who demonstrated that porcelain margin adaptation is more consistent when the metal coping contacts the shoulder, as opposed to when it is reduced short of the axiogingival line angle (Fig. 4-26).

Porcelain margins fabricated on fixed partial denture abutments can be technically challenging[73] because when porcelain margins are incorporated in a one-piece framework it has to be subjected to three additional firing cycles that may cause significant framework distortion. For three-unit fixed partial dentures with porcelain margins fabricated on both retainers, framework distortion is not clinically significant as long casting stresses are eliminated and metal finishing is kept to a minimum. Over two abutments, the technical difficulty is increased because the distortion of the shoulder porcelain material caused by the body firings is compounded with framework distortion caused by the firing shrinkage of the body porcelain. The result may be a significant marginal gap. Bridger and Nicholls[74] demonstrated on a one-piece maxillary six-unit anterior fixed partial denture supported by four abutments that framework distortion after porcelain firing leads to clinically unacceptable marginal adaptation. If those same abutments incorporate porcelain margins, this distortion would be even further aggravated by the two to three additional firings required. Lomanto and Weiner[75] demonstrated that with the shoulder porcelain technique, the increase in marginal gap during body and glaze firings may be significant enough to justify a correction firing according to the material used.

These problems may be solved by fragmenting a large restoration into smaller sections and splinting these sections with postceramic soldering after they are glazed (Figs. 4-27–4-34). Another option is to fragment a large restoration in smaller sections with a precision attachment wherever possible.

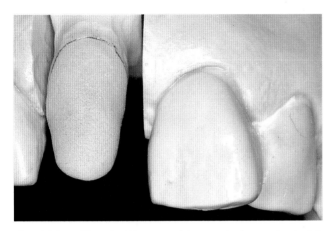

Fig. 4-24a The shoulder porcelain margin is constructed in three firings for a metal ceramic crown. The porcelain should be slightly convex at this stage to resist shrinkage caused by firing the body porcelain at the next stage.

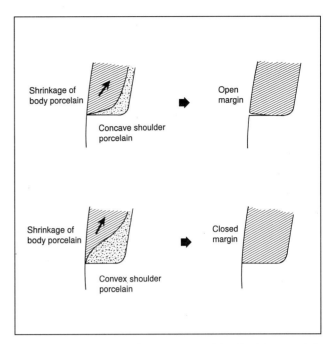

Fig. 4-24b Incidence of the convexity of the shoulder porcelain configuration on the final marginal adaptation.

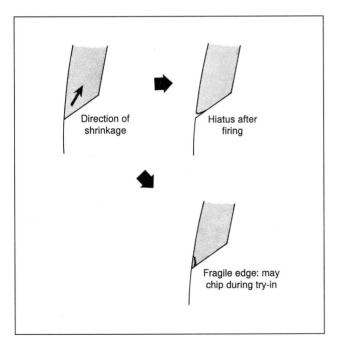

Fig. 4-24c A sloping shoulder or a chamfer finish line may result in rounded or fragile porcelain margin edges. A 90°-to-100° shoulder is the finish line of choice with porcelain margins.

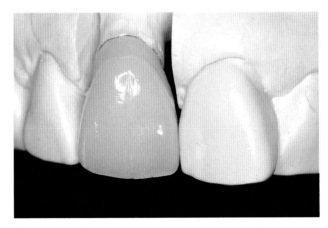

Fig. 4-24d The completed metal ceramic restoration.

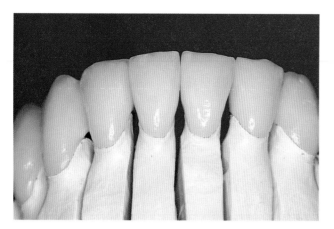

Fig. 4-25a These metal ceramic crowns incorporated porcelain margins on all eight mandibular crowns. The finish line must be a definite 90° shoulder especially if it is narrow, as typically dictated by mandibular anterior teeth.

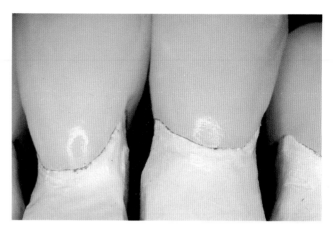

Fig. 4-25b Porcelain margin adaptation. Surface texture and color must be homogeneous at the marginal aspect.

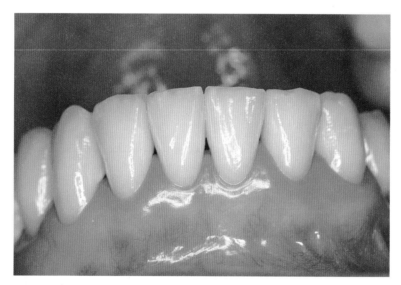

Fig. 4-25c Cemented crowns with favorable reaction of the gingival tissues.

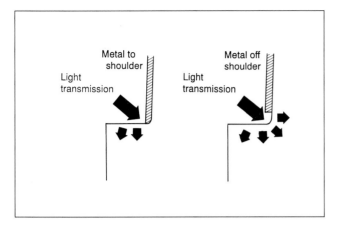

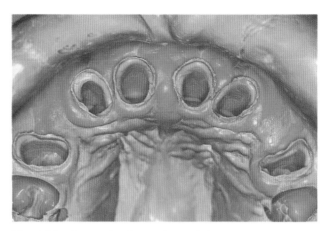

Fig. 4-26 Comparison of illumination between the metal-to-shoulder and metal-off-shoulder (Geller-Winter modification) designs for porcelain margins. The first design is technically simple but may block some light transmission and contribute to shadowing at the radicular and gingival aspects. The second design is more technique-sensitive and must be used with caution on fixed partial denture abutments, but it improves light transmission through the radicular and gingival aspects.

Fig. 4-27 Impression for an eight-unit fixed partial denture for rigid splinting of the six abutments.

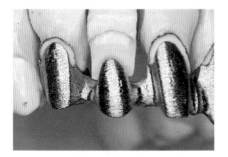

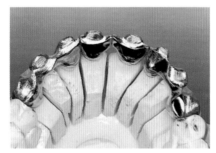

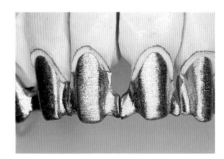

Fig. 4-28a–c All six abutments will be restored with a porcelain margin. The framework is first fragmented in four segments fabricated separately because porcelain margins can be accurately and predictably fabricated on three-unit frameworks or single units. Postceramic soldering will unite the four segments after they are glazed to minimize framework distortion.

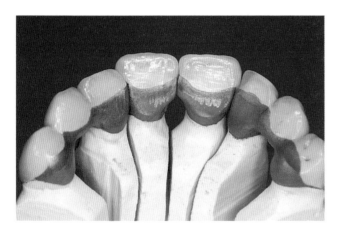

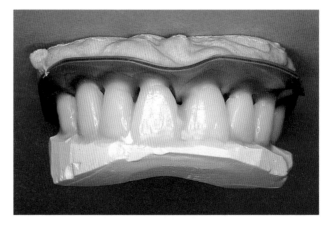

Fig. 4-29 After the bisque bake, the four segments are ready for try-in, and after esthetic and occlusal adjustments they are returned to the laboratory and glazed.

Fig. 4-30 A soldering index with fast-setting stone is then fabricated either with the four segments seated over the preparations in the mouth or over the stone dies, if the master cast is deemed accurate. The restorations should be precisely luted in position in the stone index, and a thin wax strip should be adapted over the cervical margins before the refractory investment is poured.

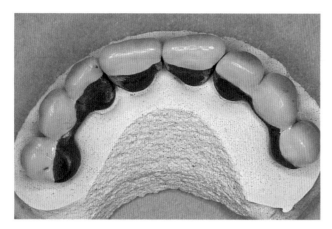

Fig. 4-31 The wax should be boiled out before the invested restorations are heated in the oven.

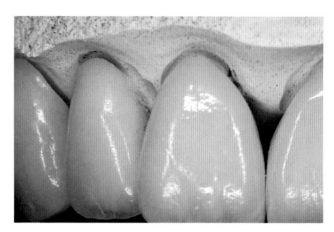

Fig. 4-32 The wax strip should cover the porcelain margins so that they do not contact the investment after the wax is boiled out.

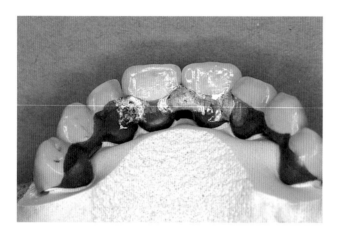

Fig. 4-33 Restorations after oven postceramic soldering.

Color rendition

Reduction thickness

An insufficiently reduced tooth preparation typically leads to an opaque and overcontoured metal ceramic restoration. Proper porcelain veneer thickness is essential because it allows for sufficient space to superimpose distinct ceramic layers for the illusion of depth in the restoration.

Recommendations for the depth of facial reduction have ranged from a minimum of 1.0 to 1.6 mm or greater,[15–18,76–80] but the only available scientific rationale is based on the research investigations of Jorgenson and Goodkind,[80] Barghi and Lorenzana,[81] Seghi et al,[82] Jacobs et al,[83] and Terada et al.[84]

1. Opaque/body porcelain thickness has a significant effect on shade rendition, thus increased porcelain thickness yields better esthetic results.
2. Thickness changes of body porcelain between 0.5 to 1.0 mm produce more significant color changes than between 1.0 and 1.5 mm.
3. The ideal thickness of opaque and body porcelain to match a given shade varies from shade to shade.
4. Opaque shade and thickness have significant influence on the final shade if opaque and body porcelain do not match and if the thickness of body porcelain is less than 1.0 mm.

In summary, approximately 1.0 mm of body porcelain thickness is necessary to match most shades; increasing body porcelain thickness above 1.0 mm is not essential. Below 1.0 mm of body porcelain thick-

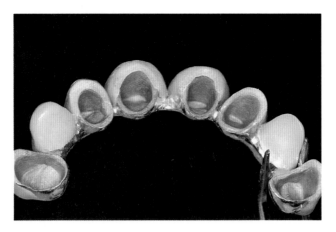

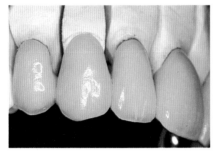 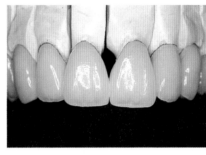 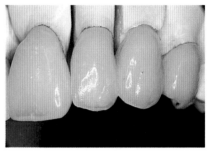

Fig. 4-34a–d Eight-unit splint incorporating six porcelain margins.

Thickness Requirements According to Shade
Dark Shade: • Facial reduction, 1.4 mm • Tooth thickness, 2.9 mm **Light Shade:** • Facial reduction, 1.7 mm • Tooth thickness, 3.2 mm

ness, every increment of thickness that can be provided in the preparation by the clinician becomes critical for the technician. Below 1.0 mm, the shade is difficult to reproduce and is influenced by the color of the opaque layer; secondary dentin[85] or highly chromatized dentin materials are required when body porcelain thickness is minimal.[86]

Measured at the junction of the incisal and middle third of the crown, which is where the opaque layer is likely to be visible with insufficient tooth reduction, the recommended facial reduction thickness with a noble porcelain alloy falls approximately within 1.4 to 1.7 mm, according to the shade considered.

A dark shade requires 0.8 mm (body porcelain) + 0.2 mm (opaque) + 0.3 mm (metal) + 0.1 mm (die relief and tolerance) = 1.4 mm ideal total reduction.

A light shade requires 1.1 mm (body porcelain) + 0.2 mm (opaque) + 0.3 mm (metal) + 0.1 mm (die relief and tolerance) = 1.7 mm ideal total reduction.

To accommodate these specifications, a natural tooth should measure in cross section at the junction of the incisal and middle third of the crown: 1.4 to 1.7 mm (facial reduction) + 0.5 mm (thickness of the preparation) + 1.0 mm (lingual reduction) = 2.9 to 3.2 mm ideal total facial-lingual thickness (Figs. 4-35 and 4-36).

Unfortunately, a significant percentage of anterior teeth measure between 2.5 to 3.1 mm and cannot accommodate these ideal reductions (Fig. 4-37). The failure to identify thin teeth is a common source of overcontouring, and the insufficient tooth thickness must be compensated for at the expense of another structure (Fig. 4-38). Thin teeth result in adequate facial reduction but insufficient lingual clearance, or in sufficient lingual clearance but inadequate facial reduction (Fig. 4-39). According to the thickness to be regained, this compensation may be achieved either simply or through a combination of several measures (Figs. 4-40–4-42).

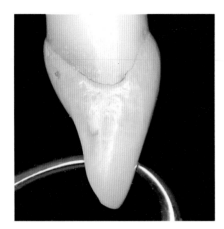

Fig. 4-35 Thin teeth measure approximately 2.5 mm labiolingually at the junction of the incisal and middle thirds. The depth of the lingual concavity also often contributes to the thin dimension of the tooth.

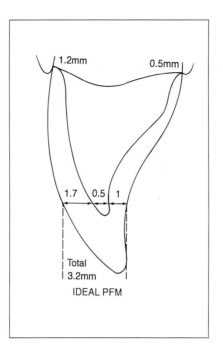

Fig. 4-36 Ideal tooth reduction for a metal ceramic (PFM) restoration of a light shade requires a thick incisor measuring 3.2 mm at the junction of the incisal and middle thirds.

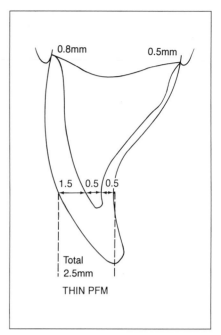

Fig. 4-37 Reduction dimensions allowed by a thin incisor measuring 2.5 mm labiolingually at the junction of the incisal and middle thirds: 1.5 mm reduction in the facial area is insufficient for lighter shades and will result in some color compromise.

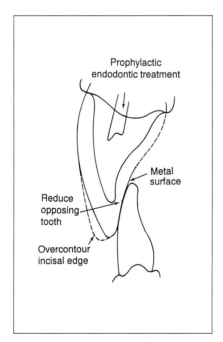

Fig. 4-38 With a thin incisor, there may be sufficient labial reduction but insufficient lingual clearance, or vice-versa; therefore, additional reduction is required at the expense of another structure. The opposing teeth may need reduction, the lingual surface may have to be restored with a selective metal design, elective endodontic therapy may be recommended or, if the patient declines these options, the crown will have to be overcontoured to a thicker labiolingual dimension.

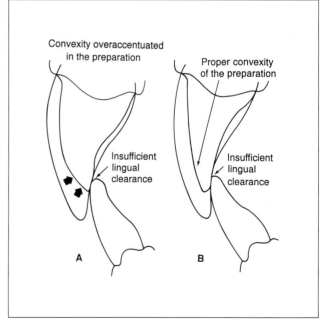

Fig. 4-39 Insufficient clearance indicates either that the incisal third was overreduced in the preparation or that the incisor is thin labiolingually.

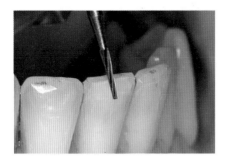
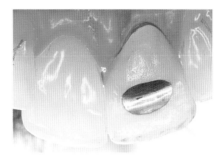
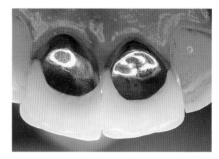

Fig. 4-40a–c   Examples of compensation for thin teeth requiring reduction of the opposing teeth, or selective lingual metal designs. These must be planned preoperatively.

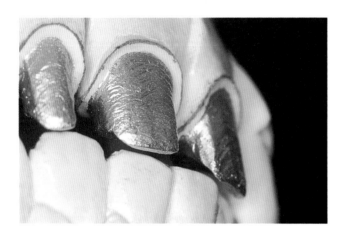

Fig. 4-41   Selective lingual metal design is required when there is minimal clearance in protrusion as dictated by the custom incisal guide table established from the provisional restorations. If porcelain were added over the metal coping in this area, it would result in a steeper anterior guidance as compared with the provisional restorations.

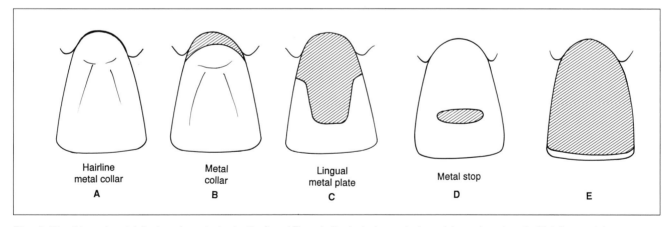

| Hairline metal collar | Metal collar | Lingual metal plate | Metal stop | |
| A | B | C | D | E |

Fig. 4-42   Lingual metal designs for anterior teeth: **A** and **B** are indicated when anterior guidance is restored with full porcelain coverage; **C** and **D** are indicated with thin teeth and minimum clearance as dictated by the required anterior guidance; **E** is unacceptable because flexure of the metal could result in porcelain fracture at the incisal edge.

Proper identification of thin anterior teeth and selection of an appropriate compensation are essential parts of diagnosis and must be explained to the patient preoperatively.

Metal type

The quality and color of the metal oxides of various porcelain alloys may effect the final shade of the restoration.[84,87–89] Shade rendition is not affected by the type of gold alloy, and high noble alloys (high gold, gold-palladium, high palladium) produce similar results. For certain shades, though, some nickel-chromium and palladium-silver alloys may cause significantly greater color changes as compared with gold and high noble alloys.

Type of Compensation for Thin Teeth

- Lingual metal design
- Coronoplasty of the mandibular incisors
- Prophylactic endodontic therapy
- Thin the incisal edge of the preparation (with cast core)

Compensations Required According to Tooth Thickness and Shade

	Thin (2.5–2.9 mm)	Medium (2.9–3.2 mm)	Thick (above 3.2 mm)
Dark Shade	Required	Not required	Not required
Light Shade	Required	Required	Not required

References

1. Potts RG, Shillingburg HT, Duncanson MG. Retention and resistance of preparations for cast preparations. *J Prosthet Dent* 1980;43:303.

2. Shillingburg HT, Jacobi R, Brackett SE. *Fundamentals of Tooth Preparations for Cast Metal and Porcelain Restorations*. Chicago: Quintessence, 1987.

3. Phillips RW. *Science of Dental Materials*, ed 9. Philadelphia: Saunders, 1991:481.

4. Gilboe DB, Teteruck WR. Fundamentals of extracoronal tooth preparation. Part I. Retention and resistance form. *J Prosthet Dent* 1974;32:651.

5. Rosenstiel E. The retention of inlays and crowns as a function of geometrical form. *Br Dent J* 1957;103:388.

6. Kaufman EG, Coelho DH, Colin L. Factors influencing the retention of cemented gold castings. *J Prosthet Dent* 1961;1:487.

7. Assif D, Azoulay S, Gorfil C. The degree of zinc phosphate cement coverage of complete crown preparations and its effect on crown retention. *J Prosthet Dent* 1992;68:275.

8. Jorgensen KD. The relationship between retention and convergence angle in cemented veneer crowns. *Acta Odontol Scand* 1955;13:35.

9. Dodge WW, Weed RM, Baez RJ, Buchanan RN. The effect of convergence angle on retention and resistance form. *Quintessence Int* 1985;3:191.

10. Ohm E, Silness J. The convergence angle in teeth prepared for artificial crowns. *J Oral Rehabil* 1978;5:371.

11. Mack P. A theoretical and clinical investigation into the taper achieved on crown and inlay preparations. *J Oral Rehabil* 1980;7:255.

12. Eames WB, O'Neal SJ, Monteiro J, Miller C, Roan JD, Cohen KS. Techniques to improve the seating of castings. *J Am Dent Assoc* 1978;96:432.

13. Noonan JE, Goldfogel MH. Convergence of the axial walls of full veneer crown preparations in a dental school environment. *J Prosthet Dent* 1991;66:706.

14. Behrend DA. Failure of maxillary canine retainers for fixed prostheses. *Int J Prosthodont* 1989;5:429.

15. McLean, JW. *The Science and Art of Dental Ceramics*, monographs I and II (1974), III and IV (1976). New Orleans: Louisiana State Univ.

16. Stein RS, Kuwata M. A dentist and a dental technologist analyze current ceramo-metal procedures. *Dent Clin North Am* 1977;21:729.

17. Shillingburg HT, Hobo S, Fisher DW. *Preparations for Cast Gold Restorations*. Chicago: Quintessence, 1974.

18. Johnston JF, Mumford G, Dykema RW. *Modern Practice in Dental Ceramics*. Philadelphia: Saunders, 1967.

19. Dawson PE. *Evaluation, Diagnosis and Treatment of Occlusal Problems*. St. Louis: Mosby, 1974.

20. Fraser F. Precision porcelain jacket crowns. *Anglo-Cont Dent Soc* 1969;21:17.

21. Oilo G, Jorgensen KD. The influence of surface roughness on the retentive ability of two dental luting cements. *J Oral Rehabil* 1978;5:377.

22. Butel EM, Campbell JC, DiFiore PM. Crown margin design: A dental school survey. *J Prosthet Dent* 1991;65:303.

23. Silver M, Klein G, Howard MC. Platinum-porcelain restorations. *J Prosthet Dent* 1956;6:695.

24. Rosner D. Function, placement and reproduction of bevels for gold castings. *J Prosthet Dent* 1960;13:1161.

25. McLean JW, Wilson AD. Butt joint versus bevelled gold margin in metal-ceramic crowns. *J Biomed Mater Res* 1980;14:239.

26. Sozio R. The marginal aspect of the ceramo-metal restoration: The collarless ceramo-metal restoration. *Dent Clin North Am* 1977;21:787.

27. Pascoe D. Analysis of the geometry of finishing lines for full crown restorations. *J Prosthet Dent* 1978;40:157.

28. Gavelis JR, Morency JD, Riley ED, Sozio RB. The effect of various finish line preparations on the marginal seat and occlusal seat of full crown preparations. *J Prosthet Dent* 1981; 45:138.

29. El-Ebrashi MK, Craig RG, Peyton FA. Experimental stress analysis of dental restorations. Part III. The concept of the geometry of proximal margins. *J Prosthet Dent* 1969;22:333.

30. Preston JD. Rational approach to tooth preparations for ceramo-metal restorations. *Dent Clin North Am* 1977;21:683.

31. McAdam DB. Preparation of a 135-degree shoulder for a ceramometal margin using an end-cutting bur. *J Prosthet Dent* 1985;54:473.

32. Lustig PL. A rational concept of crown preparation revised and expanded. *Quintessence Int* 1976;11:41.

33. Shillingburg HT, Hobo S, Fisher DW. Preparation design and margin distortion in porcelain fused to metal restorations. *J Prosthet Dent* 1973;29:276.

34. Faucher RR, Nicholls JI. Distortion related to margin design in porcelain fused to metal restorations. *J Prosthet Dent* 1981; 43:149.

35. Strating H, Pameijer CH, Gildenhuys RR. Evaluation of marginal integrity of ceramometal restorations. Part I. *J Prosthet Dent* 1981;46:59.

36. Weiss P. Towards reconciling the esthetic potential of ceramo-metal restorations with established criteria for soft tissue management. *Int J Periodont Rest Dent* 1981;1:34.

37. Stein RS. Periodontal dictates for esthetic ceramometal crowns. *J Am Dent Assoc* 1987;115:63.

38. Campbell SD, Pelletier LB. Thermal cycling distortion of metal ceramics. Part I. Metal collar width. *J Prosthet Dent* 1992; 67:603.

39. Kuwata M. *Theory and Practice for Ceramo-metal Restorations*. Chicago: Quintessence, 1980.

40. Yamamoto M. *Metal Ceramics*. Chicago: Quintessence, 1985.

41. Ando N, Nakamura K, Namiki T, Sugata T, Suzuki T, Moriyama K. Deformation of porcelain bonded gold alloys. *J Jpn Soc Appar Mater* 1972;13:237.

42. Dehoff PH, Anusavice KJ. Effect of metal design on marginal distortion of metal ceramic crowns. *J Dent Res* 1989;63:1327.

43. Campbell SD, Pelletier LB. Thermal cycling distortion of metal ceramics. Part II. Etiology. *J Prosthet Dent* 1992;68:284.

44. Buchanan WT, Svare CW, Turner KA. The effect of repeated firings and strength on marginal distortion in two ceramometal systems. *J Prosthet Dent* 1981;45:502.

45. Kulmer S, Feichtinger C, Gausch K, Sattler CO. Dimensionsanderung der Kronendurchmesser von Metallceramikkronen warhend des oxydgluhens. *Ost Z Stomat* 1978;75:408.

46. Iwashita H, Kuriki H, Hasuo T, et al. Studies on dimensional accuracy of porcelain fused to metal crowns. The influence of the porcelain to the metal coping on the porcelain fusing procedure. *Shigaku* 1977;65:110.

47. Koike K. Fabrication of ceramo-metal crowns with accurate fitness: Deformation of casting and its remedies. *Shika Giko* 1977;5:31.

48. Wise MD, Dykema RA. The plaque retaining capacity of four dental materials. *J Prosthet Dent* 1975;33:178.

49. Adamczyk E, Spiechowicz E. Plaque accumulation on crowns made of various materials. *Int J Prosthodont* 1990;3:285.

50. Koidis PT, Schroeder K, Johnston W, Campagni W. Color consistency, plaque accumulation, and external marginal surface characteristics of the collarless metal-ceramic restoration. *J Prosthet Dent* 1991;65:391.

51. Dummer RM, Harrison KA. In vitro plaque formation on commonly used dental materials. *J Oral Rehabil* 1982;9:413.

52. Tullberg A. An experimental study of the adhesion of bacterial layers to some dental materials. *Scand J Dent Res* 1986; 94:164.

53. Goldstein RE. Esthetic principles for ceramo-metal restorations. *Dent Clin North Am* 1977;21:803.

54. Chiche GJ, Radiguet J, Pinault P, Genini P. Improved esthetics for the ceramometal crown. *Int J Periodont Rest Dent* 1986; 6(1):76.

55. Miller L. A clinician's interpretation of tooth preparation and the design of metal substructures for metal-ceramic restorations. In: McLean JW (ed). *Dental Ceramics. Proceedings of the First International Symposium on Ceramics*. Chicago: Quintessence, 1983:153.

56. Zena RB, Khan Z, Fraunhofer JA. Shoulder preparations for collarless metal ceramic crowns: Hand-planing as opposed to rotary instrumentation. *J Prosthet Dent* 1989;62:273.

57. Goodacre CJ, Van Roekel NB, Dykema RW, Ullmann RB. The collarless metal-ceramic crown. *J Prosthet Dent* 1977;38:615.

58. Schneider DM, Levi MS, Mori DF. Porcelain adaptation using direct refractory dies. *J Prosthet Dent* 1976;36:583.

59. Sozio RB, Riley DJ. A precision ceramic-metal crown with a facial butted margin. *J Prosthet Dent* 1977;37:517.

60. Toogood GD, Archibald JF. Technique for establishing porcelain margins. *J Prosthet Dent* 1978;40:464.

61. Vryonis P. Improving esthetics in porcelain fused to gold restorations. *J Prosthet Dent* 1980;44:667.

62. Lahoste LH. The porcelain butt margin. *Quintessence Dent Technol* 1981;5:149.

63. Prince J, Donovan T. The esthetic metal-ceramic margin: A comparison of techniques. *J Prosthet Dent* 1983;50:185.

64. Cooney JP, Richter WA, McEntee MI. Evaluation of ceramic margins for metal-ceramic restorations. *J Prosthet Dent* 1985; 54:1.

65. West AJ, Goodacre CJ, Moore BK, et al. A comparison of four techniques for fabricating collarless metal ceramic crowns. *J Prosthet Dent* 1985;54:636.

66. Wanserski DJ, Sobczak KP, Monaco JG, et al. An analysis of margin adaptation of all porcelain facial margin ceramo-metal crowns. *J Prosthet Dent* 1986;56:289.

67. Chiche G, Pinault A. *Essentials of Dental Ceramics. An Artistic Approach*. Chicago: Mosby-Yearbook, 1988.

68. Kessler JC, Brooks TD, Keenan MP. The direct lift-off technique for constructing porcelain margins. *Quintessence Dent Technol* 1986;10:145.

69. Prince J, Donovan TE, Presswood RG. The all-porcelain labial margin for ceramo-metal restorations: A new concept. *J Prosthet Dent* 1983;50:793.

70. Pinnell DC, Latta GH Jr, Evan JB. Light-cured porcelain margins: A new technique. *J Prosthet Dent* 1987;58:50.

71. Hinrichs RE, Bowles WF, Huget EF. Apparent density and tensile strength of materials for facially butted porcelain margins. *J Prosthet Dent* 1990;63:403.

72. Belles DM, Cronin RJ, Duke ES. Effect of metal design and technique on the marginal characteristics of the collarless metal ceramic restoration. *J Prosthet Dent* 1991;65:611.

73. Hannon SM, Gunderson RB, Lorton L, Zislis T, Hondrum SO. Sequencing platinum foil matrix removal in postceramic soldering of the collarless veneered retainer. *Int J Prosthodont* 1991;4:457.

74. Bridger DV, Nicholls JI. Distortion of ceramometal fixed partial dentures during the firing cycle. *J Prosthet Dent* 1981;45:507.

75. Lomanto A, Weiner S. A comparative study of ceramic crown margins constructed using different techniques. *J Prosthet Dent* 1992;67:773.

76. Johnston JJ, Mumford G, Dykema RW. The porcelain veneered crown. *Dent Clin North Am* 1963;Nov:853.

77. McLean JW. *The Science and Art of Dental Ceramics*. Chicago: Quintessence, 1980.

78. Weiss PA. New design parameters: Utilizing the properties of nickel-chromium superalloys. *Dent Clin North Am* 1977;21:769.

79. Miller L. Framework design in ceramo-metal restorations. *Dent Clin North Am* 1977;21:699.

80. Jorgenson MW, Goodkind RJ. Spectrophotometric study of five porcelain shades relative to the dimensions of color, porcelain thickness and repeated firings. *J Prosthet Dent* 1979;42:96.

81. Barghi N, Lorenzana RE. Optimum thickness of opaque and body porcelain. *J Prosthet Dent* 1982;48:429.

82. Seghi RR, Johnson WM, O'Brien WJ. Spectrophotometric analysis of color differences between porcelain systems. *J Prosthet Dent* 1986;56:35.

83. Jacobs SH, Goodacre CJ, Moore BK, Dykema RW. Effect of porcelain thickness and type of metal ceramic alloy on color. *J Prosthet Dent* 1987;57:2.

84. Terada Y, Maeyama S, Hirayasu R. The influence of different thicknesses of dentin color reflected from thin opaque porcelain fused to metal. *Int J Prosthodont* 1989;2:352.

85. Kersten K. Spectral engineering of the thin crown. In: Preston JD (ed). *Perspectives in Dental Ceramics. Proceedings of the Fourth International Symposium on Ceramics*. Chicago: Quintessence, 1988:383.

86. Korson DL. Highly chromatised dentin porcelains. In: Preston JD (ed). *Perspectives in Dental Ceramics. Proceedings of the Fourth International Symposium on Ceramics*. Chicago: Quintessence, 1988:379.

87. Barghi N, Richardson JT. A study of various factors influencing shade of bonded porcelain. *J Prosthet Dent* 1978;39:282.

88. Brewer JD, Akers CK, Garlopo DA, Sorensen SE. Spectrometric analysis of the influence of metal substrates on the color of metal-ceramic restorations. *J Dent Res* 1985;64:74.

89. Crispin BJ, Seghi RR, Globe H. Effect of different metal ceramic alloys on the color of opaque and dentin porcelain. *J Prosthet Dent* 1991;65:351.

Chapter 5

All-Ceramic Crowns and Foil Crowns

John W McLean, Edmund E Jeansonne, Gerard Chiche, and Alain Pinault

All-ceramic crowns

Metal ceramics remain the most widely used materials in fixed prosthodontics because of their strength and predictability, and they are unlikely to be replaced by all-ceramic systems in routine situations, particularly in the posterior region, or where resistance to fatigue is needed, such as in fixed bridges.[1] However, the translucency of metal ceramic crowns is often affected by the metal coping, which restricts the transmission of light through the restoration and may increase light reflectivity of the crown. In this respect, the all-ceramic crown sets a standard in esthetics that is difficult to match by the metal ceramic crown because it permits better light transmission through the body of the tooth.[2,3] Research over the last 30 years has produced a number of reinforced porcelain crown systems according to two concepts: (1) all-ceramic crown systems with reinforced cores and/or reinforced veneering materials, and (2) foil crown systems with thin metal substructures for additional gain in porcelain thickness and ease of fabrication.

Selection

The primary advantage of using all-porcelain and foil systems is to increase the depth of translucency and light transmission in the crown either deeper into the crown or across the entire crown. Esthetic results vary from system to system, and in a laboratory setting several factors influence the choice of one crown system over another[4]: (1) strength; (2) simplicity of fabrication; (3) potential for high-volume production; (4) marginal and internal fit; (5) cost-benefit analysis; (6) personal experience; and (7) esthetic performance.

Esthetic performance

All ceramic crowns fall into two separate categories according to their esthetic performance: (1) semi-translucent; or (2) semi-opaque. Cast glass-ceramic crowns can be taken to a point of crystallization where translucency is maximal. This results in a highly translucent crown with low chroma and with a chameleon-like effect that allows it to merge with the surrounding teeth; it is also particularly useful in matching adolescent teeth (Fig. 5-1). However, when a porcelain material with low chroma is too translucent, it may appear too gray.[5] Translucency is generally better controlled when the veneering material is fabricated on a semi-opaque aluminous core (Figs. 5-2–5-4) or where dentin porcelains are specially formulated to correspond closely with the color and light transmission of the natural dentin, as in the leucite-reinforced ceramics Optec (Jeneric/Pentron, Wallingford, Conn) (Fig. 5-5) and Empress (Ivoclar, Lichtenstein). In situations with minimum porcelain thickness on the facial aspect, selection of a crown system without aluminous core and bonded with a semitranslucent composite has been advocated in order to avoid the core showing through the veneer porcelain.[6]

Intrinsic shading is demanding, time-consuming, and requires experience, but it gives the best esthetic rendition with the proper depth of color and adequate tooth reduction. Extrinsic shading eliminates the complex veneering techniques but can result, especially with cast glass-ceramic, in a painted appearance because the color is applied only on the surface of the crown.[5] To obtain maximum strength in an all-ceramic crown, the ceramic must contain a high proportion of crystalline material such as alumina, but this increases

Advantages and Disadvantages of Current Ceramic Systems*

Ceramic System	Advantages	Disadvantages
Aluminous porcelain jacket crown	Excellent esthetics Predictable with maxillary incisors Inexpensive	Moderate strength No fixed partial denture application
Hi-ceram	Improved strength over aluminous porcelain crown Core fabrication on refractory die	Core brightness No fixed partial denture application
In-ceram	Superior strength Excellent marginal adaptation Fixed partial denture applications with proper indications	Special equipment and cost Time for manufacture Need adequate reduction to mask the aluminous core
Dicor	Translucency and chameleon effect Good marginal adaptation Excellent biocompatibility	Moderate strength Special equipment and cost No fixed partial denture application
Optec H.S.P.	Good esthetics No core needed Good marginal adaptation	Moderate strength Limited fixed partial denture application
Empress	Moderate-to-good strength Excellent marginal adaptation Lost wax and vacuum-pressed technique	Special equipment and cost No fixed partial denture application
Alceram (Cerestore)	Excellent esthetics Excellent marginal adaptation	Moderate strength Special equipment and cost Availability
Metal ceramics	Maximum strength, versatility, and predictability Bridge applications Soldering possibility	Reduction thickness may require devitalization Opacity may not be suitable in situations requiring maximum translucency
Foil crowns	No casting Ease of use and low cost Thin foil for increased porcelain thickness	Exact strength mechanism needs further documentation Limited bridge applications

*Table adapted from: Wall GJ, Cipra DL. Alternative crown systems. Is the metal ceramic crown always the restoration of choice? *Dent Clin North Am* 1992;36:765.

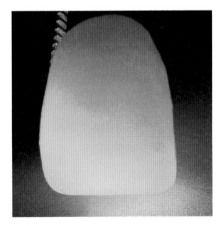

Fig. 5-1 Maximum translucency with Dicor cast glass-ceramic crown with extrinsic staining.

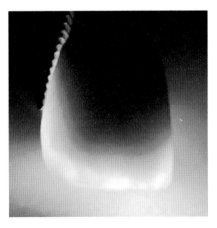

Fig. 5-2 Transillumination of an all-ceramic crown veneered on a semi-opaque aluminous core (Hi-ceram).

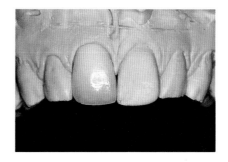

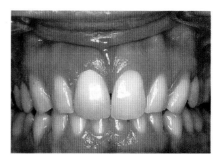

Fig. 5-3a and b Aluminous porcelain jacket crown for this single maxillary central incisor incorporates the proper balance between opacity and translucency. The semiopaque core prevents excessive translucency and graying.

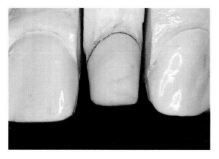

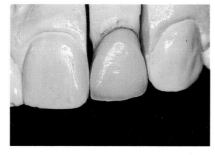

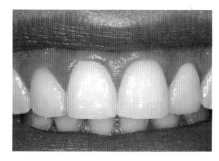

Fig. 5-4a and b Semiopaque alumina core (In-ceram) veneered with aluminous porcelain.

Fig. 5-4c Cemented crown.

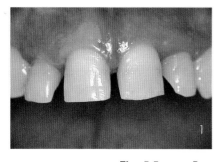

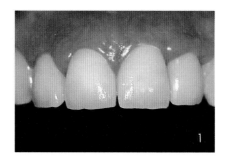

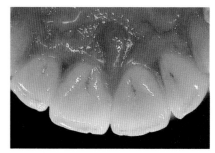

Fig. 5-5a–c Preoperative condition (a). Restoration with four bonded leucite-reinforced ceramic crowns (Optec, Jeneric/Pentron, Wallingford, CT) results in a natural appearance (b and c). (Courtesy of Dr M de Rouffignac and Mr J de Cooman.)

Fig. 5-6a and b Cast glass-ceramic cores have been veneered with aluminous porcelain to obtain adequate opacity to match the adjacent anterior teeth in this very difficult situation. (Courtesy of Dr K Malament.)

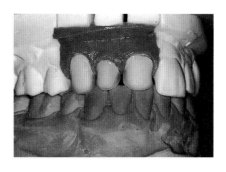

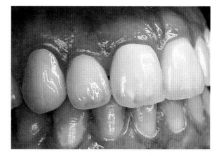

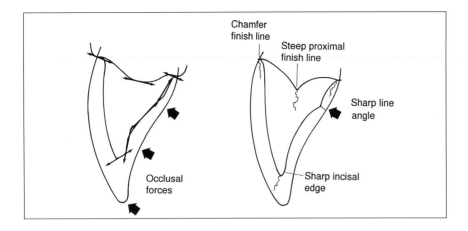

Fig. 5-7 The design of an ideal all-ceramic crown preparation is to provide maximum strength of the crown by establishing flat planes at right angles to the forces of mastication and avoiding sharp line angles. A shoulder margin is also required because it offers superior strength as compared with a chamfer.

opacity because of the mismatch in refractive index between the crystalline material and the glass matrix. Therefore, to reconcile esthetic and strength requirements, alumina crowns must use a thin coping similar in design to a metal coping over which a translucent veneer can be built.[7]

The Willi's glass crown combines the translucency of the cast glass-ceramic substructure and the shading ability of an aluminous porcelain veneered over the core[8] and yields superior esthetic results (Fig. 5-6). However, the mismatch in thermal diffusivity or incompatibility of the glass with feldspathic porcelain may increase the likelihood of breakage.

Indications

The fracture resistance of all-ceramic crowns is based on adequate support by the preparation, proper patient selection, strength of the crown material, and type of luting cement. Indications for use of all-ceramic crowns include[9]: *(1)* all anterior teeth where esthetics is of prime importance, and *(2)* adequate laboratory support and experience with the type of crown selected. Contraindications for use of all-ceramic crowns in the anterior region include[9,10]: *(1)* parafunctional activity; *(2)* insufficient support from the tooth preparation; *(3)* insufficient porcelain thickness in the lingual aspect (<0.8 mm); *(4)* opposing teeth that occlude with the cervical fifth of the crown; and *(5)* short clinical crowns.

All-ceramic crowns are highly predictable providing that the above principles and contraindications are strictly observed. When these conditions cannot be fulfilled or the patient is likely to demand some form of guarantee against breakage, then the metal ceramic restoration, even though it may compromise esthetics, is generally the material of choice. Only when the clinician is certain that the patient will accept some risk of breakage to achieve the ultimate in esthetics should all-ceramic crowns be used in high-stress-bearing areas. A further consideration should also include the possible wear of opposing natural dentition and unfavorable occlusions, such as deep horizontal overlap or parafunction, which are better treated with occlusal gold surfaces.

Preparations for all-ceramic crowns

The original porcelain jacket crown was made of feldspathic porcelain and possessed excellent esthetic qualities. However, unless it was meticulously prepared and constructed, it was prone to fracture. It was recognized early that the most frequent cause for jacket crown breakage was improper tooth preparation.[11–23] The role of the tooth preparation for a porcelain jacket crown is to provide support for the restoration with as uniform porcelain thickness as possible. Excessive porcelain bulk (caused by convergence of the preparation or coronal destruction) has an adverse effect on strength because it is not the bulk that makes the crown strong, it is the support from the preparation and the accuracy of fit. Finally, strength and support of the porcelain against the occluding stress of mastication must be provided with flat planes, adequate tooth foundation, and resistance form[13–16] (Fig. 5-7).

Length of the preparation
When a load is applied from a lingual direction, the labial shoulder is placed under compression and only the length of the preparation at the incisal lingual aspect provides significant resistance to this force.[9,23,24] Short preparations cause considerable stress[25] and may lead to fracture[21] (Fig. 5-8) even if the crown is bonded and luted with a composite cement.[26]

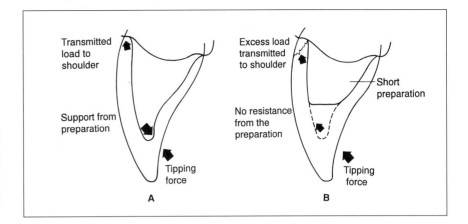

Fig. 5-8a and b **A**, The length of the preparation is important. This aspect of the preparation is essential regardless of the type of cement used. **B**, Short preparations are contraindicated with all-ceramic crowns, even luted with a resin cement, because they do not provide adequate support for the ceramic and allow it to flex.

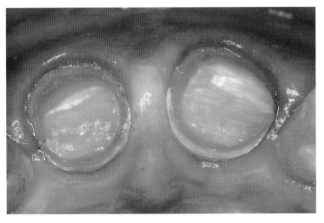

Fig. 5-9 Preparations for all-ceramic crowns. The incisal edge of the preparation should be flat, not sharp.

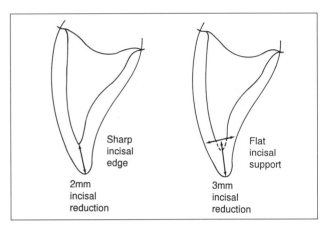

Fig. 5-10 The incisal edge may be reduced until a flat area is obtained and as long as the reduction does not exceed 3 mm.

The ideal incisal reduction ranges from 2 mm to one third of the anatomic crown,[23] according to the thickness of the incisal edge of the preparation. If it is too thin, it should be thickened and placed at a right angle to the direction of stress by reducing the preparation to a length of two thirds of the crown (Figs. 5-9 and 5-10).

Shoulder

A well-defined 90° shoulder of adequate width improves the fracture resistance of the crown[24] because it provides for additional bulk at the margins that is placed at a right angle to the direction of stress.[16] The shoulder is also required for strength at the margin because the marginal area bears much support of the crown in function. This is because the best adaptation of at least three types of all-ceramic crowns[27–33] (ie, Cerestore, Innotek Dental Corp, Lakewood, Colo; Dicor

Dentsply, York, Pa; and aluminous porcelain jacket crowns) was found at the cervical aspect, while the internal adaptation was consistently poor at the incisal aspect (with cement thickness in excess of 100 μm). This results in decreased support of the crown by the preparation and decreased strength because the more intimate the contact of a ceramic crown with the preparation, the higher the resistance to fracture under occlusal loading[27] (Figs. 5-11 and 5-12).

Shoulder versus chamfer

When the shoulder angle of the preparation to the longitudinal axis of the tooth is greater than 90°, the risk of porcelain fracture increases.[34] The internal shoulder angle should be rounded[35,36] to reduce the stress concentration factor up to 50% and because sharp internal line angles cannot be easily repro-

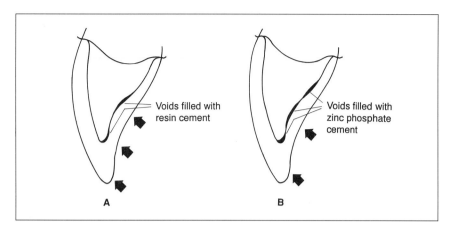

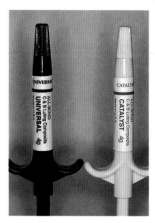

Fig. 5-11 The internal adaptation of several all-ceramic crown systems may be poor at the internal aspect (up to 100-μm voids), whereas the marginal adaptation remains satisfactory. This results with zinc phosphate cement in decreased strength because the cement may not have the required strength to support the crown under occlusal loading. The superior strength of composite resin cements and their ability to bond to porcelain and tooth structure should theoretically improve porcelain support in these areas.

Fig. 5-12 Example of composite resin cement indicated for luting of all-ceramic crowns.

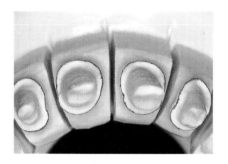

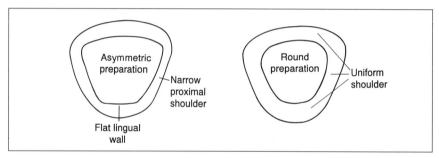

Fig. 5-13 To avoid rounding the preparation excessively, the peripheral shoulder should not be uniform. It should measure 1.0 to 1.2 mm labially and lingually, and 0.5 mm proximally.

Fig. 5-14 For additional resistance in the preparation, the lingual wall may be flattened as depicted here.

duced with porcelain.[28,37] Similarly, the internal rounded shoulder is recommended for the In-ceram crown (Vident, Baldwin Park, Calif) to facilitate the adaptation of the aluminous oxide slip on the die.[38]

A chamfer is conservative and simpler to execute and has been described as an option for cast glass-ceramic restorations,[39,40] but the fracture resistance of Dicor[30] and Cerestore crowns[41] is significantly greater for crowns produced on a shoulder than for those produced on a chamfer preparation.

Improvement in Dicor crown strength due to bonding to the tooth preparation with low-viscosity resin cements resulted in a decrease in the failure rate of resin-bonded Dicor crowns as opposed to crowns cemented with zinc phosphate or glass ionomer cement,[42] as long as there were no cement voids beneath stress-bearing areas.[43] This finding looks promising because the superior modulus of elasticity of these cements and their potential to seal internal flaws through bonding procedures could prevent crack propagation through the porcelain. Further studies, however, are warranted on the long-term clinical performance of resin cements, especially in terms of microleakage and hydrolytic instability.[44]

Shoulder width

A shoulder of uniform thickness may round the preparation excessively and compromise resistance form.[18] For a maxillary central incisor, the facial and lingual shoulder width should be 1.0 mm with a minimum of

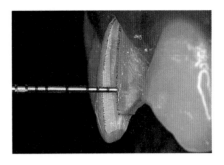

Fig. 5-15 The ideal facial reduction for an all-ceramic crown of a light shade is approximately 1.3 to 1.4 mm according to the shade considered. Careful execution for this convex tooth with a large pulp required a half-preparation controlled with a periodontal probe used as a depth gauge.

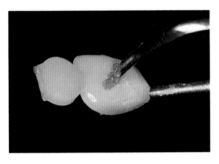
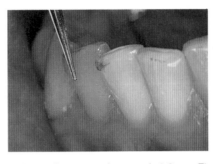
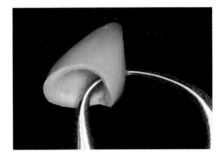

Fig. 5-16a–c The minimum allowable lingual thickness for a ceramic crown is 0.8 mm. The thickness of the provisional restoration may be measured in the lingual aspect, after protrusive adjustments, to ensure that there will be sufficient thickness in the ceramic crown. If additional reduction is needed and the preparation cannot be reduced further, the opposing tooth has to be adjusted for additional clearance. The same verification should be performed before adjusting the lingual aspect of an all-ceramic crown.

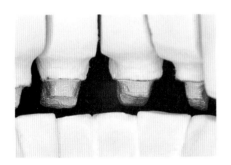
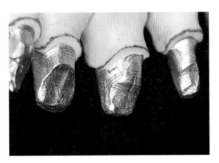

Fig. 5-17a and b A definite lingual wall is essential for stabilization of ceramic crowns. In this case, the occlusal contacts are located on the incisal third of the crowns and allow preservation of the height of the cingulum in the preparations to achieve maximum resistance form.

0.8 mm, and the interproximal width should be 0.5 mm because the proximal walls of the crown flare out and provide sufficient strength in the proximal area.[9,45] These specifications for a shoulder of nonuniform width provide for conservatism, support, and resistance of the preparation to stress (Figs. 5-13 and 5-14).

The finish line should follow a smooth curvature that is not too steep interproximally to avoid a potential V-shaped notch that could split the labial off the lingual aspect of the crown.[9,16,35,46] This is critical because the highest stresses during function occur in the interproximal area.[37] However, the danger of cutting transeptal fibers cannot be overemphasized, be-

cause deep preparations in this area are the most frequent cause of persistent inflammation of the interdental papilla and the dreaded "blue gum syndrome."

With the advent of molded and cast glass-ceramic restorations, ideal shoulder widths of 1.0 mm,[47] 1.0 to 1.5 mm,[48] and 1.2 mm[30] have also been advocated for strength.

Facial and lingual reduction

The minimum acceptable facial thickness of porcelain from an esthetic standpoint is 1.0 mm, and the ideal depth of reduction on the midfacial aspect of a typical maxillary central incisor for an aluminous porcelain jacket crown should be 1.3 mm (Fig. 5-15).[9] Facial

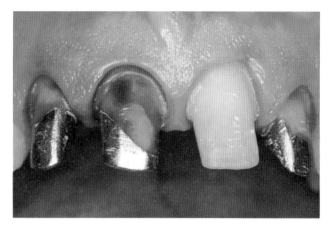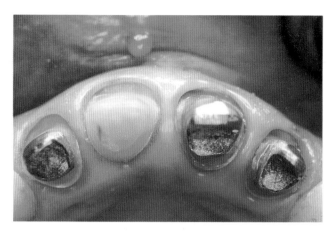

Fig. 5-18a and b The ideal total taper of the preparation should approximate 8° to 10°. This ensures maximum conservation of tooth structure and support from the preparation. The lingual walls may also be slightly flattened for additional resistance.

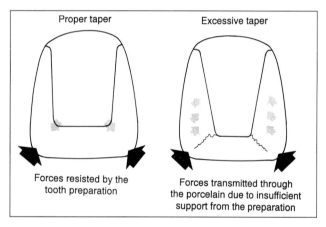

Fig. 5-19 Excessive porcelain bulk has an adverse effect on strength. It is not the bulk that gives strength to the crown, it is the resistance to flexure provided by the support from the preparation and the accuracy of fit.

depths of reduction up to 1.5 mm have also been recommended for molded, castable, and slip-cast ceramics.[47–49]

Lingual thickness values of 1.5 mm[18,24] are ideal but are difficult to achieve routinely. Practically, lingual porcelain thickness should be in the 1.0-to-1.3-mm range, and the absolute minimum should be 0.8 mm[9] (Fig. 5-16). The lingual aspect of the preparation should be shaped to avoid uneven sections in the crown[23] and sharp line angles and must incorporate, whenever occlusion and cingulum prominence allow, a

definite lingual concavity with a high lingual axial wall, as opposed to a one-plane reduction[50] (Fig. 5-17).

Taper

Minimal taper is recommended for maximum surface area and support of the preparation. Excessive taper of the preparation correlates with a reduction in breaking strength[51,52] and an increase in stress concentration in the area where support is lacking.[53,54] A 5° taper is ideal and would ensure maximum resistance form with only one path of insertion of the crown,[9] but it is also difficult to achieve without producing undercuts.[55]

The safest and most practical convergence angle of all-ceramic preparations is 10°, which represents an acceptable compromise between taper and strength (Figs. 5-18 and 5-19).

Strength of all-ceramic crown systems

New ceramic materials for esthetic dentistry have been introduced in recent years, but the objective of fabricating all-porcelain crowns is to provide the patient with lasting esthetic restorations. While new high-strength ceramics are being advocated as a replacement for metal ceramic restorations, they have various limitations in accuracy, fracture resistance, and maintenance of crack-free surfaces.[3]

The strength of dental porcelain is greatly influenced by the presence of surface flaws[56] acting as stress initiators and causing widening and propagation of microcracks through the material from the surface. Therefore dental porcelain is much weaker in tension than in compression[57] and is prone to brittle fracture. Dental porcelain is also susceptible to "static fatigue," which is generally believed to be caused by a stress-dependent chemical reaction between water vapor and the surface flaws in the porcelain restoration. This causes flaws to grow to critical dimensions, allowing spontaneous crack propagation,[58] which eventually results in a fracture with comparatively little occlusal loading, particularly over long periods (Fig. 5-20).

Surface flaws

The integrity of the ceramic surface plays a major role in the longevity of the restoration. A high-strength ceramic with a badly flawed surface may perform worse in a clinical situation than a weaker ceramic with a comparatively flaw-free surface. The fracture pattern of cast glass-ceramics (Dicor) and aluminous dental porcelains (Vitadur-N, Vita Zahnfabrik, Sackingen, Germany) is always initiated at the surface and usually at locations involving porosities.[59]

Kelly et al[59] classified porcelain defects into processing defects (eg, machining scratches, porosities, and impurity inclusions) and inherent material defects (eg, large grains, residual stresses, and microcracks).

Flaws located in surface areas were found to reach 100 μm in diameter,[60] and flaws ranging from 100 to 200 μm in size were reported on all internal surfaces of feldspathic and aluminous core porcelains fired on a platinum foil matrix.[61,62] A direct inverse relationship between the amount of porosity and the strength of porcelain jacket crowns was reported by Munoz et al[63]: the more porosity, the lower the resistance to fracture. For these reasons, the margin of safety required in ceramics is always greater than in metals.[3]

Core thickness

All dental ceramics tend to fail at the same critical strain in the order of 0.1%[64]; for this reason, any increase in strength and durability can only be achieved by an increase in the elastic modulus or elimination of surface flaws in the ceramic.[65] Increasing stiffness raises the load-bearing capacity of the ceramic, but if the porcelain is too thin (<0.5 mm), it will be more flexible and likely to reach the critical strain of 0.1%. Dentist and technician often expect a 0.5-mm section of ceramic to perform like metal, but this cannot be the case with current ceramic technology. The rigidity and thickness of the ceramic core material play an essential role in the flexural strength of the whole restoration.[66] Sections less than 1 mm should be avoided with all-porcelain crowns, and ideally the dentist should aim for cross sections of 1.5 mm.[65]

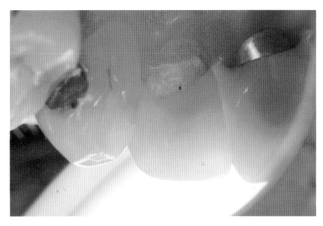

Fig. 5-20 Porcelain fracture after 12 years of service. When porcelain is subject to static fatigue, it may fracture under a comparatively light load.

To achieve maximum strength in any ceramic crown, the load-bearing areas (cervical and proximal) should be reinforced with at least 1.0-mm-thick sections of core porcelain.[2] The ideal aluminous porcelain coping for incisors should exhibit: (1) a lingual surface at least 1 mm thick; (2) a lingual collar extended proximally, similar to a metal coping; and (3) the incisal labial area thinned to 0.3 mm for esthetics.

This design is also indicated with high alumina cores because a significant reduction in flexural strength was reported when the In-ceram core thickness was reduced from 1.0 to 0.5 mm and veneered with a 0.5-mm-thick layer of Vitadur porcelain.[67]

Strengthening mechanisms

Strengthening dental porcelain for current clinical applications is achieved through four methods: enameling of metal (metal ceramic and foil crowns)[68-71]; dispersion strengthening with alumina crystals,[72] leucite crystals,[6,73-76] or with a crystallized magnesium aluminum oxide spinel[47,77,78]; dispersion strengthening by glass infusion of slip-cast alumina ceramics[79]; and crystallization of glasses.[79-84]

Current Ceramic Systems for Clinical Application

Strengthening Method	Clinical System	Characteristics
1. Enameling of metal	Metal ceramic crowns	High fracture resistance of metals Reduction in surface flaws at the metal/porcelain interface
	Foil crowns	Reduction in surface flaws at the metal/porcelain interface
2. Dispersion strengthening		Dispersion of ceramic crystals of high strength and elasticity in the glass matrix
a. Fused alumina sintered into a matched expansion glass	Aluminous porcelain jacket crown	Alumina-reinforced ceramic
	Hi-ceram (Vident, Baldwin Park, Calif)	Alumina-reinforced ceramic
b. Leucite crystals dispersed through the body of the crown	Optec (Jeneric/Pentron, Wallingford, Conn)	Leucite-reinforced ceramic
	Empress (Ivoclar, Lichtenstein)	Heat-pressed leucite-reinforced ceramic
c. Crystallized magnesium aluminum oxide spinel	Alceram (formerly Cerestore) (Innotek Dental Corp, Lakewood, Colo)	Shrink-free alumina ceramic
3. Dispersion strengthening by glass infusion	In-ceram (Vident, Baldwin Park, Calif)	High alumina coping infused with a low-fusing glass
4. Crystallization of glasses		Crystallized glass converted to a dense mass of interlocking crystals
a. Conversion by "ceramming"	Dicor (Dentsply, York, Pa)	Castable glass-ceramic with tetrasilic fluormica crystals
b. Conversion by "crystallization"	Cerapearl (Kyocera America Inc, San Diego, Calif)	Castable apatite ceramic

High alumina ceramics

McLean and Hughes[72] demonstrated that an alumina-reinforced core material consisting of 50% (by weight) fused alumina crystals in a matrix of low-fusing glass of matching thermal expansion significantly improved the transverse bending strength over conventional dental porcelain. Aluminous core porcelain is approximately twice as strong as regular porcelain.[85] This research resulted in the production of commercial aluminous porcelains, the first being Vitadur-N followed by NBK 1000 (De Trey/Dentsply, Germany) and subsequently Hi-ceram (Vita Zahnfabrik[86]). The principle of using high-strength ceramic cores has now become firmly established and has led to the further development of slip-cast alumina ceramics.

Slip casting is the art and science of preparing stable suspensions and forming ware by building up a solid layer on the surface of a porous mold that sucks up the liquid phase by means of capillary forces.[87] Sadoun, as described by Levy,[79] refined the slip-casting technique to produce a high-strength alumina coping with particle size of 0.5 to 3.5 μm destined to be veneered with aluminous-type veneer porcelain. In this technique, a pure alumina slip-cast coping is made on a special gypsum die of the tooth preparation and partially sintered in the oven. After shaping, the porous alumina is infused with a low-fusing glass of matching thermal expansion, which will melt and diffuse through the porous alumina by capillary action, resulting in a very dense alumina-glass composite structure (Figs. 5-21–5-24).

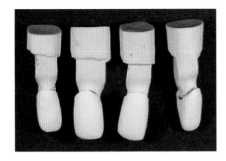

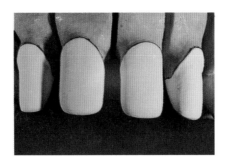

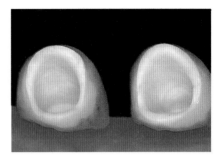

Fig. 5-21a and b In-ceram cores on shrunken plaster dies after firing (a). Copings shaped to final configuration before infiltration firing (b).

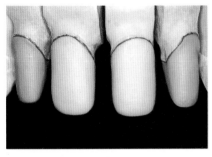

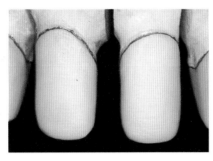

Fig. 5-22a and b Completed In-ceram copings after glass infiltration (a). Quality of the marginal adaptation (b). (In-ceram copings constructed by Mr K Hale, Vident.)

Fig. 5-23 Veneered In-ceram copings with aluminous porcelain (Alpha porcelain). The proximal shoulder may be relatively narrow (0.5 mm) because there is an adequate porcelain bulk immediately adjacent to it.

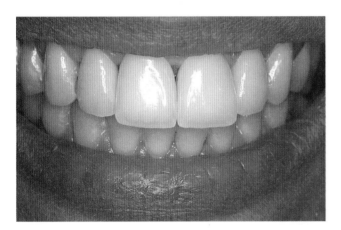

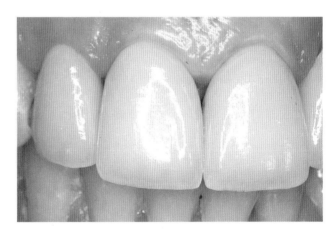

Fig. 5-24a and b Completed In-ceram crowns.

Table 5-1 Numerical Strengths of All-Ceramic Crown Systems

Type of Ceramic	Flexural Strength (MPa)*
Feldspathic porcelain	65 (S)–85 (C)
Alumina core	92 (C)–124 (S)
Glass-ceramic (Dicor)	90 (C)–124 (S)
Nonshrink alumina ceramic (Cerestore)	105 (C)–114 (C)
Leucite-reinforced ceramic (Optec)	105 (S)–120 (C)
Aluminous core porcelain (Hi-ceram)	140 (C)–141 (S)
Heat-pressed reinforced ceramic (Empress)	160 (D)–180 (D)
Slip-cast alumina ceramic (In-ceram)	400 (M)–446 (S)
High alumina, 98% purity	420 (M)–520 (M)
Gold alloy (yield strength)	350 (M)–600 (M)

*C = Campbell[66]; M = McLean[65,88]; S = Seghi et al[91]; D = Dong et al.[92]

Investigations of strength of all-ceramic crown systems

Several all-ceramic crown systems were introduced between 1982 and 1992 with various claims of superior fit, esthetics, and resistance to fracture. The comparative strengths of these ceramic crown materials were investigated on test bars through their modulus of rupture (MOR) or flexural strength, but the strength of ceramics cannot be determined reliably from "average strength" because there are wide variations in flexural strength.[88] There is also considerable controversy surrounding the strength of ceramic materials because values are affected by a variety of factors that are difficult to control and because test bars do not necessarily extrapolate to crown specimens[89] or to failures produced by delamination of the veneering glass from the core.[90] The average values listed in Table 5-1 are given for comparative purposes only and do not reflect variations among samples.

Even though test bars differ in construction from all-ceramic crowns, these absolute strength values are less important than the values relative to known standards such as the aluminous jacket crown.[66] These values tend to indicate that the clinical performance of alumina core, glass ceramic (Dicor), nonshrink alumina ceramic (Cerestore), leucite-reinforced ceramic (Optec), and aluminous core porcelain (Hi-ceram) should be relatively comparable. Besides test bars, similar results were also reported with actual crown samples where Cerestore, Dicor, and aluminous porcelain jacket crowns had approximately similar breaking strength.[28,93–95] These investigations show that within the 90-to-140 MPa range, it is difficult to select a consistently stronger system.

The safest and most predictable clinical results with all-ceramic crowns are achieved when the indications are confined to single incisor crowns or in selected cases of posterior teeth where there are no parafunctional habits and there is maximum restorative control of the occlusion.[96] With flexural strength as low as 140 MPa, the failure rate at 7 years does not seem to exceed 2% and remains acceptable in a clinical setting.[2] Long-term success can be obtained only with proper indication, adequate support from the preparation, and meticulous laboratory technique.[97]

The potential to abuse all-ceramic systems for molar crown restorations and fixed partial dentures must be analyzed in light of their comparative strength with metal ceramic crowns. The failure load of all-ceramic crowns has consistently been reported to be lower than metal ceramic crowns by a wide margin ranging from 30% to 70%.[51,52,90,91,97–101] Metal ceramics remain consistently stronger than all-ceramic systems, and ceramic systems with a flexural strength of 150 MPa or below may not yet seem adequate for routine applications for either molar crowns or for fixed partial dentures.[102] Even with slip-cast alumina, caution is recommended pending long-term clinical trials,[103] and all-ceramic fixed partial dentures should be considered only when there is ample clearance for connections of 2 mm in height and 3 mm in depth in the anterior region.

Long-term success of all-ceramic systems should be based on well-proven methods that have withstood clinical testing. All-ceramic crowns' resistance to breakage depends on several factors: adequate support from the preparation; stiffness and design of the substructure; proper thickness and stiffness of the veneering material; and skill of the dentist and technician. The future of all-ceramic crowns is very promising, and predictable long-term success should be expected with proper patient selection and good technical support.

Foil crowns

Thickness reduction

In situations where tooth reduction is minimal and there is insufficient space for a metal ceramic crown, a reduction in the thickness of the metal coping is beneficial.[97] Foil crowns provide for an additional gain in porcelain thickness at the expense of the metal coping. The first system based on metal ceramic technology consisted of adapting a tin-coated oxidized platinum foil to the die and then bonding an aluminous porcelain to the surface[69,104] (Vita-Pt., Vi-

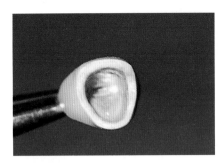
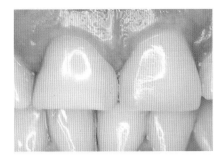

Fig. 5-25a and b Single central incisor restored with a bonded aluminous crown: an oxidized platinum foil serves as a matrix for an aluminous porcelain crown. The tin oxide coating provides for chemical bonding of the porcelain to the foil and facilitates wetting of the porcelain over the foil surface. (Laboratory work: Mr L LaHoste, CDT.)

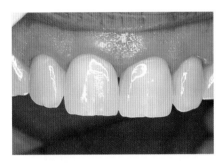
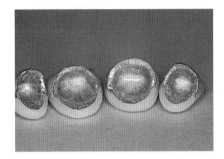

Fig. 5-26a and b Ceplatek (Renaissance) foil crowns. The main advantage of foil crowns is to provide for additional thickness of porcelain as compared with a cast metal coping, in addition to the simplicity of fabricating the foil coping. Tooth preparation should be the same as with all-ceramic crowns to provide support for the porcelain.

taZahnfabrik, Bad Sackingen, Germany). Later systems using this principle employed a prefabricated gold form by crimping, burnishing, and swaging it over a die of the preparation (eg, Renaissance/Ceplatec, Williams Gold Refining Co, Buffalo, NY; Sunrise-Tanaka Dental, Skokie, Ill).[105–109] They represent an overall time-saving procedure with no waxing, investing, and casting and with a lower investment cost compared to other all-ceramic systems. Gold foils are also claimed to be less time-consuming and to provide a more desirable color beneath the porcelain compared to platinum foils. The pioneering work of Rogers[110] on electroplated gold foils must also be acknowledged in respect to these developments.

The respective foil thicknesses are 0.025 mm (platinum-bonded aluminous crown, oxidized platinum foil) (Fig. 5-25), 0.09 to 0.159 mm (Renaissance system, 99% noble metal) (Fig. 5-26), and 0.050 mm (Sunrise System, 98% pure gold) (Fig. 5-27). This gain in porcelain thickness as compared with cast copings varies from 0.10 to 0.2 mm, allowing more depth of color. This is advantageous with minimum reduction, because any thickness increase in body porcelain between 0.5 to 1.0 mm produces significant color changes, and because below 1.0 mm of body porcelain, the color of the substrate influences the final shade. Because of their respective coefficients of thermal expansion, aluminous porcelain will be compatible with only platinum foils and feldspathic porcelain used for metal ceramic technique, with gold foil alloys. From a strength standpoint, however, aluminous porcelain is superior, particularly when used in thicker lingual sections.

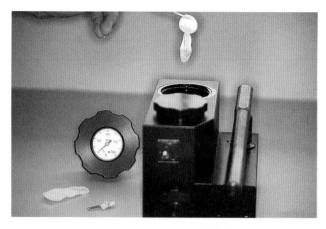
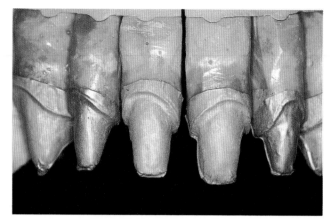
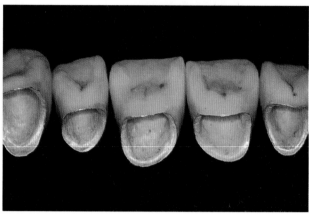
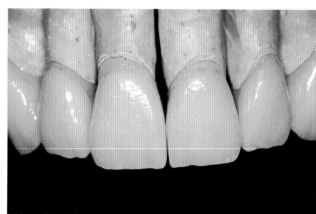

Fig. 5-27a–d Sunrise foil crowns. In the Sunrise system, the foil copings are manually adapted on the dies and further swaged onto the dies with a hydrostatic press. The copings are veneered with conventional feldspathic porcelain. (Courtesy of Mr A Tanaka and Dr H Shavell.)

Strengthening mechanism

An important feature of all dental ceramics is the nature and the quality of their surfaces; a smooth flawless surface will produce high strength. In the platinum-bonded aluminous crown, a standard platinum foil is tin-plated and then oxidized before the veneer crown is fabricated with aluminous dental porcelain. An increase of 83% in biaxial flexural strength over the conventional aluminous porcelain jacket crown was reported with chemical bonding of the tin-plated oxidized platinum foil to the porcelain[111] because of improved wetability of the porcelain over the oxidized tin layer, reducing the flaws at the porcelain/foil interface.[112]

In the Renaissance (Ceplatek or CeraPlatin) crown, a bonding agent is painted and fused on the coping by sintering. A conventional feldspathic porcelain crown is then built from this layer. The composition of the interfacial alloy powder was reported from x-ray analysis to be composed of 77% Au, 9% Ag, 5% Cu, and 9% Cl.[113] Because there was no evidence of any of the oxidizing elements usually incorporated in metal ceramic alloys to promote chemical bonding to porcelain, it was concluded that porcelain retention on the foil was purely mechanical.

Role of the foil matrix

Excellent clinical performances of foil crowns are demonstrated on anterior teeth with proper indication and adequate porcelain thickness,[114] and it is reasonable to expect from a properly constructed foil crown an intermediate resistance between a porcelain jacket crown and a metal ceramic crown.

The strength of Renaissance foil crowns was reported to be superior to that of Dicor and Cerestore systems[115] and ranges from 40% to 60%[93,115,116] of the strength of metal ceramic crowns. Stripping of the foil can cause a reduction of 24% in strength of the crown, possibly by opening up the flaws or by removing beneficial compressive stress in the porcelain.[117]

Leaving the foil in place prevents the opening of such flaws by keeping them sealed[113] and by reducing the potential for crack propagation. Nevertheless, it is safer to recommend for foil systems the same indications and preparations as with all-ceramic crowns because of the lack of strength and rigidity of the foil coping.[114]

Foil adaptation

Unlike cast metal copings, foils may be susceptible to distortion caused by porcelain firing shrinkage. The resulting contraction in the foil may result in poor fit or may generate tensile stress in the crown during or after cementation.[118] Distortion of the Renaissance foil coping after firing of the crown is due to the release of internal stresses created within the foil by swaging

in addition to the firing shrinkage of the porcelain, and internal grinding adjustments may be required to fit the crown back on the die.[119] Scores made on the opaque and the margin porcelain before firing may also reduce foil distortion and produce satisfactory marginal adaptation.[119]

Another alternative to grinding the foil internally or scoring the opaque is to simply increase the thickness of die relief because the foil could be perforated by repeated grinding adjustments. The marginal fit of the Renaissance crown was found to improve when a thick coat of die spacer (36 μm relief) was used[120]; likewise, the compressive strength of cemented Sunrise crowns was increased by approximately 40% by both the use of die relief and internal adjustments as compared with untreated dies and unmodified foils to yield a clinically acceptable marginal fit.[121,122]

References

1. Yamamoto M. *Metal Ceramics*. Chicago: Quintessence, 1985.

2. McLean JW (ed). *Dental Ceramics: Proceedings of the First International Symposium on Ceramics*. Chicago: Quintessence, 1983.

3. McLean JW. The science and art of dental ceramics. Buonocore Memorial Lecture. *Oper Dent* 1991;16:149.

4. Castellani D. Differential treatment planning for the single anterior crown. *Int J Periodont Rest Dent* 1990;10:230.

5. Campbell SD. Esthetic modification of cast dental-ceramic restorations. *Int J Prosthodont* 1990;3:123.

6. De Rouffignac M, De Cooman J. Aesthetic all-porcelain anterior restorations. *Pract Periodont Aesth Dent* 1992;4:9.

7. McLean JW. High strength ceramics. *Quintessence Int* 1987; 18:97.

8. Geller W, Kwiatkowski SJ. The Willi's glass crown: A new solution in the dark and shadowed zone of esthetic porcelain restorations. *Quintessence Dent Technol* 1987;11:233.

9. McLean JW. *The Science and Art of Dental Ceramics* monographs I and II (1974), III and IV (1976). Louisiana State Univ.

10. Shillingburg HT, Hobo S, Fisher DW. *Preparations for Cast Gold Restorations*. Chicago: Quintessence, 1974.

11. Land CH. A new system of restoring badly decayed teeth by means of an enameled metallic coating. *Independent Pract* 1886;7:407.

12. Bastian CC. The all-porcelain jacket crown by the indirect method. *Dental Cosmos* 1923;65:1285.

13. Argue JE. The preparation of teeth for porcelain jacket crowns. *J Am Dent Assoc* 1930;17:1259.

14. Vehee WD. Some basic principles underlying porcelain veneer crown technic. *J Am Dent Assoc* 1930;17:2167.

15. Oppice HW. A resumé of ideas on porcelain jacket crown preparations. *J Am Dent Assoc* 1934;21:1030.

16. Conod H. Etude sur la statique de la couronne jaquette. *Rev Mens Suisse d'Odontol* 1937;47:485.

17. Klaffenbach AO. Science, art and ceramic fundamentals involved in porcelain jacket crown prosthesis. *Aust Dent J* 1951:88.

18. Ewing JE. Atypical porcelain jacket crown preparations. *J Prosthet Dent* 1952;2:815.

19. Ewing JE. Beautiful but glum—porcelain jacket crowns. *J Prosthet Dent* 1954;4:94.

20. Bartels JC. Full porcelain veneer crowns. *J Prosthet Dent* 1957;7:533.

21. Saklad MJ. The disclosure of cleavage and fracture lines in porcelain restorations. *J Prosthet Dent* 1958;8:115.

22. Nuttall EB. Factors influencing success of porcelain jacket restorations. *J Prosthet Dent* 1961;11:743.

23. Pettrow JN. Practical factors in building and firing characteristics of dental porcelain. *J Prosthet Dent* 1961;11:334.

24. Fairley JM, Deubert LW. Preparation of a maxillary central incisor for a porcelain jacket preparation. *Br Dent J* 1958;18: 208.

25. Dérand T. Effect of variation in the shape of the core on stresses in a loaded model of a porcelain crown. *Odontol Rev* 1974;25:11.

26. Scherrer SS, de Rijk WG. The effect of crown length on the fracture resistance of posterior porcelain and glass-ceramic crowns. *Int J Prosthodont* 1992;5:550.

27. Brukl CE, Philp GK. The fit of molded, twin foil, and conventional ceramic crowns. *J Prosthet Dent* 1987;58:408.

28. Dickinson AJG, Moore BK, Harris RK, Dykema RW. A comparative study of the strength of aluminous porcelain and all-ceramic crowns. *J Prosthet Dent* 1989;61:297.

29. Davis DR. Comparison of fit of two types of all-ceramic crowns. *J Prosthet Dent* 1988;59:12.

30. Friedlander LD, Munoz CA, Goodacre CJ, Doyle MG, Moore BK. The effect of tooth preparation design on the breaking strength of Dicor crowns. Part I. *Int J Prosthodont* 1990;3:159.

31. Abbate MF, Tjan AHL, Fox WM. Comparison of the marginal fit of various ceramic crown systems. *J Prosthet Dent* 1989; 61:527.

32. Vahidi F, Egloff ET, Panno FV. Evaluation of marginal adaptation of all ceramic crowns and metal ceramic crowns. *J Prosthet Dent* 1991;66:426.

33. Weaver JD, Johnson GH, Bales DJ. Marginal adaptation of castable ceramic crowns. *J Prosthet Dent* 1991;66:747.

34. Dérand T. Analysis of stresses in loaded models of porcelain crowns. *Odontol Rev* 1974;25:189.

35. Walton CB, Leven MM. A preliminary report of photoelastic tests of strain patterns within jacket crowns. *J Am Dent Assoc* 1955;50:45.

36. El-Ebrashi MK, Craig RG, Peyton FA. Experimental stress analysis of dental restorations. Part III. The concept of the geometry of proximal margins. *J Prosthet Dent* 1969;22:333.

37. Dérand T. Analysis of stresses in the porcelain crowns. *Odontol Rev* 1974;25(suppl 27).

38. *Vita In-Ceram Technical Manual*. Baldwin Park, Calif: Vident, 1991.

39. Adair PJ, Grossman DG. The castable ceramic crown. *Int J Periodont Rest Dent* 1984;4(2):33.

40. Malament KA, Grossman DG. The cast glass-ceramic restoration. *J Prosthet Dent* 1987;57:674.

41. Sjogren G, Bergman M. Relationship between compressive strength and cervical shaping of the all-ceramic Cerestore crown. *Swed Dent J* 1987;11:147.

42. Malament KA, Grossman DG. Bonded vs non-bonded Dicor crowns: Four-year report [abstract 1720]. *J Dent Res* 1992; 71:321.

43. Anusavice KJ, Hu S, Hojjatie B. Tensile stress in glass-ceramic crowns: Effect of flaws and cement voids [abstract 1343]. *J Dent Res* 1991;70 (special issue):434.

44. Ferrari M. Cement thickness and microleakage under Dicor crowns: An in vivo investigation. *Int J Prosthodont* 1991;4: 126.

45. Dérand T. The importance of an even shoulder preparation in porcelain crowns. *Odontol Rev* 1972;23:305.

46. Lehman ML, Hampson EL. A study of strain patterns in jacket crowns on anterior teeth resulting from different tooth preparations. *Br Dent J* 1962;20:337.

47. Sozio RB, Riley EJ. Shrink-free ceramic. *Dent Clin North Am* 1985;29:705.

48. Grossman DG. Cast glass ceramics ceramic. *Dent Clin North Am* 1985;29:725.

49. Futterknecht N, Jinoan V. A renaissance of ceramic prosthesis? *QDT Yearbook* 1992;16:65.

50. Dérand T. Ultimate strength of porcelain crowns. *Odontol Rev* 1974;25:393.

51. Doyle MG, Munoz CA, Goodacre CJ, Friedlander LD, Moore BK. The effect of tooth preparation design on the breaking strength of Dicor crowns. Part 2. *Int J Prosthodont* 1990;3: 241.

52. Doyle MG, Goodacre CJ, Munoz CA, Friedlander LD, Moore BK. The effect of tooth preparation design on the breaking strength of Dicor crowns. Part 3. *Int J Prosthodont* 1990;3:327.

53. El-Ebrashi MK, Craig RG, Peyton FA. Experimental stress analysis of dental restorations. Part IV. The concept of parallelism of axial walls. *J Prosthet Dent* 1969;22:346.

54. Dérand T. Analysis of stresses in the porcelain crowns. *Odontol Rev* 1974;25(suppl 27).

55. Mack P. A theoretical and clinical investigation into the taper achieved on crown and inlay preparations. *J Oral Rehabil* 1980;7:255.

56. Griffith AA. *Philos Trans Soc Lond* 1920;A 221:163.

57. Saachi H, Paffenbarger GC. A simple technique for making dental porcelain jacket crowns. *J Am Dent Assoc* 1957;54:366.

58. Jones DW. The strength and strengthening mechanisms of dental ceramics. In: McLean JW (ed). *Dental Ceramics: Proceedings of the First International Symposium on Ceramics*. Chicago: Quintessence, 1983.

59. Kelly JR, Campbell SD, Bowen HK. Fracture analysis of dental ceramics. *J Prosthet Dent* 1989;62:536.

60. Kelly JR, Giordano R, Pober R, Cima MJ. Fracture surface analysis of dental ceramics. *Int J Prosthodont* 1990;3:430.

61. Southan DE, Jorgensen KD. Faulty porcelain jacket crowns. *Aust Dent J* 1972;17:436.

62. Southan DE, Jorgensen KD. An explanation for the occurrence of internal faults in porcelain jacket crowns. *Aust Dent J* 1973;18:152.

63. Munoz CA, Goodacre CJ, Moore BK, Dykema RW. A comparative study of the strength of aluminous porcelain jacket crowns constructed with the conventional and twin foil techniques. *J Prosthet Dent* 1982;48:271.

64. Jones DW. Chemical strengthening of three dental porcelain materials. In: Yamada HN (ed). *Dental Porcelain, The State of the Art–1977*. Los Angeles: Univ of Southern California, 1977: 342.

65. McLean JW. Long-term esthetic dentistry. *Quintessence Int* 1989;20:701.

66. Campbell SD. A comparative study of metal ceramic and all-ceramic esthetic materials: Modulus of rupture. *J Prosthet Dent* 1989;62:476.

67. Sorensen JA, Avera SP, Fanuscu MI. Effect of veneer porcelain on all-ceramic crowns [abstract 1718]. *J Dent Res* 1992;71: 320.

68. Weinstein M, Katz S, Weinstein AB. Fused porcelain-to-metal teeth. US patent 3,052,982 (1962).

69. McLean JW, Sced IR. The bonded alumina crown. 1. The bonding of platinum to aluminous dental porcelain using tin oxide coatings. *Aust Dent J* 1976;21:119.

70. Schoessow D. Die porzellan-Krone nach der cera-platin-technik. "Renaissance der Jacket-Krone." *Quintessenz Zahntech* 1983;9:645.

71. Tanaka A. Fabrication of a bridge using the Sunrise Metal Ceramics system. *QDT Yearbook* 1989;13:87.

72. McLean JW, Hughes H. The reinforcement of dental porcelain with ceramic oxides. *Br Dent J* 1966;119:251.

73. Bourelly G, Prasad A. Le procédé OPTEC HSP. Concepts et mise en oeuvre au laboratoire. *Cahiers de Prothèse* 1989; 68:93.

74. De Rouffignac M, De Cooman J. Reconstitutions céramo-métalliques des dents dépulpées destinées à recevoir des coiffes sans alliage. *RFPD Actualités* 1990;21:29.

75. Lehnner CR, Scharer P. All-ceramic crowns. *Current Opinion in Dentistry*. 1992;2:45.

76. Beham G. A new ceramic technology. *Ivoclar-Vivadent Report* 1990;6:1–13.

77. Sozio RB, Riley EJ. The shrink-free ceramic crown. *J Prosthet Dent* 1983;49:182.

78. Riley EJ, Sozio RB, Krech K. Shrink-free ceramic crowns versus ceramo-metal: A comparative study in dogs. *J Prosthet Dent* 1983;39:766.

79. Levy H. Working with the In-Ceram porcelain system. *Prothèse Dentaire* 1990;44/45:1.

80. Adair PJ, Bell BH, Pameijer CH. Casting technique of machinable glass ceramics [abstract 1024]. *J Dent Res* 1980; 59:475.

81. Adair PJ, Hoekstra KE. Fit evaluation of a castable ceramic [abstract 1025]. *J Dent Res* 1982;61:345.

82. Adair PJ, Sackett BP, Cammarato VT. Preliminary clinical evaluation of a cast ceramic full crown restoration [abstract 1500]. *J Dent Res* 1982;61:292.

83. Hobo S, Iwata T. Castable apatite ceramics as a new biocompatible restorative material. I. Theoretical considerations. *Quintessence Int* 1985;16:135.

84. Hobo S, Iwata T. Castable apatite ceramics as a new biocompatible restorative material. II. Fabrication of the restoration. *Quintessence Int* 1985;16:207.

85. Sherill CA, O'Brien WJ. Transverse strength of aluminous and feldspathic porcelain. *J Dent Res* 1974;53:683.

86. Scherrer S, Mojon P, Belser U, Meyer JM. The Vita Hi-Ceram crown system: A clinical and laboratory investigation. *J Dent Res* [abstract no. 812]. 1988;67:214.

87. Kingery WD. *Ceramic Fabrication Processes*. New York: Technology Press of Massachusetts Institute of Technology and John Wiley and Sons, Inc., 1958.

88. McLean JW. High strength ceramics. *Quintessence Int* 1987; 18:97.

89. Hondrum SO. A review of the strength properties of dental ceramics. *J Prosthet Dent* 1992;67:859.

90. Smith TB, Kelly JR, Tesk JA. Fracture behaviour of In-Ceram and PFM crowns [abstract]. *J Dent Res* 1992;71:321.

91. Seghi RR, Sorensen JA, Engelman MJ, Roumanas E. Flexural strength of new ceramic materials [abstract 1348]. *J Dent Res* 1990;69:299.

92. Dong JK, Luthy H, Wohlwend A, Schärer P. Heat-pressed ceramics: Technology and strength. *Int J Prosthodont* 1992;5:9.

93. Philp GK, Brukl CE. Compressive strengths of conventional, twin foil, and all-ceramic crowns. *J Prosthet Dent* 1984;52:215.

94. Rodrigues A, Nathanson D, Goldstein R. Fracture resistance of different porcelain crown systems [abstract]. *J Dent Res* 1990;69:270.

95. Seghi RR, Daher T, Caputo AA. Flexural strength of ceramic core materials [abstract]. *J Dent Res* 1990;69:378.

96. Wall GT, Cipra DL. Alternative crown systems. Is the metal ceramic crown always the restoration of choice? *Dent Clin North Am* 1992;36:765.

97. Vrijhoef MMA, Spanhauf AJ, Renggli HH. Axial strengths of foil, all-ceramic and PFM molar crowns. *Dent Mater* 1988; 4:15.

98. Josephson BA, Schulman A, Dunn ZA, Hurwitz W. A compressive strength study of complete ceramic crowns. Part II. *J Prosthet Dent* 1991;65:388.

99. Kang SK, Sorensen JA, Avera SP. Fracture strength of ceramic crown systems [abstract 1723]. *J Dent Res* 1992;71:321.

100. Miller A, Long J, Miller B, Cole J. Comparison of the fracture strengths of ceramometal crowns versus several all-ceramic crowns. *J Prosthet Dent* 1992;68:38.

101. Probster L. Compressive strength of two modern all-ceramic crowns. *Int J Prosthodont* 1992;5:409.

102. Christensen R, Christensen G. Service potential of all-ceramic fixed prostheses in areas of varying risk [abstract 1716]. *J Dent Res* 1992;71:320.

103. Probster L, Diehl J. Slip-casting alumina ceramics for crown and bridge restorations. *Quintessence Int* 1992;23:25.

104. McLean JW, Kedge MI, Hubbard JR. The bonded alumina crown. 2. Construction using the twin-foil technique. *Aust Dent J* 1976;21:262.

105. Schoessow D. Die porzellan-Krone nach der cera-platin-technik. "Renaissance der Jacket-Krone." *Quintessenz Zahntech* 1983;9:645.

106. Koerber KH. Metalceramik ohne Gussgerust. Die Cera-Plat-in-Folien-Krone. Ceplatec. *Quintessenz* 1985;36:617.

107. Koerber KH, Ludwig K. Ein Gerat zum Temperaturkontrollieren Diffusionsverschmermelzung von Ceraplatin-Kronengerusten. *Quintessenz Zahntech* 1985;11:997.

108. Tanaka A. Fabrication of a bridge using the Sunrise Metal Ceramics system. *QDT Yearbook* 1989;13:87.

109. Shavell HM. The bioesthetics of complete porcelain occlusal rehabilitation using the Sunrise Ceramic System: A case report. *Int J Periodont Rest Dent* 1990;10:256.

110. Rogers OW. The dental application of electro-formed pure gold. 1. Porcelain jacket crown technique. *Aust Dent J* 1979; 24:163.

111. Sced IR, McLean JW, Hotz P. The strengthening of aluminous porcelain with bonded platinum foils. *J Dent Res* 1977;56:1067.

112. Sarkar NK, Jeansonne EE. Strengthening mechanism of bonded alumina crowns. *J Prosthet Dent* 1987;45:95.

113. Sarkar NK, Chiche GJ, Pinault A. Microstructural characterization of a foil crown system. *Quintessence Int* 1991;22:113.

114. Brukl CE, Ocampo RR. Compressive strengths of a new foil and porcelain fused-to-metal-crowns. *J Prosthet Dent* 1987; 57:404.

115. Josephson BA, Schulman A, Dunn ZA, Hurwitz W. A compressive strength study of complete ceramic crowns. Part II. *J Prosthet Dent* 1991;65:388.

116. Chiche GJ, Pinault A. Données actuelles sur la réduction de l'infrastructure métallique de la couronne céramo-métallique unitaire. Actualités. *Odonto-Stomat* 1988;164:791.

117. Piddock V, Marquis PM, Wilson HJ. Comparison of the strengths of aluminous porcelain fired on to platinum and palladium foils. *J Oral Rehabil* 1986;13:31.

118. Schärer P, Sato T, Wohlwend A. Marginal fit in the Cera-Platin crown system. *Quintessence Dental Technol* 1987;11:11.

119. Schärer P, Sato T, Wohlwend A. A comparison of the marginal fit of three cast ceramic crown systems. *J Prosthet Dent* 1988;59:534.

120. Sorensen JA, Okamoto SK, Miller R, Yarovesky U. Marginal fidelity of four methods of Renaissance crown fabrication [abstract 1414]. *J Dent Res* 1987;66:283.

121. Hummert T, Barghi N, Berry T. Effect of fitting adjustments on compressive strength of a new foil crown system. *J Prosthet Dent* 1991;66:177.

122. Hummert T, Barghi N, Berry T. Postcementation marginal fit of a new foil crown system. *J Prosthet Dent* 1992;66:177.

Chapter 6

Communication with the Dental Laboratory: Try-In Procedures and Shade Selection

Gerard Chiche and Alain Pinault

Patients are increasingly aware of what constitutes an esthetic dental restoration, and dental technicians and porcelain manufacturers are meeting this demand with improved build-up procedures and porcelain materials with superior translucency, opalescence, and color diversification.[1–6] There is nothing more frustrating for the clinician and the technician than to have to modify crown contours at the try-in appointment to the point of eradicating most of the subtle effects built into the restoration. This problem can be prevented to a great extent through improved communication between dentist and dental technician.

Dentist-Technician Communication

Goals _____

- Predictable try-in
- Minimum adjustment of crown restorations

Methods of Achieving Goals _____

- Proper occlusion and orientation of the master cast
- Determination of incisal edge position
- Communication of tooth shape and arrangement
- Proper shade determination

Orientation of the master cast

Esthetic orientation

The master cast must be oriented so that the ceramist has the perspective of the patient facing him. Roach and Muia[7] state: "One of the most common errors in a restored dentition is a slanted incisal plane on the maxillary anterior teeth. Regardless of the incisal plane of the mandibular anterior teeth or even a slanted lip line, the maxillary incisal plane should be meticulously aligned with the interpupillary line." It is easy in the laboratory to misjudge horizontal and vertical alignment of the working cast, especially when restoring multiple preparations, large edentulous spaces, and implants. The worst case scenario is to construct properly aligned crowns on the articulator that in turn appear slanted at try-in and require excessive correction and subsequent remakes. This means that, at some point, the correct orientation of the master cast was not properly communicated to the technician.

A facebow transfer for anterior fixed prostheses may have adverse esthetic consequences because there is no connection between the intercondylar axis and the esthetic reference planes of the face. As Lee[8] stated, it is preferable from an esthetic standpoint when the plane of occlusion follows the lower lip line, but the esthetic plane of occlusion "is not always coincidental with the functional plane of occlusion." Because the techniques of orienting the maxillary cast on the articulator focus on anatomic or arbitrary condylar axis points for the location of an intercondylar reference plane,[9,10] their parallelism with any esthetic reference plane is only accidental (Fig. 6-1).

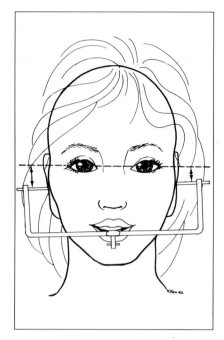

Fig. 6-1 Divergence between the interpupillary line and the intercondylar axis can lead to an unnatural cant of the maxillary cast because the facebow record transfer converts the oblique intercondylar axis to the horizontal axis of the articulator. (Adapted from Stade EH, Hanson JG, Baker CL. Esthetic considerations in the use of facebows. *J Prosthet Dent* 1982;48:253.)

Natural asymmetries of the head may result in a divergence between the interpupillary line and the intercondylar axis and lead to unnatural cants of the maxillary cast because the facebow record transfer converts these asymmetrical axis locations to the horizontal symmetrical axis of the articulator.[11] The dental laboratory technician may not recognize this problem on the bench surface, and improperly canted incisal and occlusal planes of the crown restorations may ensue at try-in.[11,12]

In addition, the working cast itself may incorporate misleading elements that could jeopardize its proper orientation in the laboratory:

Gingival plane: natural asymmetry of the gingival margins is common, and the gingival plane alignment may not be parallel with the interpupillary line.

Tooth preparation: the axis of tooth preparations does not necessarily match the axis of the original tooth or of the final crown.

Residual teeth: as the number of preparations increases, residual teeth become less-reliable guides of orientation of the master cast.

Trimming of the master cast: the way the base of the master cast is trimmed affects the perspective of its orientation. If the base of the cast is automatically trimmed perpendicular to the axis of the preparations, it will not necessarily reproduce the alignment of the preparations as the clinician sees them in the mouth.

Opposing cast: alignment to the mandibular cast may give a false perspective of alignment because the mandibular plane of occlusion may be slanted.

Orientation techniques

The most convenient landmarks for orientation on the patient are the interpupillary line and the facial midline. The ophriac line, the horizon, or any reference plane that may assist the proper horizontal and vertical perspective is also acceptable. The following guidelines are helpful:

- Take a photograph (eg, Polaroid) of the front part of the mouth after tooth preparations with the camera aligned horizontally. The technician can use the photograph to mount the master cast in the same perspective.
- Prepare the proximal walls of the central incisors parallel to the vertical axis of the face. The dentist must face the patient for best results. The master cast is then mounted using the axis of the preparations as guides.
- Draw a pencil line at the base of the working cast to indicate the orientation of the horizontal plane. This requires removal of the provisional restorations at a subsequent appointment. Alternatively, it may be conducted during framework try-in.
- Mount the preoperative casts in the proper alignment before any tooth is prepared. A pencil line may be drawn at the base of the maxillary study cast to set the horizontal plane, or its base may be trimmed parallel to the interpupillary line. When the master cast is mounted to the same opposing cast, it will automatically assume the correct orientation because it is mounted to a cast that was already properly oriented.
- Mount a cast of the impression of the provisional restorations. Score or trim this cast so that with its base held parallel to the pupillary line, the orientation of the incisal plane and the dental midline coincide in the mouth and on this cast. This cast with its opposing cast is then mounted on the articulator with its base parallel to the mounting plate and so that the mounting stone is evenly distributed for both casts. In the sagittal plane, the labial surfaces of the central incisors can be made parallel with the articulator pin for convenience. After the final impression is made, the master cast is articulated to the opposing cast and automatically assumes the proper orientation (Figs. 6-2–6-4).

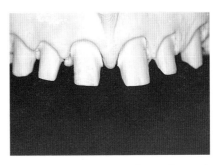

Fig. 6-2 Master cast of anterior tooth preparations. No reliable landmark on this cast indicates to the technician how to align it so that the preparations assume the same orientation on the bench that they have in the mouth.

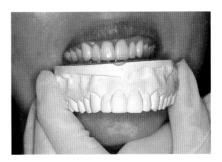

Fig. 6-3 A method for properly orienting the master cast consists of holding the cast of the provisional restorations in the same alignment as in the mouth and trimming its base until it is parallel to the interpupillary line.

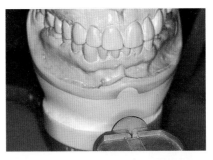

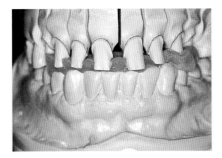

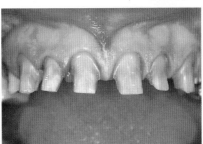

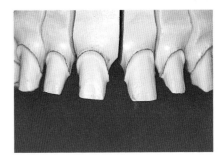

Fig. 6-4a–d Here the maxillary cast of the provisional restorations is mounted on the articulator so that its base is parallel to the mounting plate. In this fashion, the stone cast faces the technician with the same orientation as the provisional restorations face the clinician. After the mandibular cast is articulated to the maxillary cast, the master cast is in turn articulated against the mandibular cast. In this fashion, the preparations become aligned on the articulator with the same orientation of the natural preparations when the patient faces the clinician.

Occlusal orientation

Facebow transfer

With semiadjustable articulators, a facebow transfer for anterior fixed prostheses may have adverse esthetic consequences because there is no connection between the intercondylar axis and the esthetic reference planes of the face. If posterior quadrants must be restored at the same time as the anterior teeth, a facebow transfer is necessary because the condylar determinants must be transferred to the articulator.[13] The cast of the provisional restorations must be trimmed as previously described and secured on the facebow

record. The cast may be mounted on the articulator if, in this position, its base is parallel to the mounting plate.

If the base of the cast is slanted after it was secured on the facebow record, it means that the esthetic plane and the posterior occlusal plane do not coincide and that a compromise must be made. The cast must be aligned so that its base is parallel to the upper mounting plate, and this position should be secured on the facebow recording with wax before pouring the mounting stone. In this situation, the facebow relationship is altered for esthetic purposes at the expense of the proper condylar relation to the master

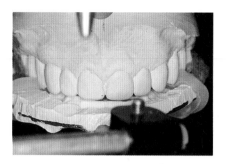

Fig. 6-5 When the anterior esthetic plane and the posterior occlusal plane do not coincide, the base of the cast that was aligned to the interpupillary line becomes slanted as it is positioned on the facebow record. The cast is realigned so that its base is parallel to the upper mounting plate and is secured with wax on the facebow recording before pouring of the mounting stone. In this situation, the facebow relationship is altered for esthetic purposes.

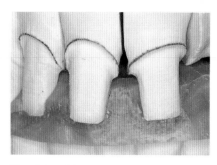

Fig. 6-6 A hard wax record is preferred over a silicone record when the casts cannot be related at all unless an occlusal record is used. Rigidity of the recording medium is essential for an exact occlusal relation, and flexibility must be avoided.

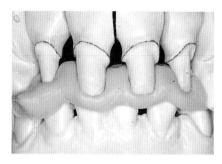

Fig. 6-7 A silicone interocclusal record is mostly accurate when the casts need only minimal additional information for an exact occlusal relation.

cast (Fig. 6-5). Therefore, some degree of intraoral adjustment in lateral excursions is to be expected.

Interocclusal recording

A proper occlusal recording should provide precise reference for accurate articulation of the dental casts with no ambiguity (Table 6-1). Injectable silicone materials offer ease of dispensing and simplicity over traditional wax materials, but their flexibility and resiliency may be a severe handicap in the laboratory as the number of preparations increases, and where more rigid materials are required (Fig. 6-6). Under optimal conditions, the minimum error caused by this resiliency during a constant load was found to be at least 61 μm.[14]

It should not be assumed that a full complement of intact posterior teeth is sufficient for an accurate occlusal relation of the casts after only the incisors have been prepared. Preparing anterior teeth results in loss of anterior stop and frequently leads to several possible intercuspations of the casts in the laboratory. In this case, a silicone record is most often all that is necessary to accurately tripodize the casts for an accurate relation (Fig. 6-7).

Anterior guidance

Anterior guidance is transferred to the final restoration through an anterior guide table constructed on the articulator. In the laboratory, the table is derived from the occlusal relation of the study casts when the original anterior guidance does not need to be altered or from the cast of the provisional restorations that served to establish a new guidance.

Table 6-1 Occlusal Records for Anterior Tooth Preparations

Restoration	Record
Single anterior restoration	No occlusal record required
Restoration of two to four incisors or anterior three-unit fixed partial denture	Silicone record
Restoration of four incisors and at least one canine	Wax record
Full-arch reconstruction	Wax record with provisional posterior fixed partial dentures serving as occlusal stop

---

Function of the Anterior Guide Table[14–16]

- Transfer the original anterior guidance or the anterior guidance established in the provisional restorations
- Determine the framework design and the type of restorative material in the lingual aspect of the restorations
- Minimize the extent of occlusal adjustment during try-in and eliminate or minimize postcementation adjustments

The established guidance accurately determines the available thickness of porcelain and/or metal available in protrusion. When comfortable and functional anterior guidance is provided in the provisional restorations, the clinician must measure the thickness of the provisional restorations along the protrusive pathways to determine the nature of the restorative material to be used in the lingual aspect of the restorations.

When the lingual thickness of the provisional restorations is measured by the clinician and falls below 0.5 mm, metal must be prescribed in the laboratory form unless provision will be made for adjustment of the opposing teeth. The anterior guide table must be constructed from casts of the provisional restorations in order to wax the metal contour to the proper concavity.

When the lingual thickness of the provisional restorations is measured by the clinician and falls above 0.5 mm, porcelain over metal may be safely prescribed in the laboratory form in conjunction with an anterior guide table for conforming the porcelain to the proper concavity.

When the lingual thickness was not measured by the clinician but a guide table can be constructed from preoperative casts or casts of the provisional restorations, the technician must select the lingual design and restorative material according to the available clearance dictated by the anterior guide table.

When the lingual thickness was not measured by the clinician and no reference is available for constructing the anterior guide table, the anterior guidance of the final restorations is arbitrary and most often developed on porcelain over metal. Patients may adapt to this guidance, but if this new envelope of function is too restricted, functional disturbances may occur in the form of pain and discomfort, tooth mobility, or posterior condylar displacement.[15–18] In severe cases, postcementation adjustment to a comfortable anterior guidance could result in eradication of the lingual anatomy in porcelain and exposure of the opaque or of the metal coping.

Incisal edge position

Preoperative casts or casts of the provisional restorations should be provided to the technician when they represent a reasonable outline of the final result. A common error is to place the incisal edge too far labially in the final restoration.[19] This is frequently due to insufficient tooth reduction: the preparation must reproduce the natural convexity of a maxillary central incisor and provide for a minimum reduction thickness of 1.5 mm at the junction of the middle and incisal thirds of the crown.[20–24] Insufficient tooth reduction is the leading cause of overcontouring of the restoration, especially at the incisal third of the central incisor.

Another common error is to drastically alter the original incisal edge position without testing it with provisional restorations fabricated from a diagnostic wax-up. When a new anterior guidance results from significant alteration in incisal edge position with new crowns, the patient should first demonstrate functional adaptation to this new position in the provisional restorations.[15] On occasion, retraction of the incisal edge position toward the lingual may create functional disturbances such as mobility, pain, or discomfort to which the patient cannot adapt. Correction to a more comfortable guidance will likely result in thinning of the incisal edges of the provisional restorations to the point that the clinician and the technician must realize that the final incisal edge position will have to be further labial than anticipated from the diagnostic waxing. Esthetics and function must be monitored and restored simultaneously when significant esthetic alterations are performed.

Horizontal overlap

In the laboratory, determination of the horizontal overlap is made either from the original overlap of the study casts or from the cast of the provisional restorations. Typically, three casts are used: the reference cast, the opposing cast, and the master cast. When the original tooth shape from the study cast serves as a reference and yields sufficient information for the final restoration, the provisional restoration is not required to have significant esthetic diagnostic value. When the cast of the provisional restorations serves as the esthetic reference, the facial thickness of the provisional restorations must be systematically measured by the clinician before final impression making[25] at the junction between the incisal third and the middle third. Tooth preparations must be further modified if there is insufficient thickness according to the type of selected ceramic crown.

A silicone index of the reference cast is especially helpful for waxing the framework. By capturing the outline of the incisal edges in the cast, it allows for predictable framework design and adequate porcelain thickness.[7] The reference cast should first be articulated with the opposing cast to achieve the proper esthetic orientation. The master cast is then mounted to the same opposing cast. Consequently, the master cast is interchangeable with the reference cast and can share the same indexing.

The allocated dimensions for the framework are precisely gauged with the silicone index to ensure

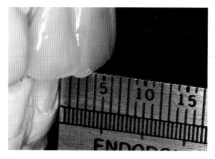
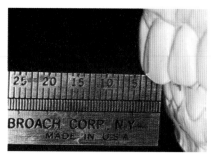

Fig. 6-8a and b   Silicone indexes are indicated for fabrication of frameworks, proper location of connectors, and to ensure that porcelain is correctly supported. They lack precision for final monitoring of incisal edge position. The horizontal overlap should be measured with a ruler on the reference cast, which is either the diagnostic cast or a cast of the provisional restorations. It should match the porcelain crown overlap because both maxillary casts are occluded against the same mandibular cast. The final overlap should be within 0.5 mm of the reference overlap at most.

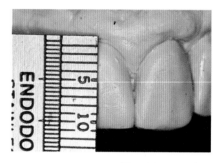
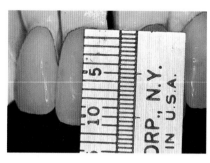
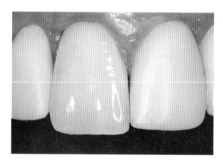

Fig. 6-9a–c   Communication of tooth length. The technician measures the length of the provisional restorations and matches it on the porcelain restoration, making allowance for subgingival penetration. This technique, although useful in most situations, may lack precision because it is not possible for the technician to know the exact depth of subgingival penetration of the preparation in the mouth. This explains why the seated porcelain crown is longer than the adjacent provisional crown that serves as a reference.

proper support of the porcelain, which is critical with long-span fixed partial dentures, overreduced preparations, or implant restorations. The thickness of porcelain veneering between abutments and pontics is controlled to achieve the same shade. Buccolingual and mesiodistal alignment of the connections is visualized against the index and allows optimal embrasure form and proximal contact position to be created. Screw emergence of implant restorations is evaluated in relation to the final crown structure.

In the porcelain construction, the horizontal overlap must be monitored with a ruler to achieve the desired incisal edge position. A silicone index is effective for framework construction but is of limited value after porcelain firing because of the flexibility of the material. The ruler is also an effective communication tool between the clinic and the laboratory because the horizontal overlap between the provisional restora-

tions and the delivered crowns can be objectively compared (Fig. 6-8).

Practically, the difference between the crowns' overlap and the reference overlap must not exceed 0.5 mm. A discrepancy of just 1 mm may make the difference between success or failure for some patients who typically report phonetic or pressure changes against the upper lip caused by the new crowns. If the patient complains of phonetic disturbances caused by the provisional restorations, and if those are too subtle to be noticed by the attentive clinician, it is safer to exactly reproduce the original incisal edge position from the study casts.

Vertical overlap

It is the dentist's responsibility to communicate sufficient information to the laboratory to achieve the de-

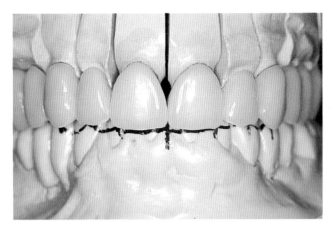

Fig. 6-10 Tooth length can be communicated by marking on the opposing cast the outline of the provisional restorations or of the original teeth from an articulated cast. The technician must ensure that the porcelain restorations match this outline; however, this technique lacks precision because variations of the angle of vision lead to several possible interpretations of crown length.

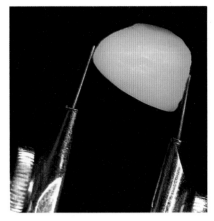

Fig. 6-11 An accurate method of communicating tooth length consists of measuring the provisional restoration after removing it from the preparation and communicating it in the prescription to the technician. The porcelain crown can in turn be precisely fabricated and measured according to this specification.

sired crown length. If the crown is found to be excessively short at try-in, precious time is wasted for firing new porcelain additions. If the crown is too long and must be reduced, the incisal color effects are obliterated and the incisal edge becomes deported further labially as it is reduced in length. Length can be monitored with any of four techniques (Figs. 6-9–6-11):

- The outline of the incisal edges of the reference cast (study cast or cast of the provisional restorations) is inscribed on the opposing cast and matched against the master cast. This technique is simple but lacks accuracy because its interpretation is subject to various angles of vision.
- The tooth length as measured on the reference cast dictates the crown length. This method is generally reliable but is subject to interpretation of the subgingival depth of the preparation by the laboratory.
- The length of the provisional restoration is measured out of the mouth by the clinician and becomes a part of the prescription. This is the most accurate technique when the length of the provisional restorations must be precisely reproduced.
- The custom guide table established from the reference cast and the opposing cast is shaped so that the articulator pin carves a precise stop in the acrylic resin in the edge-to-edge position. The crown length on the master cast is adjusted at that same border position.

Crown contour

Shape and arrangement

The involvement of the ceramist in the treatment occurs at various stages according to the imperatives of the situation.

Diagnostic waxing and/or provisional restorations

For best communication with the laboratory, the clinician should determine general tooth shape, arrangement, and alignment; all refinements envisioned are then transmitted on the prescription form to the ceramist.[26] This means that limitations are imposed on the technician, but this valuable information is determined clinically and cannot be second-guessed in the laboratory. When sufficient information is present preoperatively, the study casts serve as references either for duplication or for slight alterations of the original tooth arrangement. When there are insufficient references (eg, with deficient crowns) several possibilities exist (Figs. 6-8 and 6-12–6-15):

1. The existing crowns are sequentially removed, and changes and improvements are incorporated in the provisional restorations; these are directly fabricated intraorally with no diagnostic waxing.
2. A diagnostic waxing is fabricated on the study cast incorporating the planned modifications, and the provisional restorations are constructed intraorally from this waxing. The waxing is therefore tested and modified intraorally if necessary.

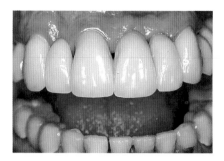

Fig. 6-12a Provisional restoration adjusted according to esthetic and functional requirements.

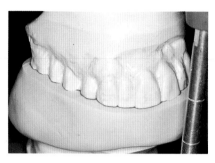

Fig. 6-12b An alginate impression of the provisional restoration is poured in stone and articulated in centric relation occlusion with the mandibular cast. A silicone index is made with the casts in occlusion.

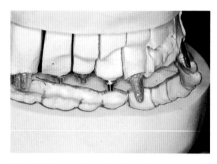

Fig. 6-12c After the final impression is made, the master cast is articulated to the same mandibular cast in centric relation. This cast and the cast of the provisional restorations are interchangeable against the same mandibular cast, hence the master cast assumes a correct orientation in relation to the silicone index. This assists the technician in waxing the framework and in developing the proper location and dimension of connectors and pontics.

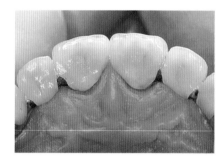

Fig. 6-12d With proper planning and use of indexes, it is possible to locate the proximal connectors lingually for proper morphology of the facial embrasures while preserving connector strength.

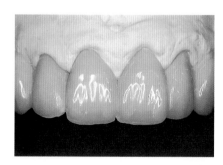

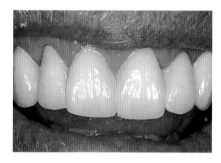

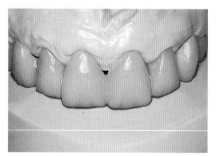

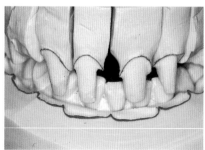

Fig. 6-13a Esthetic trial set-up with hollow ground denture facings on a preliminary cast of the preparations. The acrylic resin laminates are connected lingually with autopolymerizing resin.

Fig. 6-13b Trial set-up fitted over the preparations after minor adjustments are completed.

Fig. 6-13c The trial set-up is secured to its cast and articulated with the mandibular cast. A silicone index is made with the casts in occlusion.

Fig. 6-13d After the final impression is made, the master cast is articulated with the same mandibular cast in occlusion. The silicone index allows visualization of the relationship between the preparations and the desired result and planning of the framework design accordingly.

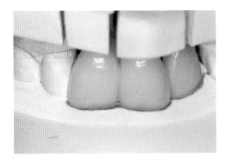

Fig. 6-14a The diagnostic waxing is directly constructed on the master cast derived from an impression of three implants. The silicone index registers the incisal outline of the waxing.

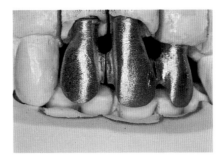

Fig. 6-14b The emergence of the abutment screws may be visualized accurately against the silicone index to ensure that it is lingual to the incisal edges through the cingulum areas. In case of eccentric emergence, preangled or custom abutments must be considered. After abutment selection is completed, the framework is waxed and checked against the silicone index so that porcelain is properly supported by the framework.

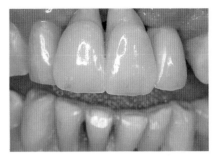

Fig. 6-14c Completed implant-retained fixed partial denture. (In collaboration with Dr R Rooney.)

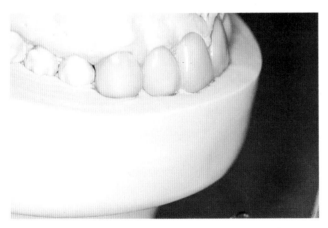

Fig. 6-15a The diagnostic waxing for porcelain laminate veneers is constructed on the diagnostic cast with the silicone index in position. This waxing is useful for fabrication of the provisional laminate restorations.

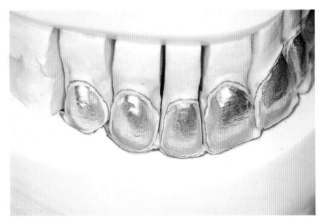

Fig. 6-15b After the final impression is made, the master cast is articulated with the same mandibular cast in occlusion. The silicone index allows visualization of the relationship between the preparations and the desired result. In the case of laminate veneers, the index serves as only a general guide due to its flexibility.

3. A diagnostic waxing is fabricated on the working cast after final impression for determination of the framework design, and indexes are made for coping and pontic patterns.[27–31] This waxing is not tested in the mouth.
4. A denture tooth set-up is fabricated on an accessory cast of the final preparations and tried in the mouth for final acceptance by the patient.

Intraoral photographs and computerized video imaging

Intraoral photographs and full-face or profile pictures can help sensitize the technician to the needs of the patient and give an improved perspective of depth and shape over stone casts. They are invaluable for assessment of shade distribution and special color effects.

Computerized video imaging allows patients to preview proposed treatment alternatives before committing to the treatment plan. It also allows the clinician to communicate to the technician the expected outcome of the treatment.[32] From the dental laboratory standpoint, computerized imaging may replace diagnostic waxing or serve to complement it according to the clinical situation. Natural tooth and soft tissue color also improve the perspective of shape over stone cast or acrylic resin restorations.[33]

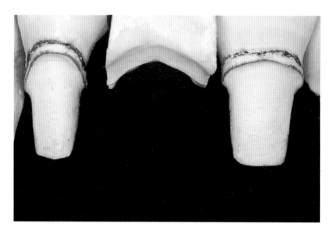

Fig. 6-16　When the root area immediately adjacent to the finish line is captured in the impression, it should be preserved during the die trimming process. It is comprised between the apical extent of the root area *(blue line)* and the margin of the preparation *(red line)*.

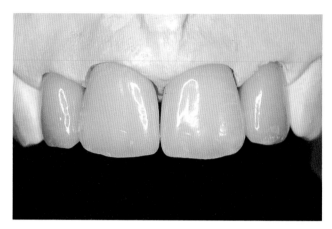

Fig. 6-17　The unsawed cast is essential for final appraisal of the crown contours and embrasure shapes and for avoiding dark triangles in the cervical embrasures. It also provides the technician with a better perspective of contours compared to the sawed cast.

Crown emergence

Crown emergence affects general tooth shape, cervical embrasures, and periodontal health.[34–40] If, to maximize periodontal health, the cervical crown emergence is too flat, the crowns will appear tapered and unnatural[41] and the cervical embrasures may be open and esthetically unacceptable. Conversely, excessive cervical convexity may be pleasing to the patient but could lead to chronic gingival inflammation. The objective is to reconcile esthetic and periodontal imperatives by restoring an anatomic curvature in the sulcus[42] with a flat or slightly convex emergence profile and closed cervical embrasures that do not jeopardize periodontal health.

Master cast

The master cast, trimmed and indexed, is used for fabricating the framework, porcelain margins, and initial porcelain build-up. If the root anatomy was captured in the impression, it must be preserved during the die-trimming process so that it is continuous with the cervical emergence of the crown restoration: this area is termed "the area of anatomic information" by Martignoni and Schonenberger[42] and should be left untouched by the bur in order to extrapolate the emergence of the crown (Fig. 6-16).

Accessory master cast

The absence of gingival tissue on the master cast of the prepared dies significantly affects the esthetic appraisal of the restoration because it is an unnatural perspective. Crown emergence, contours, and embra-sures must be refined on an unsawed cast issued from the same impression. The objective is not to systematically close the cervical embrasures but to develop a better perspective of the crown contours (Fig. 6-17).

The accessory master cast is also useful for constructing fixed partial denture connectors. The vertical height of the connectors from the papilla toward the incisal area is most critical for strength,[43–45] whereas their labiolingual placement is critical for proper contour of the facial embrasures. This may require that the connector be located toward the lingual and that metal be exposed in the lingual aspect with a trestle[40] or interrupted trestle design[46] (Fig. 6-18).

When crown contours are adjusted on the accessory master cast, gingival retraction must also be taken into account. The cervical emergence should be arbitrarily contoured so that the porcelain does not completely fill the gingival sulcus, and the proximal embrasures should be slightly opened to account for the slight depression of the interdental papilla caused by the gingival retraction. Therefore, the clinician may have to customize this emergence further according to the blanching of the marginal gingiva and the compression of the interdental papilla when inserting the crown restorations.

Several techniques are available for constructing the accessory master cast[47–53] (Figs. 6-17, 6-19, and 6-20):

- Soft tissue model: the gingival outline is replicated with a resilient silicone or resin material.
- Solid stone model: a second pour of the final impression is made in stone.

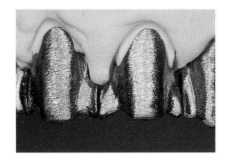
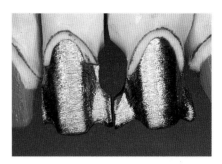

Fig. 6-18a and b The metal framework is fabricated on the master cast, but the embrasure spaces and their relation to the soft tissues must be checked against an unsawed cast, which is a second pour of the same impression.

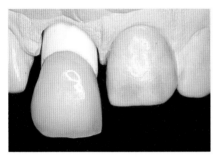

Fig. 6-19a Accessory cast for soft tissue reproduction. A resin die is poured in the preparation site, and after setting it is reshaped to eliminate any undercuts. The die is replaced in the impression and a stone base is poured. The cast incorporates a removable die with a rigid reproduction of soft tissues.

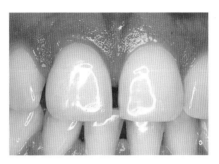

Fig. 6-19b The cemented metal ceramic crown is in harmony with the soft tissues.

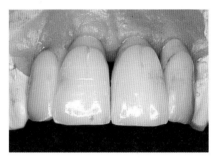

Fig. 6-20 Soft tissue casts are commonly made from a pick-up impression of the framework positioned on the preparations or, as in this case, from a transfer impression of implants.

- Solid epoxy model: a second pour of the final impression is made in epoxy resin. This method is particularly useful with single incisors for determining the proper surface texture and with single implant restorations.
- Removable die–solid stone model: a single die of the preparation is first constructed and repositioned into the final impression. The impression is poured in stone and allows for replication of the gingival outline.
- Soft tissue cast constructed after framework try-in from a pick-up impression. The main advantage of this technique is that gingival tissues are captured in an unretracted state.

Clinical try-in

The goal of a successful clinical try-in is to achieve optimum seating of the crowns, harmonious occlusion, and optimum esthetics. A segmental try-in technique where anterior crowns on one side are tried first and matched against the provisional restorations offers significant advantages:

- The incisal edge position of the final crowns may be checked against the provisional restorations.
- The occlusion established in the provisional restorations may be precisely transferred into the final crowns for the same function and immediate comfort.
- Changes and expected improvements in the final crowns can be evaluated against the provisional restorations.
- If the esthetic results are disappointing, the deficiencies can be objectively identified and corrected using the provisional crowns as reference.

By contrast, simultaneous try-in of all the final restorations does not allow precise identification of alterations and improvements incorporated in the final crowns. This is not critical when the esthetic results are satisfactory, but without a ready reference it is more difficult to proceed methodically when corrections are necessary.

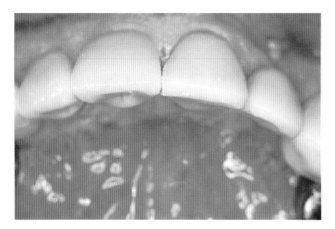

Fig. 6-21 The provisional crowns on the central and lateral incisors on one side are removed first, and the crown restorations are compared with the provisional restorations. The incisal edge position should first be evaluated in an occlusal view and should be within 0.5 mm of the incisal edge of the provisional restorations. If the discrepancy is greater than 0.5 mm, the provisional restorations may be more esthetically pleasing than the porcelain crowns, which have a straighter facial aspect.

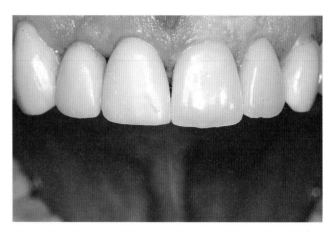

Fig. 6-22 The length between the porcelain and provisional crowns should be compared. They should align or should be within 0.5 mm of one another. If a discrepancy greater than 0.5 mm is observed at this stage, a significant departure in tooth shape and composition from the provisional restorations is to be expected.

Try-in sequence

The following sequence describes a typical situation involving four crowns for the maxillary incisors.

1. The provisional crowns on the central and lateral incisors on one side are removed first and the crown restorations are tried on the tooth preparations.
2. The seating of each crown must be evaluated with a fast-setting silicone disclosing paste, even if there seems to be adequate evidence of full seating. Christensen[54] demonstrated that the evaluation of subgingival margins was not consistently reliable. Therefore, the apparent fit of a subgingival margin cannot be fully trusted unless tested with a silicone disclosing agent.[55–58] Through successive adjustments, the silicone lining should become more translucent, indicating a closer fit of the crowns at the margins.
3. The horizontal overlap of the central incisor crown is compared with the adjacent provisional central incisor. They should be aligned when viewed occlusally, or they should be at most within 0.5 mm of one another. If a discrepancy greater than 0.5 mm is observed at this stage, it may eventually have to be corrected, unless it is deemed acceptable in the final evaluation of the four crowns (Fig. 6-21).
4. The length of the central incisor crown is compared with the adjacent provisional central incisor. They should align when facing the patient, or should be within 0.5 mm of one another. If a discrepancy greater than 0.5 mm is observed at this stage, a significant departure in tooth shape and composition from the provisional restorations is to be expected, unless it is deemed acceptable in the final evaluation of the four crowns (Fig. 6-22).
5. The shape of the central incisor crown is compared with the adjacent provisional central incisor, and it is determined whether it has been esthetically improved, is inferior, or is simply consistent with the adjacent provisional crown. The objective at this stage is not to duplicate the shape of the provisional restoration but to visualize some esthetic improvements. If there are too many discrepancies in morphology and incisal edge position, and if the esthetic results are unsatisfactory to the patient and the clinician, the provisional restorations provide a useful reference.
6. The centric occlusal contacts and the protrusive pathways of the central and lateral incisors' final crowns are refined against the provisional crowns for contact intensity and fremitus. The proprioception provided by the provisional restorations is the best guide at this stage and allows for convenient detection of occlusal interferences. Segmental adjustment of the occlusion whenever feasible allows precise transfer of the anterior guidance from the provisional restorations into the final restorations (Fig. 6-23).
7. The emergence of the crowns is customized. If there is blanching of the gingival tissues, the crown emergence should be flattened and the cervical

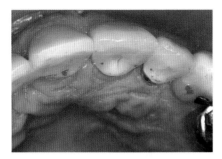 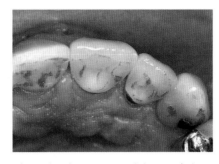 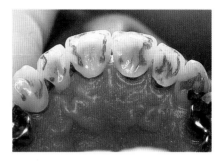

Fig. 6-23a–c The centric occlusal contacts and the protrusive pathways of the porcelain crowns are harmonized and refined against the provisional crowns. The opposing fixed partial denture is then placed and adjusted against the porcelain crowns. This segmental adjustment of the occlusion allows the transfer of the anterior guidance from the provisional restorations into the final restorations.

Fig. 6-24a and b The subgingival portion of the interproximal embrasures is customized by marking the proximal gingival margin outline on the crown surface with a pencil. The crown is reported on the die and held firmly, and the proximal portion between the pencil line and the margin is adjusted with a diamond stone into a flat or concave surface.

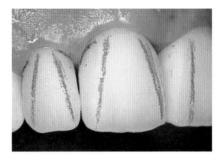 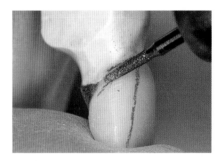

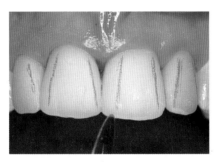 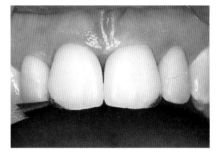

Fig. 6-25 Adjustments in length are made with the clinician facing the patient, using flexible diamond disks mounted on a straight handpiece. Adjustment of the line angles are indicated when a different perception of tooth width is required. Their desired position should first be marked on the crown surface, and the adjustments must respect the interproximal contacts.

Fig. 6-26 Fine modifications of the incisal edge outline should be previewed by masking the area to be adjusted with a pencil and squinting in order to visualize the projected outline. A decision should then be made whether these modifications are required or not.

embrasures should be adjusted so that the interdental papilla fills most of the embrasure space. This anticipates any possible papillary regeneration once the pressure exerted on the papillae by the provisional restorations is eliminated. To customize the subgingival portion of the interproximal embrasure, the proximal gingival margin outline is marked on the crown surface with a pencil. The crown is then reported on the die and held firmly, and the proximal portion between the pencil line and the margin is adjusted with a diamond stone into a flat or concave surface[53] (Fig. 6-24).

8. The provisional crowns on the incisors of the opposing side are removed and the other two crown restorations are seated following the same sequence. Finally, the occlusion is harmonized to the first two crowns.

9. The final esthetic appraisal of all four crowns is made. If they are satisfactory, they can be glazed and cemented. Esthetic corrections may be indicated if: the crowns are either too long or too short; the incisal edges are placed too far labially; the crowns are too tapered; or the crowns are either too wide or too narrow.

Adjustments are performed with diamond and green stones and flexible diamond disks (Fig. 6-25), with the clinician facing the patient,[59] and are more predictable when the modifications are first outlined in pencil on the crowns (Fig. 6-26). Polishing the line angles with a rubber wheel may also be required to achieve a correct appraisal of tooth morphology. If the line angles need to be adjusted, their desired position should be marked on the crown surface with a pencil before any adjustment is made.

Shade selection

Color has three dimensions: hue, value, and chroma. Hue is defined as the quality of sensation according to which an observer is aware of the varying wavelengths of radiant energy.[60] The primary source of natural tooth color is the dentin, and its hue is either in the yellow or yellow-red range.[61–64] Value is the quality that relates a color to a gray scale of similar brightness. It is primarily affected by the quality and transparency of the enamel. Chroma is the dimension of color that defines the intensity or concentration of the hue. It is dictated by the dentin and influenced by the translucency and thickness of the enamel.

Shade selection and color perception are affected by several variables, and some basic precautions must be met to improve consistency. The ideal light source is a balanced daylight with an average color temperature around 6,500°K.[65] The dental office and the dental laboratory should have daylight color-corrected fluorescent lamps installed so that shade selection and crown fabrication are performed in the same lighting environment.[66] Incandescent or unbalanced light sources should be avoided, and the lighting equipment should be regularly inspected to detect fluctuations in color temperature.[65]

Before shade determination, stains or deposits must be cleaned off the tooth surface. The natural tooth must be kept wet throughout the shade determination, otherwise it may lighten as it dries and will only revert back very slowly to its original condition[67] (Fig. 6-27). Similarly, the shade evaluation must not be made after anesthesia is administered, after tooth preparation is completed,[68] or after a strenuous appointment. Finally, the clinician must not stare at the tooth for more than 20 seconds or he or she will lose sensitivity to yellow.

For optimum results, shade selection must follow a logical sequence: *(1)* basic shade; *(2)* basic shade variations; *(3)* enamel shade, translucency, and location; *(4)* special effects.

Basic shade

The basic tooth shade (or hue) must first be evaluated by matching the center of the natural tooth with the closest approximating shade tab. The first impression is the most important because spontaneity gives the best results. If the base shade cannot be determined at this stage, considerable difficulties may be expected later unless a custom shade tab is fabricated.[67] Currently available shade guides offer a variety of standard colors, but because they do not cover the full color range of natural teeth,[69] it is best to expect at this stage a general impression. However, hue must be assessed correctly because hue mistakes are often made as several tabs have the same value and may appear very similar. When in doubt, the two closest matching shade tabs should be compared directly under the natural tooth for a final decision[66] (Fig. 6-28).

Shades in the A group are frequently encountered in young individuals and account for at least 65% of porcelain sales of certain manufacturers.[4] This is because their hue is well centered within the natural tooth color space[70] and because, being the closest yellow hues to orange (Fig. 6-29), they also allow for color diversification into the orange color space.[69]

Shades in the B group are closer to a pure yellow compared to shades in the A group, but they are rarely encountered in natural dentition.[4] This is probably because they are located at one extreme of the natural tooth color space[70] and as such represent only a fraction of natural hues. A false perception of yellow also occurs when the natural tooth is observed in contrast to a pink or red background, and the result is that a tooth of an A shade could be falsely perceived as more yellow and consequently matched as a B shade.[4] Various A/B combinations such as A2/B2, A3/B2, and A3/B3 are common occurrences with middle-aged patients and serve to express a hue halfway between the two groups. From a spectrophotometric standpoint, mixing between color groups is possible and results in an intermediate hue.[70]

To emphasize color difference between canines

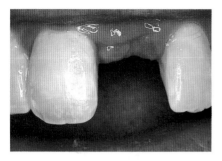 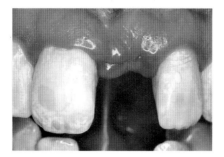 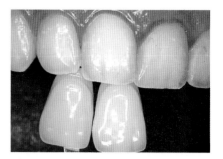

Fig. 6-27a and b It is essential to keep natural teeth wet throughout the shade determination, otherwise they lighten or become chalky as they desiccate and may revert back only very slowly to their original condition.

Fig. 6-28 The basic tooth shade (or hue) must be first evaluated against the closest approximating shade tab. The most spontaneous impression gives the best results. In this example, a mixture of two hues is confirmed by matching them simultaneously against the natural tooth.

Armamentarium for Shade Matching

- Shade guide
- Shade prescription form
- Accessory shade guides
- Instant photograph or slide
- Daylight color-corrected fluorescent lighting
- Neutral environment

The Accessory Armamentarium Includes:

- Magnifying loops
- Fluid resin stains
- Custom shade tab
- Hand mirror

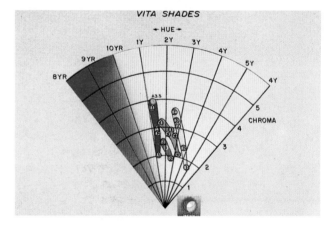

Fig. 6-29 Hue-chroma range of the four Vita-Lumin families as measured by Miller. There is a deficiency in orange (YR) hues, but also note that the A shades represent the group closest to the orange color space. (From Miller LL. Scientific approach to shade matching. In: Preston JD (ed). *Perspectives in Dental Ceramics. Proceedings of the Fourth International Symposium on Ceramics.* Chicago, Quintessence, 1988:193.

and incisors in esthetic reconstructions, central and lateral incisors should be restored with A shades and canines with a B shade, together with a decreasing value from the central incisor to the canine to emphasize individuality. For example, central incisors are restored at the mesial aspect with A1/A2 and A2/A3 at the distal aspect, lateral incisors are restored at the mesial aspect with A3 and A3.5 at the distal aspect, and canines with B4.[71]

Shades in the C group may be considered a subgroup of the B family because they have a somewhat comparable hue but a lower value.[70] Therefore, they are more frequently encountered in middle-aged and older individuals or in patients with tetracycline-stained teeth. When a shade in the B group appears to have a

higher value than the natural tooth, shade tabs in the C group should be examined and, on occasion, be deemed more appropriate.

Shades in the D group are rarely encountered but may be considered a subgroup of the A family because they have a somewhat comparable hue with a lower value.[70] When a shade in the B group appears to have a higher value than the natural tooth, shade tabs in the D group should be investigated and, on occasion, be deemed more appropriate.

Shades in the C or D group represent only isolated examples of lower value of a given hue of the B or A group, and as such do not automatically provide the expected value when an A or B tab of a lower value is desired.

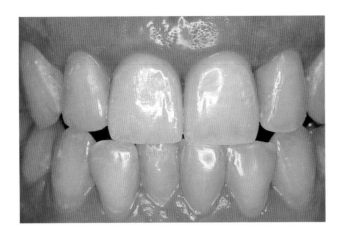

Fig. 6-30 This patient's natural dentition reveals a typical orange hue, which was replicated for these three maxillary incisor crowns with the use of M3 and M4 tabs.

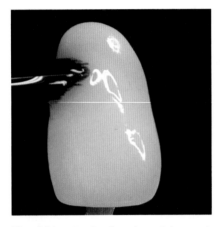

Fig. 6-31 Application of a paint-on, colored resin on the shade tab to communicate to the technician additional color or intensity of the cervical tone (Custom shading kit, Tanaka Dental Products, Skokie, IL). The stain sets within 20 seconds of being applied to the shade tab.

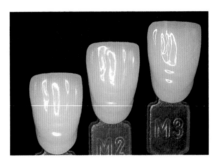

Fig. 6-32 Accessory shade tabs useful for orange variations from the basic shade are found in the Candulor shade guide (Candulor AG, Zurich, Switzerland). M tabs incorporate orange variations from shades of the A group.

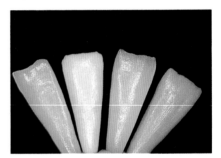

Fig. 6-33 Examples of customized tabs of dentin mamelon color.

Basic shade variations

After the basic hue is determined, the next step is to detect its variations according to the location on the tooth, the addition of orange to the basic hue, or the incompatibility with standard shade tabs.

Orange modification

Various studies[61–64] indicate that natural tooth color falls in either the yellow or orange color space. Most of the data were obtained on extracted teeth, but they may be extrapolated to natural teeth because they are consistent with daily observations. Jorgenson and Goodkind[72] and Hemendinger and Miller[69] noted that currently available porcelain shade guides do not incorporate any orange hue and are therefore confined to yellow hues only. The clinician is faced with matching yellow or orange natural teeth with yellow shade tabs only and must therefore determine whether the natural tooth is more orange than the shade tab or not.

The orange tonality is either expressed in the body of the tooth or is confined at the cervical aspect. In the latter case, the application of a fluid-colored resin on the shade tab may help visualize the quality and intensity of the cervical tone (Custom shading kit, Tanaka Dental Products, Skokie, Ill; Color Link, ADS, Anaheim, Calif) (Fig. 6-31). The stain sets within sec-

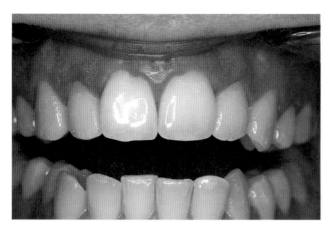
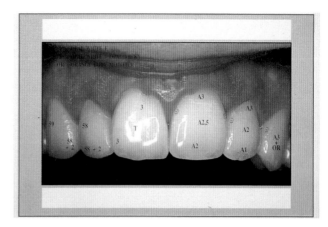

Fig. 6-34a and b   Shade determination for maxillary anterior teeth. Dentin shade (labeled on the right side of the midline) is progressively lighter from cervical to incisal aspect for the central and lateral incisors, whereas it is essentially uniform for the canine. Enamel distribution is nearly uniform on the central incisor, occupying the incisal and middle thirds of the lateral incisor and mostly the incisal third of the canine. Enamel translucency (labeled on the left side of the midline) increases from the central incisor to the canine.

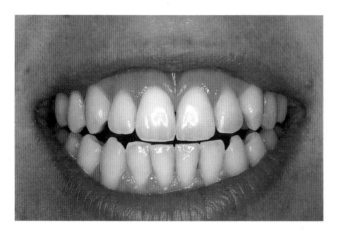
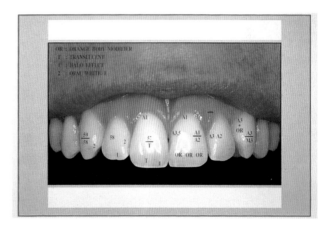

Fig. 6-35a and b   Shade determination for maxillary anterior teeth with characteristic example of orange mamelon shade *(right side)* and subtle but progressive dentin shade from central incisor to canine. The enamel shade incorporates examples of halo and translucent zones adjacent to them. Enamel progression from central incisor to canine is characterized by a subtle increase in translucency and decrease in value.

onds and is useful for communicating this type of shade modification to the technician. The Candulor shade guide (Candulor AG, Zurich, Switzerland) (Fig. 6-32) incorporates orange hues in the M group and can be used for direct evaluations of orange variations from shades in the A group: M1 = A2 + orange, M2 = A3 + orange, M3 = A3 + orange(+), M4 = A3.5 + orange, M5 = A3.5 + orange(+).

Variation according to location

Nakagawa et al[73] reported four broad categories of shade pattern according to their location on the tooth. The most frequent variation from the basic hue was observed at the incisal third. In the next most frequent category, the shade distribution was nearly uniform, resulting in a monochromatic appearance. In the third category, the color deviation from the basic hue was observed mostly at the cervical third. Finally, in the fourth group, the shade variation involved the middle aspect of the tooth. Therefore, the clinician should determine whether the basic shade is uniform or whether shade variations occur on the tooth. Accessory shade guides are also useful in this respect. Several Biodent shade tabs, for example, have a more uniform color distribution as compared with Vita shade tabs.

Cervical variations may either correspond to the cervical aspect of the shade tab or the tab of another shade guide (ie, cervical M2/body A3), or be perceived as more saturated, more orange, or lighter in comparison. Characteristics of the basic hue at the incisal third should be evaluated in terms of mamelon color (Fig. 6-33), abrasion color in case of attrition, or continuity with the basic shade if there is no enamel or translucent demarcation. Mamelon shape tends to blunt and widen with aging and take a whitish-orange hue. Examples of shade variations according to the tooth location and according to the tooth considered are depicted in Figures 6-34 and 6-35.

Nonshade guide color
Nonshade guide colors represent shades that cannot be matched with existing shade tabs.[67] According to Vryonis,[66] approximately 85% of shades can be matched with existing shade guides. The remaining 15%, however, fall outside of the hue of standard tabs and require that the technician fabricate a custom tab. This tab may be in the form of a fired dentin tab (Fig. 6-36) or a full construction of opaque, dentin and incisal porcelain.[74,75]

Laboratory considerations
In the laboratory, the basic hue is expressed in the dentin build-up. It can either be constructed according to the shade prescription, in one single dentin shade, or, to express a more pleasing diversification, with different dentin hues alternated horizontally. For example, a basic A2 hue may be constructed with bands of dentin segmented horizontally and consisting, from cervical to incisal, of A3-A1-A3-A2-A1; A3 consists of A2-A4-A2-A3-A4 following the same principle (Fig. 6-37). The control of value also starts in the dentin construction. In the Opal/Vintage porcelain system, bright shades such as A1, A2, B1, B2, and A3 or B3 of high value must preserve their value through the firing cycles. For this purpose, the selected dentin must be mixed with 10% of the corresponding Value Plus porcelain, which is a modified dentin material of high value (Fig. 6-38).

When additional brightness is required, as dictated by the shade prescription, the basic dentin may be mixed with 20% to 30% Value Plus porcelain to achieve the desired effect. With shades of lower value, such as A3.5, A4, and B4, Value Plus porcelain is used as a separate layer of opaque dentin before the basic dentin is applied. Basic shade variations may also be expressed, as dictated by local variations observed on the tooth, with modified dentins such as cervical dentin, mamelon dentin, orange modified dentin, or secondary brown or orange dentin.

Enamel shade, translucency, and location

Once the hue and its variations are determined, the clinician must separately evaluate the quality and location of the enamel overlay. Because it may range from whitish opaque to very transparent, it also affects the value of the tooth. Teeth in young patients may have white shades with high value because of the dense and highly reflective enamel. Teeth in middle-aged and elderly patients may appear duller or more orange because of the translucent or almost transparent enamel. Between these two extremes, enamel assumes a semitranslucent quality.

Enamel of the natural tooth should be analyzed by the clinician in terms of value and translucency. Compared to shade tabs, it may be perceived as similar, lighter, or grayer, and denser or more translucent. This evaluation may either be made with conventional shade tabs (Fig. 6-39), with separate enamel tabs available from the manufacturer, or with customized fired enamel samples (Fig. 6-40). The latter, however, require more clinical experience in discriminating between enamel shades. An important aspect of this evaluation is to compare the value between the natural tooth and the shade tab. The patient should either (1) hold the tab right below his tooth while the clinician stands back 2 yards for value comparison, or (2) the patient should stand in front of a mirror while the clinician stands behind the patient and makes the evaluation by looking at the mirror (Fig. 6-41). If the natural tooth has a higher value than the shade tab, a low chroma–high value dentin and an opaque and reflective enamel are required in the porcelain construction. If the value is lower than the shade tab, a high chroma–low value dentin and a more translucent enamel are required.

In the Vintage/Opal porcelain system (Shofu) (Fig. 6-42), there are four basic enamel shades ranging from 57 to 60. Enamels 57 and 58 are brighter and more reflective than enamels 59 and 60, which are more translucent. For additional brightness, opal white E and milky may be associated with the basic enamels, whereas opal T, superlucent, and amber are indicated for additional translucency and lower value, or for a softer appearance (Fig. 6-43). For maximum individuality in esthetic reconstruction, the opacity of the enamel overlay should increase when proceeding from the central incisor to the canine. For example, the enamel distribution from the central incisor to the canine may consist of 59 enamel (1 part) / opal T (2 parts), 59 enamel (1 part) / opal T (1 part), 59 enamel.

The enamel distribution, including translucent or transparent zones, should be communicated with a diagram on the shade prescription. Translucent enamel

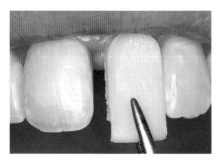

Fig. 6-36 When a shade cannot be matched with a standard shade tab and falls outside of the hues of standard tab, it requires fabrication by the technician of a custom tab, here in the form of a fired dentin tab.

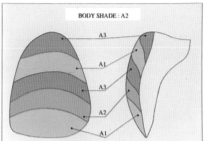

Fig. 6-37a and b Basic hue A2 and A3 is fabricated in the dentin build-up with different dentin hues alternated horizontally. This technique is systematically used for brighter shades to suggest subtle diversification.

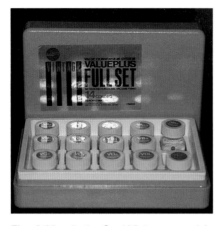

Fig. 6-38 In the Opal/Vintage porcelain system, Value Plus porcelain is a modified dentin material of high value. It serves to control or adjust the brightness of the dentin construction.

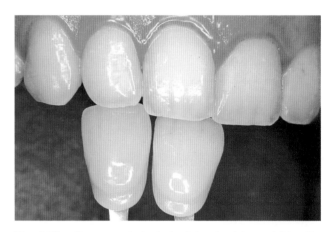

Fig. 6-39 The enamel shade is determined by matching the incisal third of the shade tab against the natural tooth. In this example, the basic enamel shade is a combination of two tabs. It could also be selected from a tab of a different dentin hue from the base shade, but with a closer matching enamel.

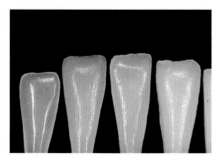

Fig. 6-40a Enamel shade determination may also be made by firing separate enamel tabs to be used intraorally. This technique requires more practice by the clinician, but it also allows more refinement in shade communication with the technician.

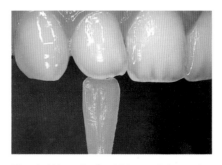

Fig. 6-40b An Opal 58 sample is used to determine enamel shade for the lateral incisor.

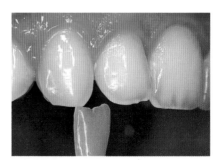

Fig. 6-40c Preliminary enamel determination for the canine with Opal amber. The final enamel composition will be two thirds Opal amber and one third Opal T to desaturate the amber shade and increase its translucency.

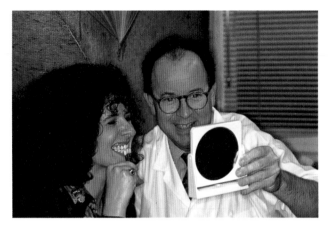

Fig. 6-41 Value control during shade matching is made with the patient looking at a mirror and the evaluator, also looking in the mirror, assessing the difference in brightness between the shade tab and the natural tooth.

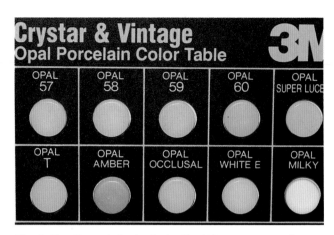

Fig. 6-42 Enamel shades in the Opal/Vintage system. Opal 57 to 60 are basic enamels recommended by the manufacturer for standard shades. Shades 57 and 58 are brighter and more reflective than 59 and 60, which are more translucent. The other enamel shades are indicated for additional effects of color and translucency.

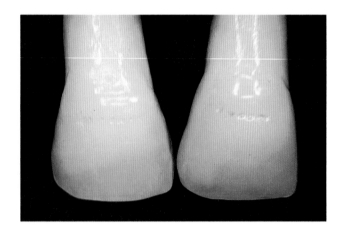

Fig. 6-43 Quality of enamel: natural tooth with a matching porcelain construction. The enamel of the middle aspect is bright and reflective, characteristic of Opal 57 or 58, whereas the incisal aspect is markedly more translucent and characteristic of Opal Super Lucent.

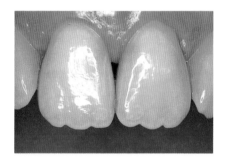

Fig. 6-44 Enamel distribution: type C enamel distribution according to Sekine, where the translucent enamel layer is distributed at both the proximal and incisal aspects. There is also a halo effect at the incisal edge, produced by total reflection of light within the incisal edge. The bluish tint of the enamel is characteristic of opalescence.

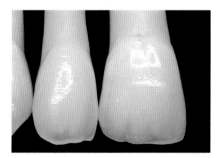

Fig. 6-45 The halo effect is replicated in these porcelain restorations with a mixture of white and orange modifiers in combination with the basic body shade. Apical to the halo, there is a transparent zone replicated with Opal Super Lucent, which highlights by contrast the dentin mamelon effect. The hue of the mamelon dentin is also part of the dentin prescription shade. This incisal pattern is characteristic of many teeth in young individuals.

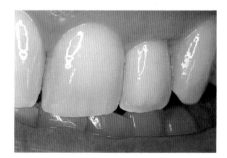

Fig. 6-46 A halo effect and adjacent enamel transparency were created for this metal ceramic restoration.

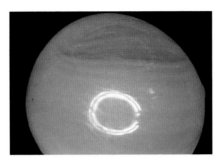

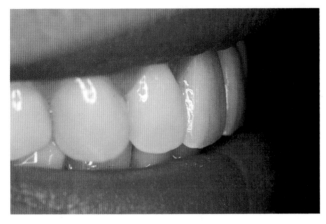

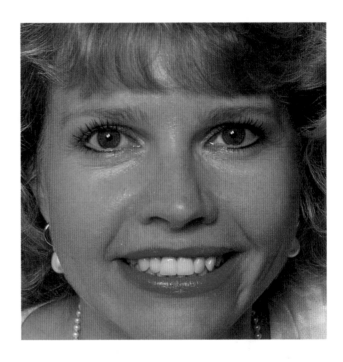

Fig. 6-47a Natural opal stone under incident light. Short wavelengths of light are selectively reflected back to the observer, which accounts for the blue tint, whereas longer light wavelengths (orange and red) are transmitted through the material. Opalescence is caused in a glass, a ceramic, or a natural tooth (see Fig. 6-44) by light scattering between two phases that have a different index of refraction. The first phase may consist of silicon dioxide, hydroxyapatite, or alumina microparticles that have a size typically ranging between 0.1 to 0.3 µm. The second phase acts as a matrix and consists of water or interprismatic substance or glass.

Fig. 6-47b and c This three-unit fixed partial denture replaces a maxillary central incisor. The bright milky-white enamel is consistent with the adjacent teeth. In a close-up view, a soft blue effect of the enamel of the natural lateral incisor is also detectable on the two central incisors constructed in opalescent porcelain. The perception of opalescence varies with the distance and angle of observation; it is a subtle effect.

zones may stand out more or less distinctly from the basic tooth color and have been classified by Sekine et al[76] into three groups. Type A are teeth in which the translucent layer cannot be discerned and teeth with a translucent layer distributed over the entire aspect of the tooth. Type B are teeth with a translucent layer at the incisal aspect only. Type C are teeth with a translucent layer at both the proximal and incisal aspects (Fig. 6-44). Additionally, a halo effect may be detected at the incisal edge. It is produced by total reflection of light within the confines of the incisal edge and results in an opaque outline.[1] It may be reproduced in the porcelain construction with a mixture of dentin powders (Figs. 6-45 and 6-46).

Opalescence is an important component of the perceived enamel color. It is produced in the enamel microstructure by the difference in refractivity be-

tween hydroxyapatite crystals and the enamel ground substance and by the ability of these crystals, acting as microparticles smaller than the wavelength of light, to scatter incident light. As a result, under incident light, longer wavelengths of light are selectively transmitted through the tooth, whereas shorter wavelengths are reflected on the enamel surface, producing the subtle bluish gleam characteristic of opalescence. This subtle effect cannot be replicated in porcelain construction with superficial or internal colorants, which would appear too artificial. In a porcelain material with opalescent properties, microparticles of a different refractive index from the ceramic are dispersed in the matrix so that the porcelain has the ability to interact with incident light in the same fashion as enamel does, without superficial colorants (Fig. 6-47).

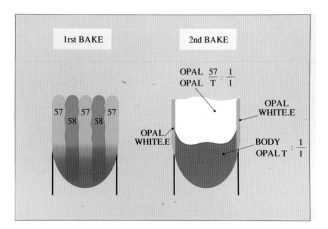

Fig. 6-48 Enamel construction according to the firing stage for an A2 shade. Before the first firing, Opal 57 and 58 are placed in alternate vertical segments for variations in translucency. Before the second firing, the enamel construction is completed with an equal combination of Opal 57 and Opal T, and the dentin is completed with an equal combination of dentin and Opal T.

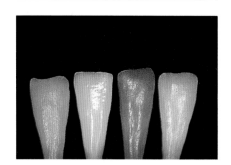

Fig. 6-49 For additional enamel effects, Opal Super Lucent may be mixed with yellow, blue, or pink modifiers.

Laboratory considerations

In the laboratory, the enamel build-up follows the same principle as in dentin construction, where several shades should be used for maximum diversification and refraction. For a young tooth with a bright and reflective enamel, 57 and 58 enamel should be selected and layered vertically in alternance. At the line angles, thicker and denser enamel should be restored with opal white E, which is a bright and reflective enamel that acts as a somewhat opaque frame that contains light within the enamel (Fig. 6-48).

When increased translucency and lower value are indicated, enamel should be mixed or overlaid with translucent or transparent powders: opal T is translucent and opalescent and serves to overlay or soften internal colored effects. Opal superlucent appears bluish gray when used at the incisal aspect without a dentin background. It also serves as a translucent overlay when applied over the dentin build-up, and for additional effects it may be mixed with blue, yellow, or pink modifiers (Fig. 6-49). Opal amber is slightly more orange than opal 60 and is used as an overlay to impart a soft orange tone to the porcelain construction. As a rule, translucent or transparent powders are mixed with enamel powders when increased enamel translucency is desired, whereas they are overlaid over the unmodified enamel in order to maintain its same degree of opacity and increase light refraction through the enamel.

Table 6-2 Luster According to Glazing Temperature and Surface Texture

Surface Texture	Temperature (C°) (rate = 55°C/min from 600°C)						
	850	855	860	890	900	910	920
Rough					Matte	Satin	Glossy
Smooth				Matte	Satin	Glossy	
Polished	Matte	Satin	Glossy				

Flagship—Jelenko oven

Value and reflectivity of the enamel may also be adjusted by varying the surface texture and luster according to the glazing temperature and the adjunction of mechanical polishing with pumice or diamond paste if a high gloss is desired (Table 6-2).

Table 6-3 depicts basic shade variations that are useful to the clinician for expressing variations from a standard shade tab. Their incorporation into the porcelain construction is described for shades A1, A2, and A3.

Figures 6-50–6-52 depict examples of shade prescription for single maxillary central incisors, with their translation in the porcelain construction.

Table 6-3 Basic Variations for Standard Shades A_1, A_2, A_3 and Translation in the Porcelain Construction

DENTIN			
Standard shade	A_1	A_2	A_3
Cervical third			
Lighter	A_1 + VA_1 or A_1 + white modifier or A_1 + opal milky	A_2 + VA_2	A_3 + VA_3
Darker	A_1 + opal T or A_2	A_2 + A_3	A_3 + $A_{3.5}$
More orange	A_1 + orange modifier + white modifier	A_2 + orange modifier + white modifier	A_3 + orange modifier
More saturated	A_1 + 716 or A_1 + A_C	A_2 + 716 or A_2 + A_C	A_3 + 716 or A_3 + A_C
Middle third			
Lighter	A_1 + white modifier	A_1	A_2 + A_1
Darker	A_1 + gray modifier + opal T	A_2 + gray modifier + opal T	A_3 + gray modifier
Red-brown	A_1 + orange modifier + brown modifier + opal T	A_2 + brown modifier + pink modifier + opal T	
Incisal third			
Lighter	A_1 + VA_1	A_2 + VA_2	A_3 + VA_3
Mamelons	EF_1 (light pink/orange) or EF_2 (dark pink/orange) or opal milky + opal white E (white mamelons) or opal milky + opal yellow (yellow mamelons)		
More orange	A_1 + orange modifier + white modifier	A_2 + orange modifier + opal T	A_3 + orange modifier + brown modifier + opal T

ENAMEL			
Standard shade	A_1	A_2	A_3
First bake			
As a light coat over whole body	opal 57	opal 58	opal 59
Second bake			
Only on incisal half			
No modification	opal 57 + opal T	opal 58 + opal T	opal 59 + opal T
Whiter or more opaque	opal 57 + opal milky / opal 57 + opal white E / opal 57 + opal occlusal	opal 58 + opal white E / opal 58 + opal occlusal	opal 58 + opal white E / opal 57 + opal occlusal
More violet	opal 57 + pink modifier + blue modifier + opal T	opal 58 + pink modifier + blue modifier + opal T	opal 59 + pink modifier + blue modifier + opal T
More translucent	opal 57 + opal T	opal 58 + opal T	opal 59 + opal superlucent
Grayer	opal 57 + gray modifier + opal T	opal 58 + gray modifier + opal T	opal 59 + gray modifier + opal T
More orange	opal 57 + opal amber / opal 57 + orange modifier	opal 58 + opal amber / opal 58 + orange modifier	opal 59 + opal amber / opal 59 + orange modifier / opal 60 or opal amber
Bluer	opal 57 + blue modifier + opal T	opal 58 + blue modifier + opal superlucent	opal superlucent
More yellow	opal 57 + yellow modifier + opal T	opal 58 + yellow modifier + opal T	opal 59 + yellow modifier + opal T
Third bake			
Halo effect	orange modifier + white modifier + body A_1	orange modifier + white modifier + body A_2	orange modifier + white modifier + body A_3
Surface characterizations	opal milky	opal milky + opal white E	opal 57 + white modifier

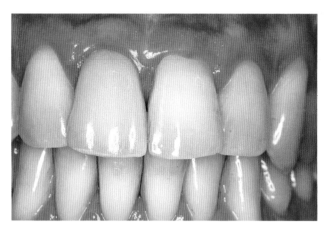

Fig. 6-50a This single maxillary central incisor was restored with a metal ceramic crown.

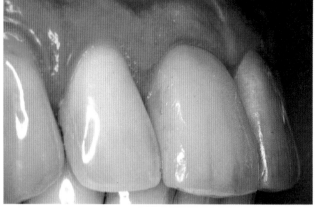

Fig. 6-50b The lateral aspect of the crown has a typical opalescent bluish tint. The natural central incisor in the background incorporates a similar blue tone at the surface, and there is an orange gleam in the depressions of the facial aspect. This is a result of the light beam transmitted laterally through the enamel ridges and its longer wavelength exiting in the fossa between the ridges.

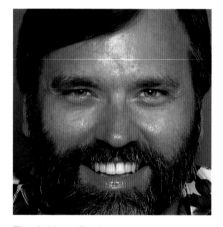

Fig. 6-50c Final result.

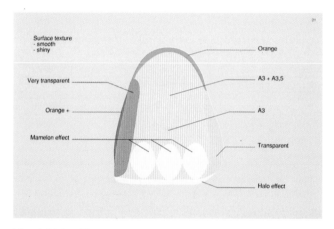

Fig. 6-50d There is a dentin shade progression of decreasing value toward the cervical aspect. The orange mamelon shade and the incisal halo effect are subtle. The transparent enamel ridges are thick faciolingually but do not extend toward the proximal contacts.

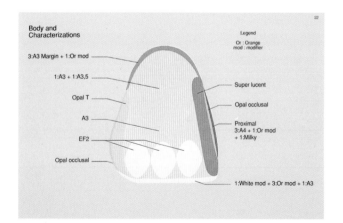

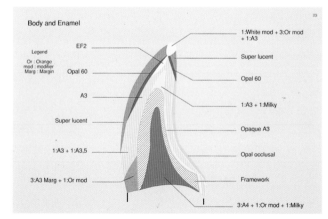

Fig. 6-50e and f Translation of the shade prescription in the porcelain construction. The shoulder porcelain is mixed with orange modifier and results here in a lower value. If an orange effect of higher value had been desired, it would have been necessary to incorporate white modifier in addition to the orange. The proximal enamel ridges are restored with Opal T or Opal Super Lucent according the desired translucency. Proximally, the opacity is increased with incorporation of Opal Milky to avoid graying.

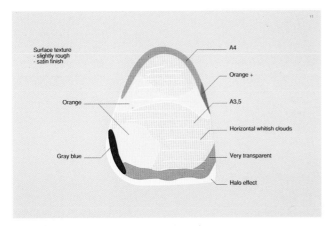

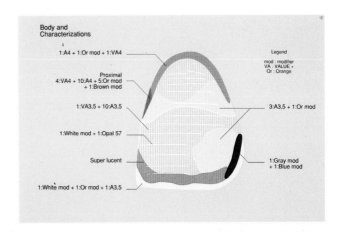

Fig. 6-51a Central incisor restored with a Maryland bridge for a young patient. The shade was matched with the metal framework in place.

Fig. 6-51b The incisal aspect incorporates a characteristic halo effect, with a transparent zone apical to it, highlighting the mamelon outline. Two orange zones and a gray-blue variation must be precisely outlined on the shade prescription diagram.

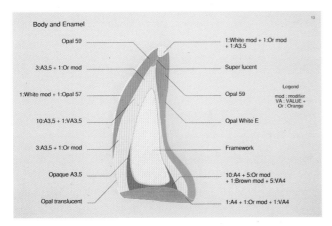

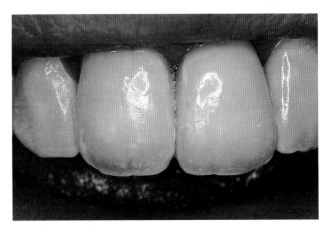

Fig. 6-51c and d Translation of the shade prescription into the porcelain construction. The basic dentin shade is A3.5 mixed with VA3.5 to maintain its brightness and with orange modifier in the two orange zones. The enamel opacity is increased with white modifier, and the transparent incisal area is replicated with Super Lucent without any dentin background. This porcelain construction required three firings: first firing—dentins and very little enamel; second firing—enamels and transparent; third firing—halo effect and whitish surface characteristics.

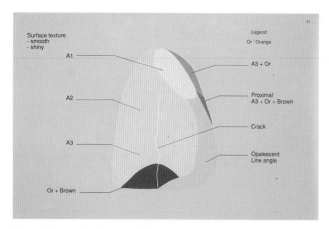

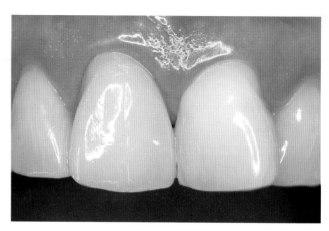

Fig. 6-52a Single central incisor restored with a ceramic restoration. The rotation of the tooth and the root exposure must be taken into consideration.

Fig. 6-52b Shade prescription: the dentin progression is subtle, but it is important to note the lighter cervical aspect.

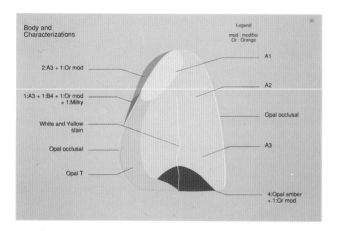

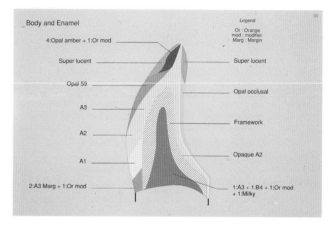

Fig. 6-52c and d Translation of the shade prescription into the porcelain construction. The dentin progression follows the shade prescription, and the root effect is obtained with an orange saturation. Opal 59 is used unmodified, the distal enamel aspect is restored with Opal T, but a background of Opal Occlusal is necessary to block light transmission and avoid graying in the interproximal areas.

References

1. Yamamoto M. *Metal Ceramics*. Chicago: Quintessence, 1985.

2. Geller W, Kwiatkowski SJ. The Willi's Glass crown: a new solution in the dark and shadowed zone of esthetic porcelain restorations. *Quintessence Dent Technol* 1987;11:233.

3. Yamamoto M. A newly developed "Opal" ceramic and its clinical use, with special attention to its refractive index. *QDT Yearbook* 1989;13:9.

4. Yamamoto M. The value conversion system and a new concept for expressing the shades of natural teeth. *QDT Yearbook* 1992;16:9.

5. Rinn LA. *The Polychromatic Layering Technique*. Chicago: Quintessence, 1990.

6. Winter R. Achieving esthetic ceramic restorations. *J Calif Dent Assoc* 1990;Sept:21.

7. Roach RR, Muia PJ. Communication between dentist and technician: An esthetic checklist. In: Preston JD (ed). *Perspectives in Dental Ceramics. Proceedings of the Fourth International Symposium on Ceramics*. Chicago: Quintessence, 1988: 445.

8. Lee R. Esthetics and its relationship to function. In: Rufenacht CR (ed). *Fundamentals of Esthetics*. Chicago: Quintessence, 1990:137.

9. McCollum BB, Stuart CE. *A Research Report*. South Pasadena, Calif: Scientific Press, 1955:54–58.

10. Teteruck WR, Lundeen HC. The accuracy of an ear face-bow. *J Prosthet Dent* 1966;16:1039.

11. Stade EH, Hanson JG, Baker CL. Esthetic considerations in the use of face-bows. *J Prosthet Dent* 1982;48:253.

12. Shavell HM. Dentist-laboratory relationships in fixed prosthodontics. In: Preston JD (ed). *Perspectives in Dental Ceramics. Proceedings of the Fourth International Symposium on Ceramics*. Chicago: Quintessence, 1988:429.

13. Guichet NF. *Principles of Occlusion*. Anaheim, Calif: Denar Corp, 1970.

14. Breeding LC, Dixon D. Compression resistance of four interocclusal recording materials. *J Prosthet Dent* 1992;68:876.

15. Dawson PE. *Evaluation, Diagnosis and Treatment of Occlusal Problems*. St Louis: Mosby, 1974.

16. Schuyler CH. The function and importance of incisal guidance in oral rehabilitation. *J Prosthet Dent* 1963;13:1011.

17. D'Amico A. Functional occlusion of the natural teeth in man. *J Prosthet Dent* 1961;11:899.

18. Farrar WB, McCarthy WL. *A Clinical Outline of Temporomandibular Joint Diagnosis and Treatment*, ed 7. Normandie Study Group for TMJ dysfunction. Montgomery, Walker Printing Co, 1983.

19. Dawson PE. Determining the determinants of occlusion. *Int J Periodont Rest Dent* 1983;3(6):17.

20. Jorgenson MW, Goodkind RJ. Spectrophotometric study of five porcelain shades relative to the dimensions of color, porcelain thickness and repeated firings. *J Prosthet Dent* 1979;42:96.

21. Barghi N, Lorenzana RE. Optimum thickness of opaque and body porcelain. *J Prosthet Dent* 1982;48:429.

22. Seghi RR, Johnson WM, O'Brien WJ. Spectrophotometric analysis of color differences between porcelain systems. *J Prosthet Dent* 1986;56:35.

23. Jacobs SH, Goodacre CJ, Moore BK, Dykema RW. Effect of porcelain thickness and type of metal ceramic alloy on color. *J Prosthet Dent* 1987;57:2.

24. Terada Y, Maeyama S, Hirayasu R. The influence of different thicknesses of dentin color reflected from thin opaque porcelain fused to metal. *Int J Prosthodont* 1989;2:352.

25. Fillastre AF. The Esthetic Restorative Practice. New Orleans, March 1982.

26. Shelby DS. Communication with the laboratory technician. In: Yamada HN, Grenoble PB (eds). *Dental Porcelain the State of the Art–1977*. Los Angeles: Univ of Southern California, School of Dentistry, 1977:269.

27. Wohlwend A. The Kuwata School of Tokyo (I). Experiences in a 6-month course. *Quintessence Dent Technol* 1983;7:169.

28. Wohlwend A. The Kuwata School of Tokyo (II). Experiences in a 6-month education course. *Quintessence Dent Technol* 1983;7:233.

29. Wohlwend A. The Kuwata School of Tokyo (III). Experiences in a 6-month education course. *Quintessence Dent Technol* 1983;7:291.

30. Wohlwend A. The Kuwata School of Tokyo (IV). Experiences in a 6-month education course. *Quintessence Dent Technol* 1983;7:363.

31. Wohlwend A. The Kuwata School of Tokyo (V). Experiences in a 6-month education course. *Quintessenz Zahntech* 1983;8:417.

32. Ganz CH, Brisman SA, Tauro V. Computer video imaging: Computerization, communication, and creation. *QDT Yearbook* 1989;13:64.

33. Rogé M, Preston JD. Color, light and the perception of form. *Quintessence Int* 1987;18:391.

34. Waerhaug J. Tissue reactions around artificial crowns. *J Periodontol* 1953;24:172.

35. Larato DC. Effect of cervical margins on gingiva. *J South Calif Dent Assoc* 1969;45:19.

36. Silness J. Periodontal conditions in patients treated with dental bridges. *J Periodontol Res* 1970;5:60.

37. Newcombe GM. The relationship between the location of subgingival crown margins and gingival inflammation. *J Periodontol* 1974;45:151.

38. Parkinson CF. Excessive crown contours facilitate endemic plaque niches. *J Prosthet Dent* 1976;34:424.

39. Wagman S. The role of coronal contour in gingival health. *J Prosthet Dent* 1977;37:280.

40. Stein RS, Kuwata M. A dentist and a dental technologist analyze current ceramo-metal procedures. *Dent Clin North Am* 1977;21:729.

41. Seluk LW, Brodbelt RHW, Walker GF. A biometric comparison of face shape with denture tooth form. *J Oral Rehabil* 1987;14:139.

42. Martignoni M, Schonenberger A. *Precision Fixed Prosthodontics: Clinical and Laboratory Aspects*. Chicago: Quintessence, 1990.

43. Berger RP. Esthetic considerations in framework design. In: Preston JD (ed). *Perspectives in Dental Ceramics. Proceedings of the Fourth International Symposium on Ceramics*. Chicago: Quintessence, 1988:237.

44. Miller L. Framework design in ceramo-metal restorations. *Dent Clin North Am* 1977;21:699.

45. Miller L. A clinician's interpretation of tooth preparation and the design of metal substructures for metal-ceramic restorations. In: McLean JW (ed). *Dental Ceramics. Proceedings of the First International Symposium on Ceramics*. Chicago: Quintessence, 1983:153.

46. McLean JW. *The Science and Art of Dental Ceramics. Vol. II: Bridge Design and Laboratory Procedures in Dental Ceramics*. Chicago: Quintessence, 1980.

47. Bugugnani R, Landez C. Les empreintes en Prothèse Conjointe. Cahiers de Prothèse 1979.

48. Wasmer H. La précision des modèles fragmentés avec socle en plastique, vu part l'utilisateur. *Technique Dentaire* 1981;39:17.

49. Zeiser M. Modell-System mit Kunststoff-Sockelplatte jetzt auch fur kleine Labors. *Dent Lab* 1982;30:489.

50. Muia P. *The Four Dimensional Tooth Color System*. Chicago: Quintessence 1982.

51. Flocken JE. Electrosurgical management of soft tissues and restorative dentistry. *Dent Clin North Am* 1980;24:247.

52. Nevins M, Skurow HM. The intracrevicular restorative margin, the biologic width, and the maintenance of the gingival margin. *Int J Periodont Rest Dent* 1984;4(3):31.

53. Martin D. Soft tissue master cast. *Int J Periodont Rest Dent* 1982;2(4):34.

54. Christensen GJ. Marginal fit of gold inlay castings. *J Prosthet Dent* 1966;16:297.

55. Davis SH, Kelly JR, Campbell SD. Use of an elastomeric material to improve the occlusal seat and marginal seal of cast restorations. *J Prosthet Dent* 1989;62:288.

56. Sorensen JA. Improving seating of ceramic inlays with a silicone fit-checking medium. *J Prosthet Dent* 1991;65:646.

57. White SN, Sorensen JA, Kang SK. Improved marginal seating of cast restorations using a silicone disclosing medium. *Int J Prosthodont* 1991;4:323.

58. Campbell SD. Comparison of conventional paint-on die spacers and those used with all-ceramic restorations. *J Prosthet Dent* 1990;63:151.

59. Goldstein RE. Esthetic principles for ceramo-metal restorations. *Dent Clin North Am* 1977;21:803.

60. Preston JD, Bergen SF. *Color Science and Dental Art. A Self-Teaching Program*. St Louis: Mosby, 1980.

61. Clark EB. Tooth color selection. *J Am Dent Assoc* 1933;20:1065.

62. Hayashi T. *Medical Color Standard. V. Tooth Crown*. Tokyo: Japan Color Institute, 1967.

63. Sproull RC. Color matching in dentistry. Part II. Practical applications of the organization of color. *J Prosthet Dent* 1973;29:556.

64. Lemire PA, Burk BB. *Color in Dentistry*. Bloomfield, Conn: Ney, 1975.

65. Jinoian V. The importance of proper light source in metal ceramics. In: Preston JD (ed). *Perspectives in Dental Ceramics. Proceedings of the Fourth International Symposium on Ceramics*. Chicago: Quintessence, 1988:229.

66. Vryonis P. Aesthetics in ceramics: Perceiving the problem. In: Preston JD (ed). *Perspectives in Dental Ceramics. Proceedings of the Fourth International Symposium on Ceramics*. Chicago: Quintessence, 1988:209.

67. Kato T, Kuwata M, Tamura K, Yamamoto M. The current state of porcelain shade guides: A discussion. *Quintessence Dent Technol* 1984;8:559.

68. Hegenbarth EA. *The Creative Color System*. Chicago: Quintessence, 1989.

69. Hemendinger H, Miller LL. In: Preston JD, Bergen SF (eds). *Color Science and Dental Art, A Self Teaching Program*. St Louis: Mosby, 1980.

70. Miller LL. Scientific approach to shade matching. In: Preston JD (ed). *Perspectives in Dental Ceramics. Proceedings of the Fourth International Symposium on Ceramics*. Chicago: Quintessence, 1988:193.

71. Geller W. Esthetic Ceramic Restorations, Paris, April 1983.

72. Jorgenson MW, Goodkind RJ. Spectrophotometric study of five porcelain shades relative to the dimensions of porcelain thickness and repeated firings. *J Prosthet Dent* 1979;42:96.

73. Nakagawa Y, et al. Analysis of natural tooth color. *Shikai Tenbo* 1975;46:527.

74. Riley EJ, Filipancic JM. Ceramic shade determination: Current technique for a direct approach. *Int J Prosthodont* 1989;2:131.

75. Sorensen JA, Torres TJ. Shade determination and communication: A team approach. In: Preston JD (ed). *Perspectives in Dental Ceramics. Proceedings of the Fourth International Symposium on Ceramics*. Chicago: Quintessence, 1988:279.

76. Sekine M, et al. Translucent effects of porcelain jacket crowns. 1. Study of translucent layer patterns in the natural teeth. Shika Giko 1975;3:49.

Chapter 7

Tissue Management for the Maxillary Anterior Region

James D Harrison, Gerard Chiche, and Alain Pinault

Tooth preparations

Anterior tissues are delicate, and a healthy facial crevice in the anterior region is shallow; therefore, the potential for trauma to the gingival tissues is great.[1] Subgingival crown restorations, as opposed to supragingival restorations, are directly responsible for adverse inflammatory periodontal reactions because of increased retention of bacterial dental plaque.[2-10] Several factors are responsible for these adverse reactions: *(1)* the roughness or porosities found at the surface of the restorative materials[11-14]; *(2)* the roughness of the tooth-restorative material interface with voids, imperfections, and exposed cement and aggravated by defective marginal fit or overhanging margins[15-22]; *(3)* the depth of the margin and its inaccessibility to toothbrushing[23,24]; *(4)* increased pathogenicity of the subgingival dental plaque[25,26]; *(5)* defective crown contours[27-30]; and *(6)* invasion of the biologic width.[31,32] Because subgingival placement of full-coverage restorations is necessary for esthetic purposes, anterior tooth preparations must adhere to strict guidelines for predictability and stability at the gingival margin.

Fit

Waerhaug[33] and Renggli and Regolati[34] have shown that even a well-fitting restoration will harbor plaque and bacteria because of the irregularities on the restorative material and because its interfacial voids are filled with cement.[18,22] Poor dentistry plays a significant role in both plaque accumulation and periodontal breakdown, and Felton et al[35] found a direct rela-

tionship between the degree of marginal discrepancy of a subgingival crown margin and the severity of periodontal inflammation. Conversely, well-fitting restorations with no overhanging margins produce only slight gingival reactions[36,37]; and with well-fitting margins and meticulous oral hygiene, gingival inflammation is not axiomatic.[25,38,39] The stability of the subgingival margins of full-coverage restorations was followed over a 10-year period on regularly supervised patients; of the 150 buccal crown margins located subgingivally at the time of cementation, 60% were located subgingivally after 1 year and only 29% at 10 years.[40-42] This demonstrates that even though well-fitting margins are essential, other factors are involved in the successful management of delicate anterior gingival tissues.

Biologic width

Gargiulo et al[43] demonstrated in human autopsy specimens a proportional dimension relationship between the dentogingival junction and the other tooth-supporting tissues. The mean sulcular depth was 0.69 mm, the mean length of the junctional epithelium was 0.97 mm, and the more consistent finding of 1.07 mm with a range of 1.06 to 1.08 mm was noted for the connective tissue attachment.

The combined width of the connective tissue attachment and the junctional epithelium averaged 2.04 mm and has been called the "biologic width." It can vary from tooth to tooth as well as from surface to surface, and average measurements do not necessarily reflect any one clinical situation.[44] However, the biologic width is always present.[31] Therefore, a restor-

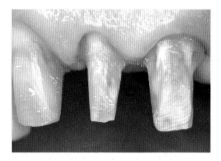
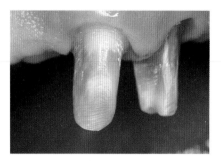
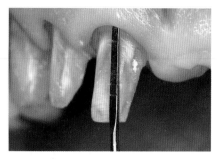

Fig. 7-1a and b When anterior gingival tissues are healthy preoperatively, the final impression needs only be deferred by approximately 3 weeks after completion of the tooth preparations. This delay should anticipate possible marginal tissue recession, and gingival levels should be stable at this stage.

Fig. 7-2 The crevice should be probed to reassess the level of the preparation margin in respect to the crevice depth. In isolated facial areas, the finish line may have become juxtagingival and require that it be delicately reprepared further apically within the crevice if a slight gingival recession has occurred. It is critical to avoid violation of biologic width in the shallow anterior sulcus.

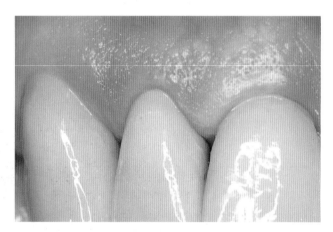
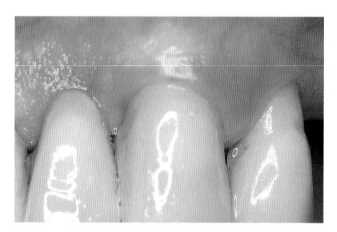

Fig. 7-3a and b Magnified view of the same gingival areas after final restoration with metal ceramic crowns with porcelain margins.

ative margin must maintain a distance from the alveolar crest that respects the biologic width; otherwise, gingival recession or pocket formation and periodontal disease may ensue,[31] depending on the thickness of the keratinized gingiva and the underlying bone. Invasion of the biologic width may result in apical migration of the dentogingival unit with gingival recession and may be self-limiting.[45] With relatively thicker bone, it may result in apical migration of the dentogingival attachment and intrabony pocket formation.[46] When restorative margins are placed adjacent to the osseous crest, fully violating the supracrestal gingival attachment, gingival inflammation, osseous resorption, and occasionally root resorption[47,48] have been observed, and thin facial plates have been especially vulnerable to destruction.[49]

Intracrevicular dentistry

Intracrevicular restorative margins are defined as those placed and confined within the gingival crevice.[31] Final intracrevicular margin placement should take place only in a healthy crevice[1,46] or it should be delayed until gingival tissues are healthy (Figs. 7-1–7-3). This is because healthy gingival tissues are stable and less prone to shrinkage and because they can be more accurately probed[46] or prepacked for accurate margin placement. In a healthy sulcus, the probing measurement closely relates to the anatomic sulcus depth with a margin of error around 0.5 mm.[50–53] On the other hand, inflamed tissues offer little resistance to probe penetration because of the loss of cohesiveness of junctional epithelial cells infiltrated with in-

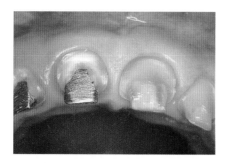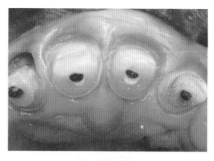

Fig. 7-4a and b The integrity of the col area is critical. The anatomic soft tissue col is normally concave, and because it is not keratinized it is more vulnerable to inflammation. With proper interproximal contact anatomy and adequate oral hygiene, the col area will often keratinize and become convex (a). Root proximity in this other situation (b) mandates careful management of these interproximal zones with concave cols in terms of oral hygiene, interproximal contours of the restorations, and location of the interproximal contacts.

flammatory cells and because of the partially destroyed connective tissue fibers just apical to it. With inflamed tissues, the probe tip proceeds through the junctional epithelium to the connective tissue and stops at the level of intact connective tissue fibers[50,51] according to the degree of inflammation.[52]

Level of margins

Waerhaug[36] believed that well-adapted subgingival margins could be tolerated as long as they did not come closer than 0.4 mm to the bottom of the crevice. Newcomb[24] demonstrated with anterior veneer crowns a positive correlation between gingival inflammation and the level of the crown margin below the gingival crest. Inflammation increased as the crown margin approached the base of the crevice. The healthy crevice, however, is very shallow[32] and generally varies in depth from 0.5 to 1 mm on the facial aspect of anterior teeth,[24,53,54] rarely extending beyond 1.5 mm[46]; the margin of safety is thus small and the potential for invasion of the biologic width during tooth preparation is great.[1] Margin placement must respect the junctional epithelium and allow for some margin of error. This means that the crevice should be entered no deeper than 0.5 mm[1] to 0.7 mm (which meticulous toothbrushing can still reach).[55] Where there has been no previous periodontal attachment loss, the gingival margin, the cementoenamel junction (CEJ), the bottom of the gingival crevice, and the alveolar crest tend to be parallel to each other, and the tooth preparation should follow this natural scallop.[56] Interproximally, the CEJ and the alveolar crest of anterior teeth follow a deep scallop,[57] whereas the anatomic soft tissue col is concave and does not mimic the underlying bone crest, which is normally flat or convex.[58] This explains why it is comparatively easier to violate the biologic width during proximal tooth preparation

(Fig. 7-4). Such violation could result in facial inflammation and recession because the inflammatory process proceeds through the circular gingival fibers, especially with thin scalloped facial gingiva (Figs. 7-5–7-7).[27]

Intracrevicular preparation technique

Mechanical insults to the supracrestal gingival attachment are reversible[2] as long as the restoration does not invade the biological width.[22] In theory, if the junctional epithelium or the gingival fiber apparatus are not disturbed, the level of the alveolar crest and the gingival margin levels should remain stable over time.[32] If the tooth preparation is extended below the base of the crevice and a temporary crown is cemented at that level, there is a rapid reformation of the dentogingival unit at 2 weeks with facial bone resorption.[45] This indicates that a rapid gingival reaction may be activated by the placement of a subgingival crown margin impinging on the junctional epithelium.[45]

A buffer zone remaining between the finish line of the prepared tooth and the bottom of the gingival crevice is highly recommended,[46] because even in the most skilled hands some violation of the junctional epithelium appears inevitable. Dragoo and Williams[54] found that when the junctional epithelium was not protected, and despite the operators' extreme care to avoid tissue trauma, a small portion of the junctional epithelium was destroyed and the connective tissue was damaged.

Prepacking healthy tissues before tooth preparation[1,54] with a nonimpregnated retraction cord and preparing to the cord provides a buffer zone in respect to the junctional epithelium during high-speed cutting and prevents laceration of the tissues.[1] Prepacking nonimpregnated retraction cords in a healthy sulcus before tooth preparation was shown to cause

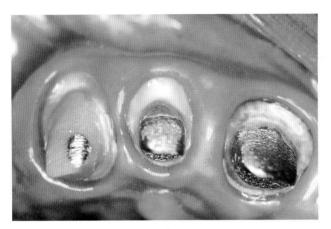
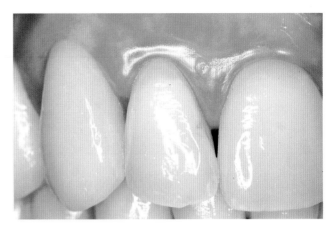

Fig. 7-5a and b With proper initial preparation and adequate oral hygiene, it is possible to achieve convex keratinized col areas that are more resistant to interproximal inflammation. Margin placement must respect the junctional epithelium and enter the crevice no deeper than 0.5 mm to 0.7 mm. The proximal margins had to be prepared subgingivally because of previous crowning, and the patient is maintaining them well.

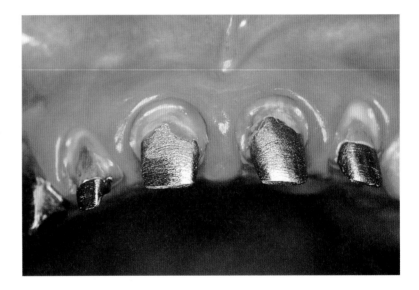

Fig. 7-6a Preparations prior to final cementation.

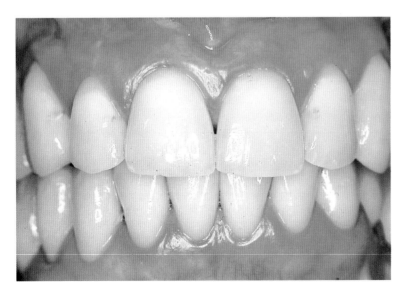

Fig. 7-6b Completed restoration. All these crowns incorporate porcelain margins.

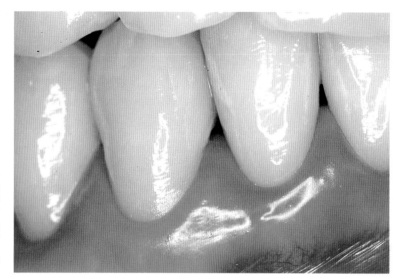

Fig. 7-7a–c Magnified view of the mandibular anterior restorations. In order to respect the integrity of the interdental papilla, it is imperative that a small space be left incisal to the papilla tip. This may be precisely monitored in the laboratory by checking the crowns on an unsawed stone cast, but it also must be customized by the clinician during crown try-in. It accounts for minor depression of the papilla by the provisional restorations and leaves some room for regeneration of the papilla.

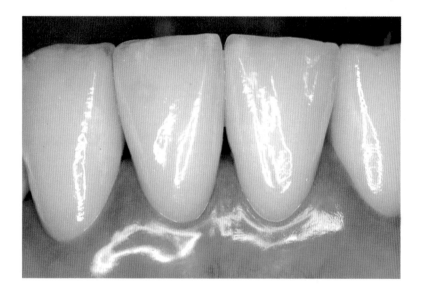

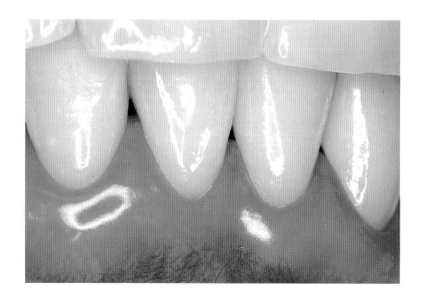

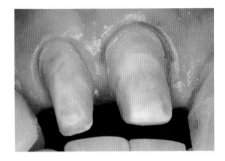

Fig. 7-8 The intracrevicular preparation should respect the fragility of the junctional epithelium and remain away from the base of the crevice to avoid violation of the biologic width. Before subgingival preparation, the crevice should be probed delicately. A 1-mm probing depth is common with healthy facial tissues in the anterior region, and this is why it is easy to violate the biologic width in the anterior region. The depth of the intracrevicular preparation should not exceed 0.5 mm. This is achieved either by probing and locating the depth of the finish line as it is prepared, or by prepacking the gingival tissues with a retraction cord. With either option, a slight ulceration of the inner lining of the crevice is to be expected.

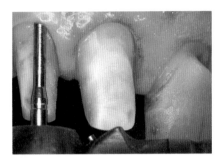

Fig. 7-9 The shoulder should be planed with a tissue protecting end diamond bur of the appropriate diameter to avoid laceration of the marginal tissues.

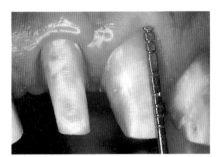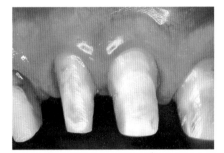

Fig. 7-10a and b Three weeks postoperatively, the sulcus lining is fully healed and the gingival apparatus more resistant to the mechanical trauma that will be caused by the retraction process. The gingival tissues are stable, and the finish line is at the desired intracrevicular depth. The potential for bleeding during impression making is virtually eliminated.

little or no damage to the epithelium and the connective tissue attachment when left up to 30 minutes, beyond which slight injury occurred, and healed within 10 days.[59] Caution must be exerted when packing, however, because Löe and Silness[60] demonstrated that even with normal pressure, strings had the potential to be pushed into the supracrestal connective tissue. Under these conditions, taking the preparation to these strings would invade the biologic width. Probing the crevice depth, especially when it is very shallow, before and during tooth preparation is also a good alternative to prepacking and essentially fulfills the same objectives (Figs. 7-8–7-10).[46,61]

Rationale for delaying impression procedure for anterior teeth

Initial tooth preparation—healthy tissues

Thin anterior gingival tissues are delicate and susceptible to traumatic recession caused by preparations or overcontoured provisional restorations. With high-speed techniques and with the potential of the periodontal probe tip or prepacked retraction cords to pierce the junctional epithelium, the crevice depth can only be presumed because the coronal extent of the junctional epithelium is difficult to identify.[32] It may

be inadvertently violated, and a rapid marginal tissue recession may occur within 2 weeks after tooth preparation, possibly leading to a supragingival margin on the day of final cementation. Therefore, marginal tissue reaction may be unpredictable after preparation and temporization because the gingival tissues may stabilize to a different level. It is preferable with anterior preparations to anticipate this problem by systematically deferring the final impression at least 2 weeks,[46] and in some cases 4 to 6 weeks,[1] to reappraise the level of the finish lines and refine them if necessary.

Deficient crowns

Marginal shrinkage may be unpredictable when the gingival complex is afflicted with periodontal disease. When deficient full-coverage restorations preexist, they must be removed as part of the initial preparation, which also includes meticulous root planing, curettage, fabrication of sound provisional restorations, and prescription of antibacterial mouthrinse.[62] The objective is to stabilize the tissues before definitive margin placement and to determine whether residual periodontal defects are still present after initial preparation (Figs. 7-11–7-13).

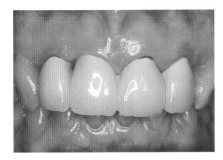

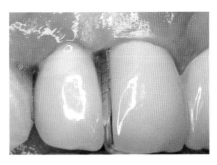

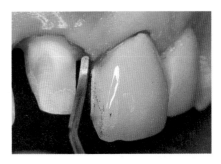

Fig. 7-11a and b When anterior gingival tissues have been chronically inflamed for several years, it must be assumed that they have been distorted in shape and must be returned to a normal architecture. This isolated 5-mm pocket resolved following tissue shrinkage after initial preparation.

Fig. 7-12 After removal of the old crowns, initial preparation consists of a thorough debridement of the area, scaling and root planing, and properly contoured provisional restorations.

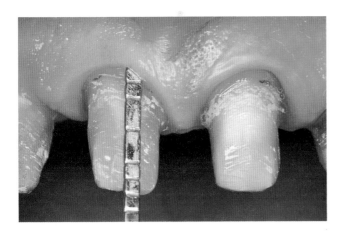

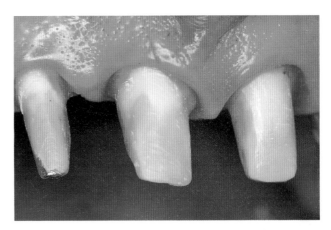

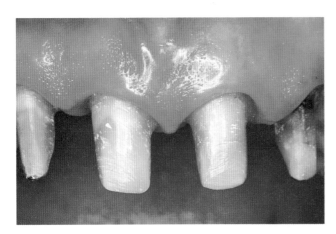

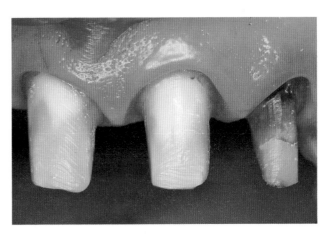

Fig. 7-13a–d The final impression should be deferred until the gingival tissues are healthy and stable. The final location of the finish lines ideally should be away from the base of the crevice as confirmed with delicate probing, and there should be no remaining periodontal defects. Return to a healthy situation not requiring surgery takes from 1 to 3 months in severe situations. Note the convex col formations.

Gingival Management—Impression Timing

Virgin Teeth

Gingivitis

1. Initial preparation, debridement with scaling and root planing, oral hygiene supervision
2. Wait 4 weeks prior to tooth preparation

Healthy gingiva: fibrous or thick-scalloped type

1. Prepare as atraumatically as possible; prepack or probe sulcus depth during tooth preparation
2. Make final impression on same day if no hemorrhage
3. Delay final impression for 3 weeks if hemorrhage

Healthy gingiva: thin-scalloped type

1. Prepare as atraumatically as possible; prepack or probe sulcus depth during tooth preparation
2. Temporize, wait 3 to 4 weeks
3. Reassess tissue levels, reprepare cervical margins where gingival recession occurred, make final impression when gingival tissues are deemed stable and healthy
4. Consider gingival augmentation when markings on intrasulcular periodontal probe can be visualized through the marginal gingiva

Deficient Crowns

1. Initial preparation: remove crowns, root plane, and scale; do not drop margins further into the crevice; fabricate provisional restorations
2. Reevaluate at 4–8 weeks, then weekly; probe gently to ensure absence of bleeding and monitor pocket depth and level of margin from a fixed reference point when possible
3. Evaluate necessity for esthetic periodontal surgery once the architecture stabilizes; thin gingiva undergoing recession may require gingival augmentation procedures:
   - If pocket is > 3 mm and/or inflammation persists, or restorative margins impinge on the biologic width, surgery may be indicated
   - If pocket is < 3 mm and the restorative margins may be placed at an ideal level respecting the biologic width, prepare margins to final level
4. Reevaluate weekly after 3–4 weeks; make final impression when tissues are deemed stable

---

Inflammation is typically associated with a dense inflammatory cellular infiltrate in the connective tissue, accounting for some distortion of the gingival architecture, and it must be reversed before crown restorative procedures are started (Figs. 7-14 and 7-15).[63,64] If gingival tissues were chronically irritated by crown restorations for several years, it would be safe to assume that the return to a fully reformed gingival architecture against sound provisional restorations will take several weeks at the minimum. Gingival tissues may also be fibrotic and irreversibly distorted; in such cases, only gingival surgery will correct the deformities.

After initial therapy, reduction in initial probing depths should be expected and is attributable to some new attachment formation, but mostly tissue shrinkage with marginal recession. With deficient crowns, it may take one month or more before healing and collagen maturation have established a resilient gingival fiber structure.[65,66] The full stabilization to a healthy architecture takes from 1 to 3 months, during which time the provisional restorations must be periodically monitored.[1] No attempt should be made at this stage to extend the finish line into the crevice unless this was dictated by caries removal. Rodriguez-Ferrer et al[67] evaluated the effect of the removal of subgingival

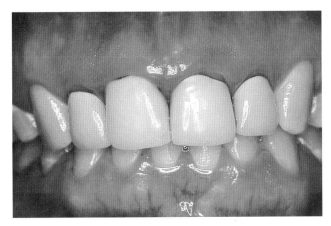

Fig. 7-14a Initial situation with overcontoured crowns and chronic gingival inflammation.

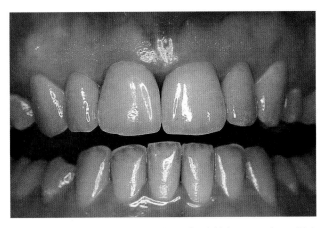

Fig. 7-14b Final crown restorations after initial preparation, which took 6 weeks.

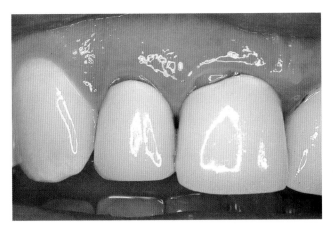

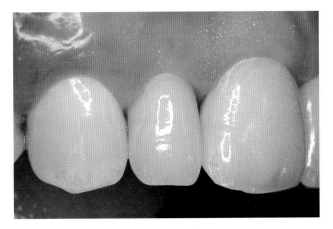

Fig. 7-15a and b Compare the scallop of the gingival tissues between the two conditions. The healthy gingiva has a knife-edge configuration with a semilunar outline around the central incisors; the healthy gingival margins around the lateral incisors have developed a steeper outline. This healthy gingival outline must be developed in the provisional restorations before final impressions are made.

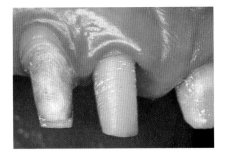

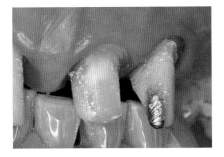

Fig. 7-16a and b Periodontal condition of a patient after 4 to 6 weeks of initial preparation. Residual periodontal defects such as deep interproximal margins with violation of biologic width, high frenum insertion, and gingival recession will have to be resolved surgically.

overhanging margins of amalgam restorations on the healing of gingival tissues. The greatest change took place during the first month of the study, but significant improvements also took place over the following 2 months. A significant proportion (53%) of subgingival restorations became supragingival within 8 weeks of initial therapy and amalgam contouring, which suggests that gingival levels may take up to 3 months to fully stabilize after initial preparation.

After initial therapy with the provisional restorations, periodontal surgery may be necessary to resolve residual problems that are not expected to improve any further (Fig. 7-16), such as: (1) intrabony pockets; (2) deep subgingival finish line violating the biologic width because of recurrent decay, decalcification, or preexisting deep margin; (3) inadequate keratinized tissues and active marginal tissue recession; (4) residual esthetic defects such as gingival recession and edentulous ridge defects; (5) gingival asymmetries; and (6) root proximity, managed either with strategic extraction or "combined preparation technique" to reduce root concavities and enhance tooth emergence profiles and gingival embrasures.[68–71]

Systematic guidelines

To improve the predictability of the final esthetic and gingival results, special attention to details is necessary because gingival facial margins are delicate and highly susceptible to mechanical trauma. With the guidelines described below, the predictability of impressions is improved and the prevention of gingival recessions is enhanced.

Subgingival contours

According to Wheeler,[72] the ridge located on the buccal surfaces of all teeth usually measures about 0.5 mm greater than the diameter of the tooth at the CEJ. It serves two purposes: (1) to hold the gingival tissues under definite tension, and (2) to deflect food materials. Weisgold[27] differentiated between subgingival and supragingival convexities.

Supragingival convexity
Overcontouring the supragingival convexity may cause plaque retention as well as inflammatory and hyper-

---

Guidelines for Predictable Tissue Management

Objectives of Initial Preparation _____
- Return to stable normal gingival architecture
- Shallow probing depth
- Knife-like marginal contours
- Absence of bleeding upon gentle probing

Prerequisites for Placing Finish Line Into the Crevice _____
- Firm dentogingival unit resistant to probing and prepacking
- Establishment of a buffer zone for the biologic width

Precautions _____
- Do not place a finish line in an inflamed gingival crevice
- Use a reference when placing a finish line in the crevice
- Probe or prepack during tooth preparation
- Use a beveled end-cutting bur when planing the facial shoulder
- Delay the final impression to anticipate gingival recession
- Assess gingival margins outline after properly fitting provisionals are constructed

plastic changes of the marginal gingiva.[28,29,73] Undercontouring and reducing the supragingival cervical bulges is preferable because plaque removal is facilitated,[28–30] but slight alterations in either direction are tolerable as long as good oral hygiene persists.[74]

Subgingival convexity

Weisgold[27] recommends evaluating the need for subgingival support by the cervical portion of the crown as a guide to the subgingival emergence of the crown (Figs. 7-17 and 7-18): (1) When the gingival margin is incisal to the CEJ, there should be a gradual curvature of the crown in the sulcus; (2) When the gingival margin is at the CEJ, the crown emergence should be flat in the sulcus and immediately convex above the gingival margin; (3) When the gingival margin is apical to the CEJ, the crown emergence should be flat subgingivally and supragingivally. Attempts were also made to correlate the prominence of the gingival tissues and of the alveolus with the degree of sub-

gingival convexity of the crown.[27,61,75] Therefore, to determine the amount of subgingival convexity to restore in the crown: (1) the location of the CEJ should be probed prior to tooth preparation; (2) during tooth preparation the clinician must observe whether the finish line narrows as it is prepared subgingivally; and (3) the gingival morphology must be considered: scalloped, thin gingival tissues dictate subtle cervical convexities[27] (Fig. 7-19). Overcontouring highly scalloped thin tissues may cause inflammation leading to recession, while undercontouring may cause a rolled, slightly inflamed gingival margin. Thin and prominent gingival tissues are more delicate and require less support and flat contours because of their fragility.[27] Flat, thick gingival tissues possibly dictate distinct cervical crown convexities.[27] Overcontouring flat, thick tissues may cause inflammation and subsequent pocketing. Undercontouring the flat, thick area may cause highly reddened and spongy marginal tissue because of collapse.[61]

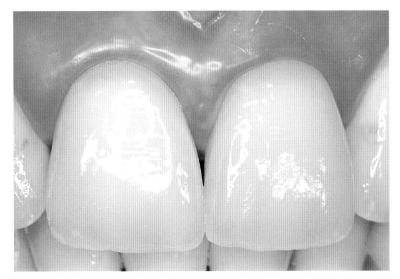

Fig. 7-17 Healthy gingival reaction to crown restorations is a result of adequate plaque control, proper marginal integrity, and respect of biologic width and physiologic contours. The subgingival aspect of these crowns is slightly convex because the finish line was narrowing as it was being prepared, which meant that it was located on the cervical convexity of the tooth.

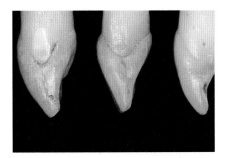 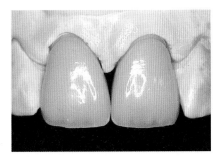 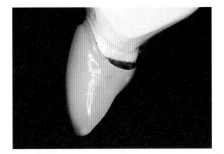

Fig. 7-18a–c Subgingival margins are either located on the cervical convexity, at the cementoenamel junction or on the root area. According to Weisgold,[27] the morphology of the subgingival crown emergence is dictated by the location of the margin in respect to the cementoenamel junction. In this example, the CEJ was located at the base of the sulcus and dictated a flat subgingival emergence followed by a mild convexity.

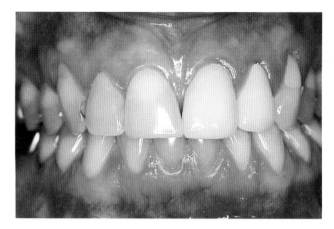

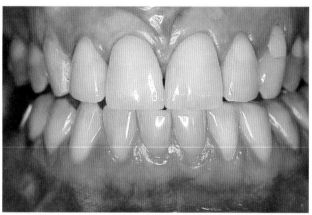

Fig. 7-19b The crown restorations were completed when it was determined that no surgery was needed to reestablish the biologic width.

Fig. 7-19a The gingival inflammation in the case of these two crowns may be caused by several factors. After crown removal and initial preparation, which took 2 months, inflammation seemed resolved, which indicated that these crowns were likely overcontoured for these scalloped, thin gingival tissues because plaque control was adequate on all the other teeth. It was also critical to ensure that the biologic width was not violated despite seemingly healthy tissues.

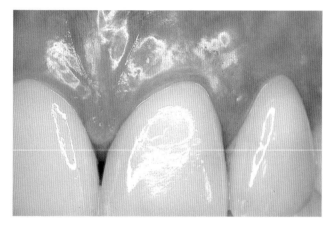

Fig. 7-19c Magnified view of the corrected gingival condition. Note the subtle facial cervical convexity dictated by the scalloped, thin marginal tissues.

Marginal precision with provisional restorations

Supracrestal injuries to the dentogingival attachment caused by tooth preparation, gingival retraction, impression technique, and placement of provisional restorations may be reversible provided that the lesions are allowed to heal against a clean tooth surface. If the interim restoration is properly polished, well fitting, and properly contoured, mechanical insults will be reversible and reattachment to the root should not be affected by common crown and bridge restorative procedures.[2,59,60,76,77] Therefore, in most cases involving anterior preparations, it is preferable to make the impression 2 to 3 weeks after biologically sound provisional restorations have been placed. Tissues should be healthy and more manageable during impression making[46] and the connective tissue attachment should be more resistant to string packing.[54]

When defective anterior crowns are replaced, sound provisional restorations fulfill two main objectives. First, they restore the inflamed gingival tissues to good health and accurate healthy dimensions after initial preparation; tissue shrinkage and remodeling may be significant once gingival architecture is restored to health. Second, they help the clinician visualize the anticipated final crowns and determine the need for esthetic periodontal surgery. Residual periodontal defects are best assessed after this initial preparation and when gingival inflammation is reduced.

These goals can be practically applied only with proper oral hygiene measures and with provisional restorations that do not irritate the gingival tissues. Improvement—not worsening—of gingival health is expected by delaying the final impression as long as necessary, and this purpose should not be defeated with faulty provisional restorations. Any factor contributing to increased plaque accumulation in the gingival aspect must be avoided.

Silness and Hegdahl[18] calculated that the area of exposed rough luting material may amount to several square millimeters around a single restoration. As stated previously, a direct relationship was found between the degree of marginal discrepancy of a subgingival crown margin and periodontal inflammation.[35] Therefore, obtaining the best possible marginal adaptation of provisional restorations is essential. It is, however, difficult to obtain and verify adequately because of polymerization shrinkage of the acrylic resin and because of the difficulty of maintaining firm adaptation of the resin against the finish line of the preparation during the setting.[78]

In the direct method of fabricating provisional restorations, the bulk of self-curing resin polymerizes on the preparations intraorally, whereas in the indirect method self-curing resin is allowed to set on a stone duplicate of the preparations.[79] Barghi and Simmons[78] found that provisional crowns constructed with a direct method did not demonstrate well-adapted margins unless they were vented and relined after their first polymerization. Many clinicians, however, prefer the simplicity of a direct technique.[80]

With either the direct or indirect technique, marginal accuracy also varies significantly with the selection of the resin material.[81] Mean marginal adaptation may vary from 25 to 157 µm according to the brand used.[82,83] According to the resin material selected, an indirect technique may yield superior marginal accuracy over a direct technique,[81,84,85] and additional relining is usually required with a direct technique.[78]

Complete cure of the resin material against the finish line of the preparation gives satisfactory marginal accuracy with the direct technique.[80,86] If the resin is allowed to harden off the preparation (bench cure), it results in poor marginal adaptation ranging from 280 to 800 µm.[87] The potential trauma of the direct technique caused by the heat of polymerization and the presence of free monomer from the resin is significant, however, and varies according to the following: (1) Type of resin. Polymethyl methacrylate produces the highest thermal release, followed by vinylethyl methacrylate and bis-acryl composite resin;[88] (2) Type of matrix. Vacuum-formed matrix produces the highest thermal release, followed by the siloxane impression matrix and the shell reline technique;[89] (3) Method of cooling. Bench curing, external air/water spray on the resin while curing on the preparations, or external air/water spray in combination with regular removal from the preparations are equally effective in minimizing pulpal temperature rise.[90]

Many clinicians prefer the ease of fabrication and the shorter chair time involved with the direct technique.[80] It is a practical option when combined with a preformed or heat-processed shell,[91] and the marginal adaptation may be significantly improved with the multiple reline technique discussed in the next section.

Single shell technique

A polycarbonate crown of the appropriate size is selected and trimmed to conform as closely as possible to the arch and the tooth preparation. It is filled with a mix of self-curing resin and placed over the preparation that has been lubricated with an insulating agent. Once the crown is fully seated, it is removed from the preparation. A mix of self-curing resin of a thinner consistency is prepared and delicately applied over the margins while the first fill is still in the doughy stage. The crown is seated over the preparation with pressure and is once again removed as soon as it is fully seated. A very thin wash of self-curing resin is then prepared and applied over the margins, and the crown is seated on the preparation and remains in position. To avoid locking into minor irregularities or undercuts, and to eliminate excess monomer and so that thermal injury to the pulp is minimized, the crown must be lifted 1 to 2 mm from the preparation every 20 to 30 seconds and the preparation must be copiously sprayed with water.[92] The crown must be firmly held in position between the irrigations until the acrylic resin fully hardens. After polymerization, the margins must be marked with a sharp lead pencil, the excess flash trimmed with a sandpaper disk, and the axial surfaces polished with flour of pumice. No further relining is usually necessary. This method offers specific advantages (Figs. 7-20 and 7-21): (1) The two relining procedures are performed without venting during the doughy phase of the initial filling, not after it is cured. This allows for significant time saving over separate relining and curing procedures. (2) Clinically superior margins are produced because the acrylic resin wash is pressured onto the finish line in the same way as a putty wash impression and is allowed to completely cure against it.

Multiple shell technique

The shell technique was originally described by Amsterdam and Fox[93] and further documented by Schluger et al[94] and Yuodelis and Faucher.[92] It consists of a laboratory-processed shell fabricated from a diagnostic waxing that is relined intraorally after the preparations are completed. This technique could be assimilated to a direct procedure because the relining material is allowed to polymerize intraorally. Advan-

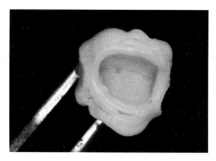

Fig. 7-20a Single shell technique for improved marginal adaptation and gingival tissue health: a trimmed polycarbonate crown is filled with a mix of self-curing resin, seated over the preparation, and removed from the preparation while the resin is still in the doughy stage. The margins are poorly registered at this stage.

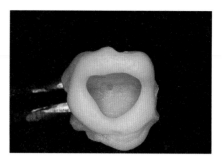

Fig. 7-20b A mix of self-curing resin of a thinner consistency is prepared and applied over the margins. The crown should be seated over the preparation with pressure and removed once again. The relining process should be repeated once again with a very thin wash of self-curing resin. The crown must be firmly held into position between regular irrigations until the acrylic resin fully hardens.

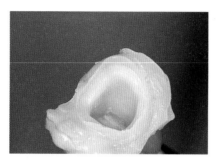

Fig. 7-20c The two relining procedures are performed before polymerization takes place and superior margins are produced because the acrylic resin wash is pressured onto the finish line in the same way as a putty wash impression. These two examples demonstrate the fidelity and accuracy of the multiple reline procedure.

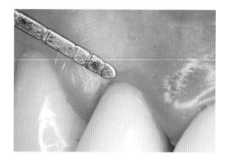

Fig. 7-20d Final marginal accuracy.

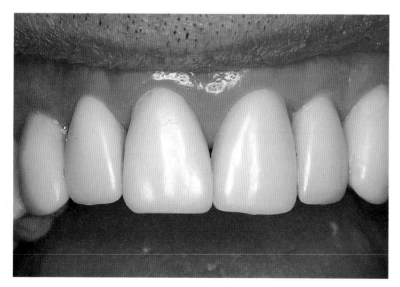

Fig. 7-21 Single provisional restorations fabricated with the multiple reline technique. Gingival tissues are conditioned by the proper contours and marginal adaptation, allowing the final impression to take place in optimal conditions.

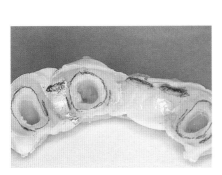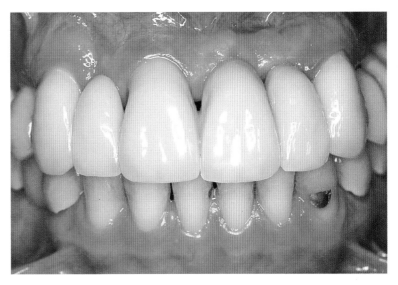

Fig. 7-22a and b The multiple reline technique is applicable to heat-processed, self-curing shells or vacuum-formed clear plastic matrixes. As with single shells, a wash of self-curing acrylic resin is applied to the margins while the bulk of resin is still in the doughy stage. With fixed partial dentures, speed is critical. To maintain control of the acrylic resin, the reline resin may need to be injected with a syringe or chilled to retard the setting. The final health of the gingival tissues is an indicator of the marginal accuracy of these provisional restorations.

tages of this technique include: *(1)* Minimal chairside involvement: chairside time is devoted to relining, reducing, and polishing the cervical areas; *(2)* Minimal occlusal adjustment: the relining procedure is performed under occlusal pressure at the vertical dimension of occlusion; *(3)* Optimal control of axial contours and occlusal morphology: the diagnostic waxing that prefigures the shell is delegated to the laboratory; *(4)* Acrylic resin shrinkage and the potential thermal trauma are minimized because the bulk of acrylic resin curing over the preparations is reduced.

Modified shell technique[91]

A preformed shell is constructed from a preoperative diagnostic wax-up. The shell may either be heat processed or fabricated of self-curing resin. After the abutments are prepared intraorally, the shell is filled with silicone disclosing material and seated on the abutments. Binding areas are marked with a lead pencil, and both the provisional fixed partial denture and the abutments are reduced accordingly until the restoration fully seats under occlusal pressure. The endentulous ridge must be protected with adhesive foil, and the shell is filled with acrylic resin and inserted over the preparations as soon as the gloss is lost.

It is seated onto its final position under occlusal pressure at the vertical dimension of occlusion, and only gross excess resin is eliminated with an explorer. The shell is removed from the preparations with a needle holder secured onto the pontic, and the mar-

gins are inspected. At this stage they typically exhibit some rounding and lack of definition. A fresh wash of acrylic resin is prepared and delicately adapted over the margins with a camel-hair brush. While the bulk of acrylic resin is still in the doughy stage, the shell is pressed back onto the abutments with moderate pressure until it is fully seated. The marginal excess is left undisturbed. The occlusal relation must be rechecked to ensure proper seating. The restoration is removed once more and, if time allows, the margins are relined with a very thin wash of acrylic resin.

After the restoration has been seated into final position, it must be lifted 1 to 2 mm from the preparations every 20 to 30 seconds while the preparations are copiously sprayed with water.[92] The bridge must be firmly held into position between the irrigation procedures until the acrylic resin fully hardens. Although cooling prolongs the resin's curing time, it also causes lower temperature elevation.[95] After polymerization, the margins must be marked with a sharp lead pencil, the excess flash trimmed with sandpaper disks, and the axial surfaces polished with flour of pumice. No further relining is usually necessary.

This technique is applicable to heat-processed shells or vacuum-formed clear plastic matrices. The marginal accuracy of provisional restorations fabricated with a direct method is improved when a wash of self-curing acrylic resin is applied to the margins while the bulk of the resin is still in the doughy stage. This technique has proven valuable in improving the marginal precision of provisional restorations and promoting gingival health (Fig. 7-22).

References

1. Shavell HM. Mastering the art of tissue management during provisionalization and biologic final impressions. *Int J Periodont Rest Dent* 1988;8(3):25.

2. Löe H. Reaction of marginal periodontal tissues to restorative procedures. *Int Dent J* 1968;18:759.

3. Larato D. The effect of crown margin extension on gingival inflammation. *J South Calif Dent Assoc* 1969;23:476.

4. Silness J. Periodontal conditions in patients treated with dental bridges. *J Periodont Res* 1970;5:60.

5. Silness J. Periodontal conditions in patients treated with dental bridges. II. The influence of full and partial crowns on plaque accumulation, development of gingivitis and pocket formation. *J Periodont Res* 1970;5:219.

6. Silness J. Periodontal conditions in patients treated with dental bridges. III. The relationship between the location of the crown margin and the periodontal condition. *J Periodont Res* 1970;5:225.

7. Mormman W, Regolati B, Renggli HH. Gingival reaction to well-fitted subgingival proximal gold inlays. *J Clin Periodontol* 1974;1:120.

8. Maruyama T, Simoosa T, Ojima H. Morphology of gingival capillaries adjacent to complete crowns. *J Prosthet Dent* 1976;35:179.

9. Leon AR. The periodontium and restorative procedures: A critical review. *J Oral Rehabil* 1977;4:105.

10. Jameson LM. Comparison of the volume of crevicular fluid from restored and nonrestored teeth. *J Prosthet Dent* 1979;41:209.

11. Waerhaug T. Effect of rough surfaces upon gingival tissue. *J Dent Res* 1956;35:323.

12. Swartz ML, Phillips RW. Comparison of bacterial accumulations on rough and smooth enamel surfaces. *J Periodontol* 1957;28:304.

13. Zander HA. Effect of silicate cement and amalgam on the gingiva. *J Am Dent Assoc* 1957;55:111.

14. App RGR. Effect of silicate, amalgam and cast gold on the gingiva. *J Prosthet Dent* 1961;11:522.

15. Waerhaug J. Current basis for prevention of periodontal disease. *Int Dent J* 1967;17:267.

16. Waerhaug J. Periodontology and partial prosthesis. *Int Dent J* 1968;18:101.

17. Glyn Jones JC. The success rate of anterior crowns. *Br Dent J* 1972;132:399.

18. Silness J, Hegdahl T. Area of the exposed zinc phosphate cement surfaces in fixed restorations. *Scand J Dent Res* 1970;3:163.

19. Leon A. Amalgam restorations and periodontal disease. *Br Dent J* 1976;140:377.

20. Saltzberg DS, Ceravolo FJ, Holstein F, Groom G, Gottsegen R. Scanning electron microscope study of the junction between restorations and gingival cavosurface margins. *J Prosthet Dent* 1976;5:518.

21. Janenko C. Anterior crowns and gingival health. *Aust Dent J* 1979;24:225.

22. Silness J. Fixed prosthodontics and periodontal health. *Dent Clin North Am* 1980;24:317.

23. Marcum J. The effect of crown marginal depth upon gingival tissue. *J Prosthet Dent* 1967;17:479.

24. Newcomb GM. The relationship between the location of subgingival crown margins and gingival inflammation. *J Periodontol* 1974;45:151.

25. Lang NP, Kiel RA, Anderhalden K. Clinical and microbiological effects of subgingival restorations with overhanging or clinically perfect margins. *J Clin Periodontol* 1983;10:563.

26. Flores-de-Jacoby L, Zafiropoulos GG, Ciancio S. The effect of crown margin location on plaque and periodontal health. *Int J Periodont Rest Dent* 1989;9:197.

27. Weisgold AS. Contours of the full crown restoration. *Alpha Omegan* 1977;December:77.

28. Perel ML. Axial crown contours. *J Prosthet Dent* 1971;25:642.

29. Perel ML. Periodontal considerations of crown contours. *J Prosthet Dent* 1971;26:627.

30. Yuodelis RA, Weaver JD, Sapkos S. Facial and lingual contours of artificial crown restorations and their effects on the periodontium. *J Prosthet Dent* 1973;29:61.

31. Maynard GJ, Wilson RD. Physiologic dimensions of the periodontium fundamental to successful restorative dentistry. *J Periodontol* 1979;50:107.

32. Nevins M, Skurow HM. The intracrevicular restorative margin, the biologic width, and the maintenance of the gingival margin. *Int J Periodont Rest Dent* 1984;4(3):31.

33. Waerhaug J. Histologic considerations which govern where the margins of restorations should be located in relation to the gingiva. *Dent Clin North Am* 1960;March:161.

34. Renggli H, Regolati B. Gingival inflammation and plaque accumulation by well-adapted subgingival and supragingival proximal restorations. *Helv Odontol Acta* 1972;159:99.

35. Felton DA, Kanoy BE, Bayne SC, Wirthman GP. Effect of in vivo crown margin discrepancies on periodontal health. *J Prosthet Dent* 1991;65:357.

36. Waerhaug J. Tissue reactions around artificial crowns. *J Periodontol* 1953;24:172.

37. Karlsen K. Gingival reactions to dental restorations. *Acta Odontol Scand* 1970;28:895.

38. Richter WA, Ueno H. Relationship of crown margin placement to gingival inflammation. *J Prosthet Dent* 1973;30:156.

39. Koth DL. Full crown restorations and gingival inflammation in a controlled population. *J Prosthet Dent* 1982;48:681.

40. Valderhaug J, Birkeland JM. Periodontal conditions in patients 5 years following insertion of fixed prostheses. *J Oral Rehabil* 1976;3:237.

41. Valderhaug J, Heloe LA. Oral hygiene in a group of supervised patients with fixed prostheses. *J Periodontol* 1977;221.

42. Valderhaug J, Birkeland JM. Periodontal conditions and carious lesions following the insertion of fixed prostheses. A 10-year follow-up study. *Int Dent J* 1981;30:296.

43. Garguilo AW, Wentz FM, Orban B. Dimensions and relations of the dento-gingival junction in humans. *J Periodontol* 1961;32:261.

44. Ingber JS, Rose LF, Coslet JG. The "biologic width"—a concept in periodontics and restorative dentistry. *Alpha Omegan* 1977;10:62–65.

45. Tarnow D, Stahl SS, Magner A, Zamzok J. Human gingival attachment responses to subgingival crown placement-marginal remodeling. *J Clin Periodontol* 1986;13:563.

46. Wilson RD, Maynard G. Intracrevicular restorative dentistry. *Int J Periodont Rest Dent* 1981;1(4):35.

47. Parma-Benfenati S, Fugazzotto PA, Ruben MP. The effect of restorative margins on the postsurgical development and nature of the periodontium. Part I. *Int J Periodont Rest Dent* 1985;5(6):31.

48. Tai H, Soldinger M, Dreiangel A, Pitaru S. Responses to periodontal injuries in the dog: Removal of gingival attachment and supracrestal placement of amalgam restorations. *Int J Periodont Rest Dent* 1988;8(3):45.

49. Parma-Benfenati S, Fugazzotto PA, Ruben MP. The effect of restorative margins on the postsurgical development and nature of the periodontium. Part II. Anatomical considerations. *Int J Periodont Rest Dent* 1986;1:65.

50. Lisgarten MA, Mao R, Robinson PJ. Periodontal probing and the relationship of the probe tip to periodontal tissues. *J Periodontol* 1976;47:511.

51. Lisgarten MA. Periodontal probing: What does it mean? *J Clin Periodontol* 1980;7:165.

52. Armitage GC, Svanberg GK, Löe H. Microscopic evaluation of clinical measurements of connective tissue attachment levels. *J Clin Periodontol* 1977;4:173.

53. Robinson PJ, Vitek RM. The relationship between gingival inflammation and the probe resistance. *J Periodont Res* 1975; 14:239.

54. Dragoo MR, Williams GB. Periodontal tissue reactions to restorative procedures. *Int J Periodont Rest Dent* 1981;1(1):9.

55. Waerhaug J. Temporary restorations: Advantages and disadvantages. *Dent Clin North Am* 1982;24:305.

56. Ross SE, Garguilo A, Crosseti HW, Phillips DJ. The surgical management of the restorative alveolar interface (II). *Int J Periodont Rest Dent* 1983;4:9.

57. Kois J. The conceptual basis for creating periodontal and restorative harmony. Presented at the American Academy of Esthetic Dentistry, 16th Annual Meeting, August 9, 1991, Santa Barbara, Calif.

58. Nevins M. Interproximal periodontal disease—the embrasure as an etiologic factor. *Int J Periodont Rest Dent* 1982;2(6):9.

59. Harrison JD. Effect of retraction materials on the gingival sulcus epithelium. *J Prosthet Dent* 1961;11:514.

60. Löe H, Silness J. Tissue reactions to string packs used in fixed restorations. *J Prosthet Dent* 1963;13:318.

61. Kay H. Criteria for restorative contours in the altered periodontal environment. *Int J Periodont Rest Dent* 1985;5(3):43.

62. Flemmig TF, Sorensen JA, Newman MG, Nachnani S. Gingival enhancement in fixed prosthodontics. Part II. *J Prosthet Dent* 1991;65:365.

63. Benjamin SD, Coleman HL. Periodontal considerations in gingival retraction procedures. *J South Calif Dent Assoc* 1970;38:823.

64. Nemetz H. Tissue management in fixed prosthodontics. *J Prosthet Dent* 1974;31:628.

65. Ramfjord SP, Ash MM. *Periodontology and Periodontics*. Philadelphia: Saunders, 1979.

66. Wunderlich RC, Caffesse RG. Periodontal aspects of porcelain restorations. *Dent Clin North Am* 1985;29:693.

67. Rodriguez-Ferrer HJ, Strahan JD, Newman HN. Effect on gingival health of removing overhanging margins of interproximal subgingival amalgam restorations. *J Clin Periodontol* 1980; 7:457.

68. Ross SE, Garguilo A. The surgical management of the restorative alveolar interface. *Int J Periodont Rest Dent* 1982;2(3):9.

69. Ross SE, Garguilo A, Crosseti HW, Phillips DJ. The surgical management of the restorative alveolar interface (II). *Int J Periodont Rest Dent* 1983;3(4):9.

70. Carnavale G, Sterrantino SF, DiFebo G. Soft and hard tissue wound healing following tooth preparation to the alveolar crest. *Int J Periodont Rest Dent* 1983;3(6):37.

71. DiFebo G, Carnavale G, Sterrantino SF. Treatment of a case of advanced periodontitis: Clinical procedures utilizing the "combined preparation technique." *Int J Periodont Rest Dent* 1985; 5(1):53.

72. Wheeler RC. Complete crown form and the periodontium. *J Prosthet Dent* 1961;11:722.

73. Sackett BP, Guldenhuys RR. The effect of axial crown overcontour on adolescents. *J Periodontol* 1976;47:320.

74. Ehrlich J, Hochman N. Alterations of crown contour—effect of gingival health in man. *J Prosthet Dent* 1980;44:523.

75. Wagman S. Role of coronal contour in gingival health. *J Prosthet Dent* 1977;37:280.

76. Duncan JD. Reaction of marginal gingiva to crown and bridge procedures. Part I. *J Mississippi Dent Assoc* 1979;2:35.

77. Dragoo MR, Williams GB. Periodontal tissue reactions to restorative procedures. Part II. *Int J Periodont Rest Dent* 1982; 2(2):35.

78. Barghi N, Simmons W. The marginal integrity of the temporary acrylic resin crown. *J Prosthet Dent* 1976;36:274.

79. Fisher DN, Shillingburg HT, Dewhirst RB. Indirect temporary restorations. *J Am Dent Assoc* 1971;82:160.

80. Tjan AHL, Tjan AH, Grant BE. Marginal accuracy of temporary composite crowns. *J Prosthet Dent* 1987;58:417.

81. Richards ND, Mitchell RJ. Effects of materials and techniques on accuracy of temporary fixed partial dentures [abstract 1484]. *J Dent Res* 1984;63:336.

82. Wang RL, Moore BK, Goodacre CJ, Swartz ML, Andres CJ. A comparison of resins for fabricating provisional fixed restorations. *Int J Prosthodont* 1989;2:173.

83. Koumjian JH, Holmes JB. Marginal accuracy of provisional restorative materials. *J Prosthet Dent* 1990;63:639.

84. Crispin BJ, Watson JF, Caputo AA. The marginal accuracy of treatment restorations: A comparative analysis. *J Prosthet Dent* 1980;44:283.

85. Monday JL, Blais D. Marginal adaptation of provisional acrylic resin crowns. *J Prosthet Dent* 1985;54:194.

86. Kaiser DA. Accurate acrylic resin temporary restorations. *J Prosthet Dent* 1978;39:158.

87. Robinson FB, Hovijitra S. Marginal fit of direct temporary crowns. *J Prosthet Dent* 1982;47:390.

88. Driscoll CF, Woolsey G, Ferguson WM. Comparison of exothermic release during polymerization of four materials used to fabricate interim restorations. *J Prosthet Dent* 1991;65:504.

89. Moulding MB, Teplitsky PE. Intrapulpal temperature during fabrication of provisional restorations. *Int J Prosthodont* 1990; 3:299.

90. Moulding MB, Loney RW. The effect of cooling techniques on intrapulpal temperature during direct fabrication of provisional restorations. *Int J Prosthodont* 1991;4:332.

91. Chiche G. Improving marginal adaptation of provisional restorations. *Quintessence Int* 1990;21:325.

92. Yuodelis RA, Faucher R. Provisional restorations: An integrated approach to periodontics and restorative dentistry. *Dent Clin North Am* 1980;April:285.

93. Amsterdam M, Fox L. Provisional splinting principles and techniques. *Dent Clin North Am* 1959;March:73.

94. Schluger S, Yuodelis RA, Page RC. *Periodontal Disease*. Philadelphia: Lea & Febiger, 1977:638–656.

95. Grajower R, Shaharbani S, Kaufman E. Temperature rise in pulp chamber during fabrication of temporary self-curing crowns. *J Prosthet Dent* 1979;41:535.

Chapter 8

Impressions for the Anterior Dentition

Gerard Chiche and Alain Pinault

Impressions for natural teeth

Gingival retraction

Gingival tissues in the anterior region deserve special attention because they are fragile and vulnerable to mechanical trauma. For esthetic reasons it is essential to maintain the level of the free gingival margins and to avoid a permanent gingival recession. Therefore, retraction materials and techniques should be selected to create as little tissue trauma as possible and ideally to avoid irreversible loss of tissue height.[1,2] Yet tissue deflection must be sufficient and provide for adequate horizontal displacement and adequate vertical access and prevent hemorrhage or seepage[1-3]; a slight marginal recession in the order of 0.1 mm is expected after gingival retraction but should not be critical.[4]

Mechanical-chemical method

Nonmedicated plain retraction cords placed in the gingival sulcus are safe when left up to 30 minutes,[4] but they have poor retraction ability compared with medicated cords.[5,6] Popular chemicals and drugs currently used for gingival deflection include aluminum chloride (buffered), aluminum sulfate, potassium sulfate (alum), and ferric sulfate.[1] They are effective and safe if left for limited time in the sulcus and used at proper concentrations or in a buffered form such as Hemodent solution (buffered 14% aluminum chloride, Premier Dental Products, Norristown, Pa).[4-9] Tissue injury caused by gingival retraction techniques with plain cords or cords impregnated with alum, buffered aluminum chloride, or 8% racemic epinephrine will

heal completely between 6 and 10 days when cords are left in place up to 15 minutes.[4,5,10,11]

Weir and Williams[7] demonstrated that the hemostatic success of plain cords, aluminum sulfate cords, and R-epinephrine cords was approximately doubled when they were soaked in Hemodent solution. They also showed that when the impression was made on the same day of preparation, the success rate of Hemodent-soaked cords ranged from 70% to 95%. With polyvinyl siloxane impressions, a plain cord saturated with Hemodent solution is a safe and effective retraction method, and according to Albers[12] aluminum chloride is the chemical of choice to prevent recession of thin delicate gingival tissues in the anterior region. Even though racemic epinephrine was popular in a survey, several investigators advise against it because of its unpredictable absorption and the potentially dangerous systemic reaction that may result depending on the medical status of the patient, with various degrees of tissue laceration and the number of preparations involved.[4,5,13] Aluminum sulfate has also been suspected of possibly inhibiting the setting reaction of polyvinyl siloxane impression materials.[12,14]

Retraction techniques for the anterior region

Nevins and Skurow[15] emphasized the need to respect the fragility of the junctional epithelium and the attachment of the supracrestal fibers during gingival retraction procedures. Packing must be delicate and as atraumatic as possible, because Löe and Silness[10] showed that with normal pressure, strings had the potential to be pushed into the supracrestal connective tissue. Similarly, Dragoo and Williams[16] demonstrated that retraction cord placement following subgingival preparation often tore the epithelial and connective tissue attachments from teeth. By delaying the final impression 2 to 3 weeks in cases involving anterior preparations, tissues should be firmer and more resistant to string packing.[17]

The potential for permanent gingival recession is greater when a cord is left in a thin facial crevice for more than 15 minutes or if two cords are packed on top of one another with uncontrolled pressure within a shallow crevice. For this reason, the facial crevice in the anterior region should be delicately packed with one string whenever possible.

Single string technique

The single string technique is the simplest and least traumatic option. It is, therefore, indicated when gingival tissues appear healthy and do not bleed as the string is packed. To achieve optimum saturation of the cord by the chemical, plain knitted cords (eg, Ultrapak no. 0 and no. 00, Ultradent Products, Salt Lake City, Utah) can be permanently soaked in buffered aluminum chloride solution. Knitted cords do not shred easily and maintain their shape during handling.[18] Before impression making, the cord is retrieved from the solution and is sequentially packed from the mesial aspect to the lingual aspect to the distal aspect and finally on the buccal aspect of the preparation.

This sequence allows the string to be well secured in the sulcus before engaging the shallow facial crevice, so that packing the thin facial area is facilitated. Lateral deflection for elastomeric materials should be approximately 0.5 mm.[12] Lateral deflection is frequently insufficient interproximally with only one string because the tissue may collapse over the cord. This usually requires that the same cord be packed once more in the mesial, lingual, and distal aspects. In this fashion, however, the delicate and shallow facial crevice remains packed once whereas, when indicated, the interproximal and lingual aspects are deflected with two-string thicknesses. For optimal results, the string should remain in place for approximately 10 minutes (Figs. 8-1–8-4).[12,19]

Selective double string technique

The selective double string is recommended when spontaneous bleeding of the gingival crevice is likely to occur during impression making. A bleeding crevice is the major obstacle to an accurate impression and is usually caused by laceration laterally or apically during tooth preparation. It is also associated with plaque accumulation in marginal defects of the provisional restorations or with deep margins.

Whether the impression is made immediately following tooth preparation or at a subsequent appointment, the likelihood of gingival bleeding during the impression procedure must be assessed before or during packing. After the provisional restoration is removed or as the temporary cement is eliminated, spontaneous bleeding of the free gingival margin may occur. If the gingival sulcus appears erythematous or bleeds spontaneously, the retraction sequence should be modified. The hemostatic success of commercially available string preparations and chemical agents is variable,[7] especially when tooth preparation and impression making occur during the same appointment. Therefore, whenever there is a suspicion of spontaneous bleeding during impression making, selective prepacking of an extra-thin string is recommended as a safety precaution. Typically, the interproximal or lingual aspects of the crevice are more prone to localized inflammation, whereas the facial sulcus remains relatively healthier. With the selective double string technique, prepacking of the facial crevice is usually avoided; it is packed only once to minimize the risk of tearing the epithelial and connective tissue attachments from the tooth.

A braid of extra-thin cord (eg, Ultrapack no. 00) impregnated with buffered aluminum chloride is prepacked and confined to the inflamed portion of the crevice only. The excess braid should be sectioned with thin scissors and the excess seepage and coagulum wiped with a cotton pellet. A thin impregnated knitted cord (eg, Ultrapack no. 0) is then packed into the crevice according to the sequence previously outlined for the single string technique. Before the impression material is injected, the thin cord should be removed, but the extra-thin braid is left in place for hemostatic effect. It may get caught in the impression but should be left undisturbed when the impression is poured (Fig. 8-5).

Double string technique

As more hemorrhage control is required, the retraction process becomes more aggressive. If gingival tissues are highly inflamed, obtaining an accurate impression is technically feasible, but the gingival healing and reattachment are unpredictable.[19] The double string technique should ideally be reserved for situations where the whole gingival crevice is prone to bleeding. This typically occurs with gingival laceration due to aggressive tooth preparation or after the wearing of faulty provisional restorations with overhanging margins.

In this technique, an extra-thin cord (eg, Ultrapack no. 00) impregnated with buffered aluminum chloride is prepacked into the entire crevice and sectioned so

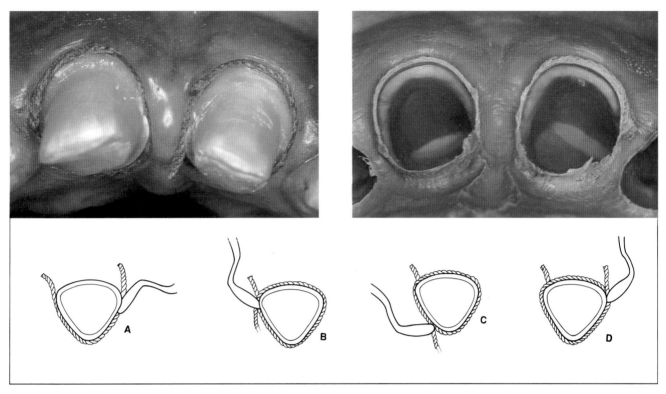

Fig. 8-1 The single retraction cord technique is indicated with healthy gingival tissues. A cord impregnated with buffered aluminum chloride solution is sequentially packed from the mesial to the lingual aspect, distal **(A)** and finally on the buccal aspect of the preparation **(B)**. If there is insufficient lateral deflection at this stage, the same cord should be packed once more in the mesial, lingual, and distal aspects **(C and D)**. The facial crevice may remain packed once if there is sufficient lateral deflection, otherwise it will require additional packing. The final impression should faithfully reproduce the continuity of the marginal areas without tear or voids. (Express, 3M Dental, St Paul, MN)

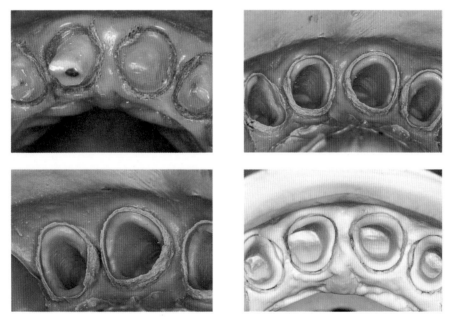

Fig. 8-2a–d The single retraction cord technique is the simplest and least traumatic retraction for delicate facial gingival tissues. However, tooth proximity may require systematic double packing of the proximal aspect for adequate deflection. Note on the stone cast the extent of proximal deflection as compared with facial deflection.

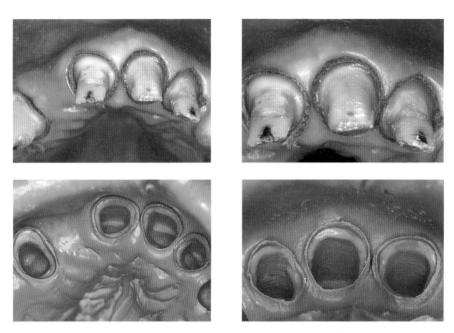

Fig. 8-3a–d Another clinical example where proximal deflection obliterates the interdental papillae because of tooth proximity. The retraction cords must be packed as atraumatically as possible and the adaptation of the provisional restorations must be optimum for the interdental papillae to fully recover.

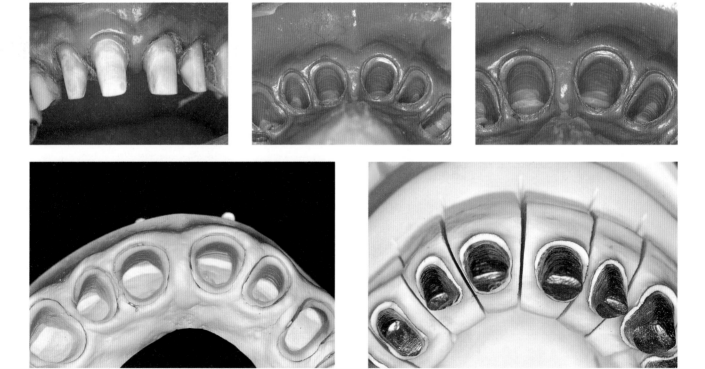

Fig. 8-4a–e With situations involving at least six preparations, it is recommended that the healthiest possible gingival condition be obtained before making the final impression. In this fashion a single cord technique may be used. If tissue bleeding was caused by gingival inflammation, a double cord technique would be indicated but would also be much more time-consuming.

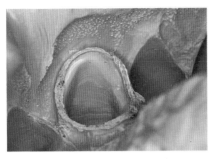

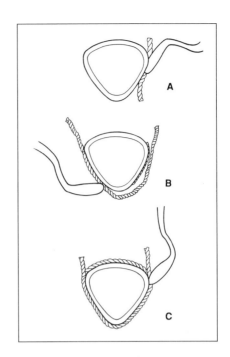

Fig. 8-5a and b The selective double cord technique is recommended when spontaneous bleeding of the gingival crevice is likely to occur during impression making. Selective prepacking of an extra-thin cord into the inflamed portion of the crevice (**A**) is followed by packing of a thin impregnated braided cord (**B and C**), which will be removed before the impression material is injected. The extra-thin braid is left in place in the crevice for hemostasis and was picked up in this impression.

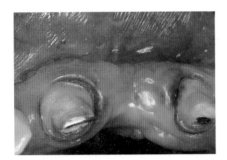

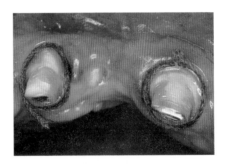

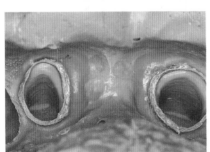

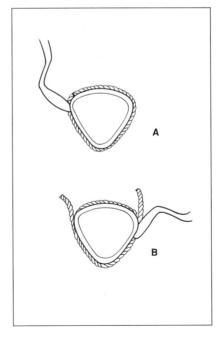

Fig. 8-6a–d The double cord technique is reserved for situations where the entire gingival crevice is prone to bleeding. Considering that the anterior gingival crevice is usually shallow, this is a relatively aggressive technique. An impregnated extra-thin cord is prepacked into the entire crevice (**A**) followed by a thin impregnated cord on top of it (**B**), which is removed before the impression material is injected. The extra-thin cord is left in place for hemostasis. Here it was picked up in the impression, and loose segments were sectioned off prior to pouring the impression.

Retraction Procedures for the Anterior Region			
Technique	Indication	Advantages	Disadvantages
Single string	Healthy tissues	Simple Least traumatic Little potential for gingival recession	Impression material may tear if lack of lateral displacement
Selective double string	Healthy tissues with localized irritation	Control of bleeding Good lateral displacement	Additional time for placement of cord
Double string	Inflamed tissues	Control of bleeding Excellent lateral displacement	Time-consuming Potentially traumatic Least predictable gingival response

that its two extremities meet at right angles without overlapping. If gingival bleeding still occurs, as would happen with exposed connective tissue, the papilla may need to be injected with 2% lidocaine solution with 1/50,000 epinephrine to cause local vasoconstriction. The crevice may also be very delicately rubbed with aluminum chloride, ferric sulfate, or hydrogen peroxide solution. A thin impregnated knitted cord (eg, Ultrapack no. 0) is then packed into the crevice according to the sequence outlined for the single string technique, and before the impression material is injected it is removed, while the extra-thin cord is left in place for hemostasis. It may get caught in the impression, but only loose segments should be sectioned off before the pouring of the impression. The double string technique controls gingival hemorrhage effectively and yields excellent tissue displacement. However, it has greater potential for gingival recession because packing two cords into a facial crevice in the anterior region may tear the connective tissue attachment from the root (Fig. 8-6).

Accuracy of impression procedures

Dimension of stone die

Elastomeric materials commonly used for impressions in fixed prosthodontics have comparable accuracy as long as they are used properly.[20–25] The excellent dimensional stability of addition reaction silicones and polyethers allows for delayed pouring of the impression with no loss of accuracy and accounts in part for their popularity.[22,23,26,27]

However, predicting the effect of even minute dimensional changes of a given elastomeric impression material on the fit of the casting is difficult, because several variables are involved. With addition reaction silicones or polyethers, the size of the stone die may increase or decrease compared with the original tooth preparation, even within the same category of impression material. This deviation varies according to the selected impression product, the rigidity and type of tray, the delay in pouring the impression, the stone expansion, and the type of viscosities used.[22–24,26–31]

Measured in percent deviation from the original preparation, variations in size of stone dies may range from −0.3% to 0.97% in occlusogingival height and from −0.07% to 0.79% in mesiodistal or buccolingual width.[21–24,26–29] These variations affect the amount of die relief required to produce a consistent fit of the casting over the preparation in the mouth. In the anterior region, there is little latitude to consistently achieve proper stability of the crown over the tooth preparation because of the relatively reduced surface area of the tooth preparation.

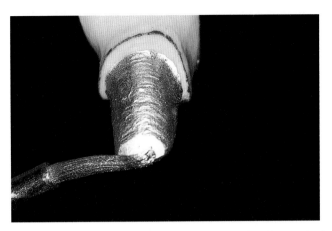 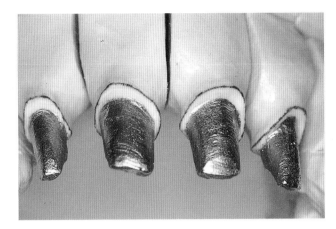

Fig. 8-7a and b   With a given impression/stone die combination, the stability of the crown in the mouth depends on the amount of die relief on the die of the preparation. For example, with Express (3M Dental) and Die Keen (Columbus Dental, Columbus, OH) three coats of spacer should be applied at the incisal aspect and a single thin coat on the axial walls. This compensates for the slightly shorter and wider die resulting from this specific combination.

Causes of Size Deviation of Stone Dies	
Discrepancy With the Tooth Preparation	**Compensation on the Stone Die**
Wider and higher	One coat of die spacer over the incisal edge
Narrower and higher	Three coats of die spacer over the axial surfaces and the incisal line angles and one coat over the incisal edge
Wider and shorter	Three coats of die spacer over the incisal edge and one coat over the axial walls
Narrower and shorter	Three coats of die spacer over the axial walls and the incisal edge

Practically, the clinician must evaluate the fit and stability of the crown in the mouth with a given impression tray/stone/die relief combination and relay this information to the technician. The application of die relief should be adjusted in the laboratory until a stable and passive fit of the crown is consistently achieved clinically with this combination of materials. Williams et al[22] observed that changes in impression material dimensions are complex because they may be beneficial to the fit in one portion of the casting but have an adverse effect in another. They recommended applying casting relief in the appropriate locations on the stone die. Compared with the original tooth preparation, the size of the stone die may deviate in four different ways[22–24,26–30] that should be compensated precisely on anterior preparations (Fig. 8-7).

Disclosing of the casting

Marginal discrepancy of the crown restoration may be caused by abrasion of the incisal edge of the stone die, casting nodules inside the incisal aspect, or insufficient relief at the incisal line angles.[32] Marginal discrepancies in subgingival areas are difficult to detect and evaluate visually.[33] Therefore, the fit of subgingival margins should not be deemed clinically acceptable unless tested intraorally with a disclosing medium. Silicone disclosing pastes have proven simple and reliable for the intraoral detection of internally binding areas. In the anterior region, incisal or lingual line angles are frequently disclosed with this method. Reduction of these areas that impede the full seating of the crown on the preparation is mandatory because it will improve the marginal seal and seating of restorations from 40% to 70%[34–36] (Fig. 8-8).

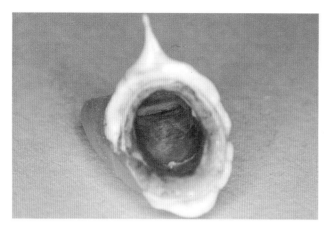

Fig. 8-8a Besides adequate die relief for predictable crown stability, it is essential to disclose at the try-in appointment any possible internal binding areas in the crown with a silicone disclosing paste (Fit Checker, GC International, Scottsdale, AZ). Incisal or lingual line angles are frequently disclosed in anterior crown restorations with this method. To avoid perforating the metal, the corresponding area in the mouth should be delicately reduced.

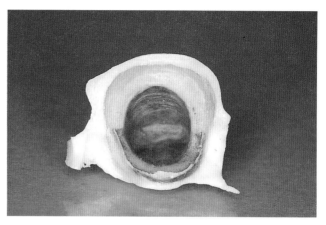

Fig. 8-8b After the binding areas that impede full seating of the crown on the preparation have been reduced, the seating of the restoration will be significantly improved as evidenced by the reduced silicone film thickness at the margins.

Tray selection for impressions in the anterior region

There is a wide selection of impression techniques, especially because addition reaction silicones are now available with various viscosities. Even though these materials are accurate and dimensionally stable, they are vulnerable to permanent deformation if an unsuitable tray is used for the type of procedure or if a poor adhesive treatment is used.

Manufactured stock plastic trays (polystyrene). These trays are popular because of their convenience and low cost[37] and because they can be used for impressions of one or two single units for addition reaction silicones, polyethers, and polysulfides, provided the tray has sufficient rigidity and the preparations are well enclosed in the tray.[31] With stock plastic trays, die height is accurate for all three types of impression materials, but die width is accurate only with addition reaction silicones and is greater with polysulfides and polyethers.[38] Die relief may, therefore, have to be adjusted accordingly. This type of tray is universally contraindicated with fixed bridgework because its flexibility adversely affects interpreparation, cross-arch, and anteroposterior dimensions, resulting in poorly fitting fixed partial dentures.[38–41]

Acrylic resin custom trays. The primary purpose of these trays is to provide uniform thickness of material because dimensional changes that occur during the setting of elastomeric impression materials are proportional to their thickness. The recommended thickness of spacer varies from 2 to 4 mm according to the impression material.[42–44]

A custom tray must be precisely fabricated, or the thickness of impression material may end up being the same as with a stock plastic tray.[37] The tray must be as rigid as possible and must be designed to fully enclose the preparations. A tray adhesive must be properly used on a clean uncontaminated tray surface.[21,45,46] Custom trays are especially recommended for fixed bridgework with elastomers, either monophasic or in any combination of heavy-medium-light viscosity.

Stock metal trays. Coated steel or stainless steel trays combine the convenience of stock plastic trays with the rigidity of custom trays. Dimensional accuracy between perforated metal and custom trays appears to be comparable,[47] but perforated metal trays are especially indicated with putty-light impressions because the adhesion of polyvinylsiloxane putty to its impression adhesive is time-dependent and may not be as reliable as with other viscosities. Because a weak bond between acrylic resin or polystyrene coated with adhesive and polyvinylsiloxane putty material has been reported,[48–50] it may be safer with putty-light impressions to rely on the mechanical retention of rigid metal trays in addition to the adhesive.

Tray Selection for Impressions in the Anterior Region		
Material	One or Two Single Units	Multiple Units and Fixed Bridgework
Polysulfide	Custom tray or stock plastic tray	Custom tray
Polyether	Custom tray or stock plastic tray	Custom tray
Addition silicone monophasic heavy-light heavy-medium medium-light	Stock plastic tray	Custom tray
Addition silicone putty-light putty-medium	Stock plastic tray or perforated metal stock tray	Perforated metal stock tray

Impressions for laminate veneers

An elastomeric material of sufficient tear strength must be selected for impressions for porcelain laminate veneers.[51] This property is essential for accurate registration of cervical and interproximal undercut areas without tearing or distorting the impression material. Various combinations of putty, heavy- and medium-viscosity polyvinylsiloxanes (Figs. 8-9 and 8-10), or heavy and light polysulfides are well suited for this purpose. Before impression making, deep interproximal undercuts must be partially blocked out with orthodontic wax, as long as this does not prevent the technician from sectioning the cast into individual dies. It may also be necessary at this stage to accentuate the separation between the veneer preparations with a high-speed flame bur while preserving the lingual aspect of the proximal contacts. In this fashion, the dies will be easily sawed in the laboratory, after lingual contact areas have been undermined on the working cast with the extremity of a sharp, curved scalpel blade.

The two most common methods of porcelain veneer fabrication are the platinum foil technique and the refractory die technique. Individual dies can be fabricated with either technique, and both methods produce clinically acceptable veneers[51] according to the preference and expertise of the technician. Single refractory dies are a better alternative than a solid refractory cast in minimizing the volumetric distortion of refractory investments.[52] Sorensen et al[53] compared the accuracy of the two techniques and reported that the platinum foil veneers had significantly better marginal fidelity (187 μm) than the refractory die veneers (292 μm). They also, however, had significantly more overcontouring than the refractory die veneers. The potential for damage of individual stone dies during veneer fabrication is another significant consideration. It is recommended with either veneer technique that additional master casts be fabricated for final marginal corrections and adjustments.[54] Finally, an unsawed cast is also useful for final adjustment of the proximal contacts and of the cervicoproximal embrasures (Figs. 8-11–8-14).

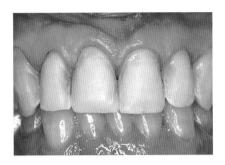

Fig. 8-9 Continuous cord packed in the sulcus before an impression for laminate veneers.

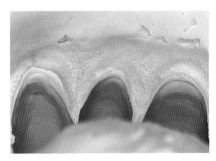

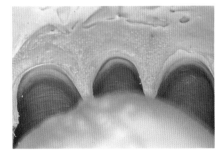

Fig. 8-10a and b A medium-body elastomeric material of sufficient tear strength must be selected for accurate registration of cervical and interproximal undercut areas without tear or distortion of the impression material. In this example, a combination of Express putty and Imprint 2:5 (3M Dental) was selected and two impressions were made.

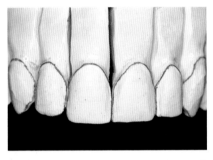

Fig. 8-11 These two impressions will serve to fabricate three casts in the laboratory. The potential for damage of individual stone dies during veneer fabrication dictates construction of additional casts for final marginal corrections and adjustments. The first cast consists of a conventional stone master cast with individual dies.

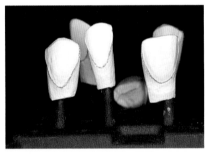

Fig. 8-12a and b The second cast is fabricated after duplicating the individual stone dies in refractory material, replacing them in the first impression, and pouring a silicone and stone base. This master cast incorporates removable single refractory dies. This technique is a variation of the single refractory die technique described by Sheets.[54] The porcelain laminate veneers are initially built and fired on this cast.

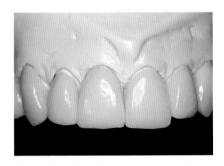

Fig. 8-13 The third cast is an unsawed cast made from the first pour of the second impression. It is used for final adjustment of the proximal contacts and of the cervicoproximal embrasures, and for a more accurate perspective of tooth shape.

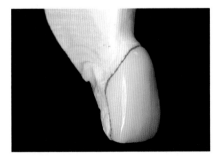

Fig. 8-14a Final porcelain veneer adaptation.

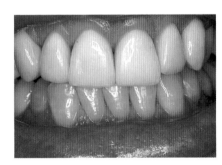

Fig. 8-14b Porcelain laminate veneers cemented in place.

Impressions of implants

Impressions of implant-retained crowns and fixed partial dentures rely on two options. The first option is to transfer a replica of the implant to the master cast.[55] In this technique, a post fastened to the implant is picked up in an elastomeric impression and, after removal of the impression, the post is secured to the implant replica and a master cast is poured. The second option is the transfer of a replica of the selected abutment to the master cast.[56,57] A transfer coping fastened to the implant is picked up in an elastomeric impression, and after removal of the impression the coping is secured to the abutment replica and a master cast is poured. In addition, according to the implant system used, the transfer copings may remain in the impression when it is removed from the mouth or may be replaced in the impression after its removal.[55–58] All these techniques involve some error in the transfer process.

In fabricating an implant-retained superstructure, a primary objective is to fabricate a passively fitting casting that generates no stress to the abutment fixtures and the supporting bone in the unloaded state.[59–62] This ideal objective is difficult to fully realize clinically because of the potential for distortion of the master cast, which is caused by a combination of dimensional errors and positional errors in the transfer process of the replicas[59] and also because framework adaptation may change when the retaining screws are tightened.[60] The tolerable discrepancy of a framework over several implants is not known, but because discrepancies of less than 30 μm in the fit of an implant-retained framework on multiple abutments cannot be detected clinically by experienced operators, this figure could serve as a criterion between acceptable and unacceptable frameworks.[60]

Factors responsible for inaccuracy of the master cast include polymerization shrinkage of the cold-curing resin used for splinting abutments,[62] reposi-

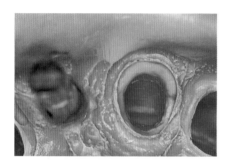
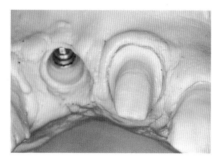

Fig. 8-15a and b Master cast options with implant impressions. The implant impression involves transfer to the master cast of an implant replica. The impression was poured in stone. The main inconvenience of this material is the fragility of the stone margin around the implant, which is prone to chipping during the laboratory manipulations, causing the level of the gingival margin to possibly be lost. (In collaboration with Dr D Palmisano.)

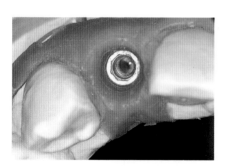

Fig. 8-16 Flexible tissue cast. The gingival mask was constructed after the stone cast was poured and the stone margin eliminated around the implant (GI Mask, Coltene). This popular technique allows for preservation of the gingival margin during crown fabrication, but the flexibility of the material allows for some degree of interpretation of the exact gingival margin height.

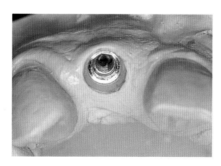

Fig. 8-17 Epoxy resin cast. The silicone impression is directly poured in epoxy resin, which has a superior resistance to abrasion and chipping compared to stone. The height of the gingival margin is precisely preserved throughout crown fabrication. With implant restorations, the ideal indication of this material is with single units.

Try-in Options and Verification for Implant Impressions

Type of Implant	Verification	Accessory Cast
Single unit	No verification needed: adjust crown on delivery appointment	None
Fixed partial restoration: short span	Framework try-in requires no soldering	None
	Presoldering required	Remount cast from soldering index before soldering
	Postsoldering required	Remount cast from splinted gold copings
Fixed partial restoration: long span (over three-unit)	Framework try-in	Remount cast from splinted gold copings
	Presoldering required	Remount cast from soldering index before soldering
	Postsoldering (indicated whenever porcelain firing may cause framework distortion)	Remount cast from splinted gold copings
Fixed bridge over mesostructure	Mesostructure try-in satisfactory	None
	Presoldering of the mesostructure required	Remount cast of soldered mesostructure

tioning of the transfer coping in the impression, excessive tightening of the copings to their analogs, and residual distortion of the impression material due to insufficient elastic recovery. The comparative accuracy of master casts fabricated with various implant impression techniques was tested with transfer copings replaced back into the impression, unsplinted undercut copings remaining in the impression, or splinted undercut copings remaining in the impression. Reports[59–62] on the accuracy of these three techniques demonstrate a certain amount of error in the transfer process in each technique and do not agree on a transfer method consistently superior to the others.

Assif et al[60] showed, however, that the accuracy of master casts is satisfactory if the shrinkage of the cold-curing resin used to splint transfer posts before the impression can be controlled. When the resin is left to polymerize for 24 hours before uniting the transfer posts, the accuracy of the master cast is significantly improved. While this modification is not directly clinically applicable to the first transfer impression, it may be applied to an accessory cast derived from copings preassembled on the first master cast, which serve as additional verification.

The minor accuracies involved in the fabrication process of single-tooth implants may be corrected on the final delivery appointment (Figs. 8-15–8-17). For transfer impressions of implant fixed partial dentures, it is recommended as a rule to systematically test the accuracy of the master cast with either a metal framework try-in or a verification try-in of the splinted gold copings before porcelain veneering. Postceramic soldering[63–71] may also be used for final splinting after porcelain veneering, according to individual preference (Figs. 8-18–8-24).

The selection between preceramic or postceramic soldering is made according to the type of alloy, the restoration design, and the potential for distortion of the framework after porcelain firing.[71] Due to the variables involved and the fact that technical difficulty increases with the number of units and length of the span, there is no decisive agreement favoring soldered restorations over one-piece castings.[72–78] Therefore, the decision rests with the preference and experience of the technician on a case-by-case basis according to the fit of the implant-retained framework.

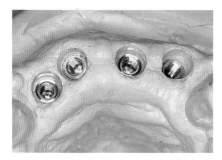

Fig. 8-18 Master cast fabricated from an implant impression. Minor discrepancies in repositioning of the transfer coping in the impression (with snap-on copings), excessive tightening of the copings to their analogs, and minor distortion of the impression material because of insufficient elastic recovery result in some imprecision of the master cast. All these factors mandate framework try-in, with possibly a pick-up impression of the soldered framework.

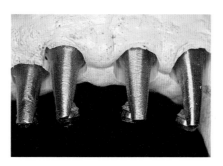

Fig. 8-19 With splinted implant restorations, it is preferable to fabricate the restoration in several sections before try-in. Four single implant restorations will be constructed over these customized abutments, incorporating accessory transversal screws. (Abutments: Implants Innovations, West Palm Beach, FL.) The crowns are constructed individually in the laboratory.

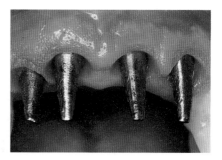

Fig. 8-20a The abutments are screwed in the implants, and the single crowns are adjusted according to the occlusal and esthetic requirements and are glazed.

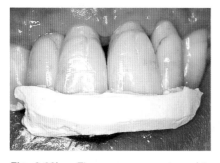

Fig. 8-20b The crowns are returned to the mouth, and a postsoldering matrix is fabricated. Splinting was required because of the long clinical crowns and to further stabilize the primary and secondary abutment screws.

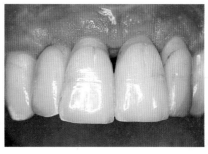

Fig. 8-21 Splinted implant crowns after oven soldering. The master cast served for individual crown fabrication only and was not deemed precise enough for the final splinting relation.

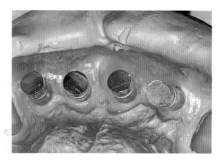

Fig. 8-22 Impression of four anterior implants.

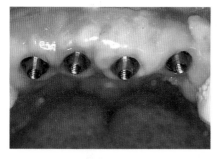
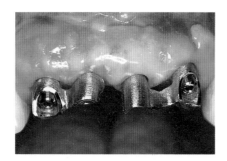

Fig. 8-23a and b Implant divergence required fabrication of a mesostructure before fabrication of the metal ceramic suprastructure. The mesostructure fabricated on the master cast must be tried intraorally to test the accuracy of the master cast. If adaptation is satisfactory, the same master cast will be used for fabrication of the suprastructure. If soldering of the mesostructure is required, a pick-up impression will be necessary for construction of a new master cast before fabrication of the suprastructure.

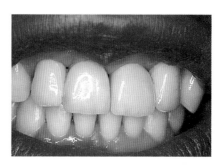

Fig. 8-24 Completed implant restorations. (In collaboration with Dr J Ortiz.)

References

1. Ramadan FA, Harrison JD. Literature review of the effectiveness of tissue displacement materials. *Egypt Dent J* 1970;16:271.

2. Nemetz EH, Seibly W. The use of chemical agents in gingival retraction. *Gen Dent* 1990;March/April:104.

3. Donovan TE, Gandara BK, Nemtz H. Review and survey of medicaments used with gingival retraction cords. *J Prosthet Dent* 1985;53:525.

4. Harrison JD. Effect of retraction materials on the gingival sulcus epithelium. *J Prosthet Dent* 1961;11:514.

5. Woycheshin FF. An evaluation of the drugs used for gingival retraction. *J Prosthet Dent* 1964;14:769.

6. Anneroth G, Nordenram A. Reaction of the gingiva to the application of threads in the gingival pocket for taking impressions with elastic materials. *Odontol Rev* 1969;20:301.

7. Weir DJ, Williams BH. Clinical effectiveness of mechanical-chemical tissue displacement methods. *J Prosthet Dent* 1984;51:326.

8. Ramadan FA, El-Sadeek M, Hassanein ES. Histopathologic response of gingival tissues to Hemodent and aluminum chloride solutions as tissue displacement materials. *Egypt Dent J* 1973;19:35.

9. Mokbel AM, Mohamed YR. Local effect of applying aluminum chloride on the dento-gingival unit as a tissue displacement material. Part I. *Egypt Dent J* 1973;19:35.

10. Löe H, Silness J. Tissue reactions to string packs used in fixed restorations. *J Prosthet Dent* 1963;13:318.

11. de Gennaro GG, Landesman HM, Calhoun JE, Martinoff JT. A comparison of gingival inflammation related to retraction cords. *J Prosthet Dent* 1982;47:384.

12. Albers HF. *Impressions. A Text for Selection of Materials and Techniques*. Santa Rosa, Calif: Alto Books, 1990:21.

13. Malamed SF. *Handbook of Local Anesthesia*, ed 3. St Louis: Mosby–Year Book, 1990.

14. Gendusa NJ. *An Illustrated Guide to Impression Troubleshooting. Special Report No. 29*. Farmingdale, NY: Parkell Products, 1992.

15. Nevins M, Skurow HM. The intracrevicular restorative margin, the biologic width, and the maintenance of the gingival margin. *Int J Periodont Rest Dent* 1984;3:31.

16. Dragoo MR, Williams GB. Periodontal tissue reactions to restorative procedures. *Int J Periodont Rest Dent* 1981;1(1):9.

17. Wilson RD, Maynard G. Intracrevicular restorative dentistry. *Int J Periodont Rest Dent* 1981;1(4):35.

18. Shavell HM. Mastering the art of tissue management during provisionalization and biologic final impressions. *Int J Periodont Rest Dent* 1988;8(3):25.

19. Nemetz H, Donovan T, Landesman H. Exposing the gingival margin: A systematic approach for the control of hemorrhage. *J Prosthet Dent* 1984;51:647.

20. Stauffer JP, Meyer JM, Nally JN. Accuracy of six elastic impression materials used for complete-arch fixed partial dentures. *J Prosthet Dent* 1976;35:407.

21. Lacy AM, Fukui H, Bellman T, Jendresen M. Time-dependent accuracy of elastomer impression materials. Part II: Polyether, polysulfides and polyvinylsiloxane. *J Prosthet Dent* 1981;45:329.

22. Williams PT, Jackson G, Bergman W. An evaluation of time-dependent dimensional stability of eleven elastomeric impression materials. *J Prosthet Dent* 1984;52:120.

23. Johnson GH, Craig RG. Accuracy of four types of rubber impression materials compared with time of pour and a repeat pour of models. *J Prosthet Dent* 1985;53:484.

24. Price RB, Gerrow JD, Sutow EJ, MacSween R. The dimensional accuracy of 12 impression material and die stone combinations. *Int J Prosthodont* 1991;4:169.

25. Dounis GS, Ziebert GJ, Dounis K. A comparison of impression materials for complete-arch fixed partial dentures. *J Prosthet Dent* 1991;65:165.

26. Marcinak CE, Draughn A. Linear dimensional changes in addition curing silicone impression materials. *J Prosthet Dent* 1982;47:411.

27. Panichuttra R, Jones RM, Goodacre C, Munoz CA, Moore BK. Hydrophylic poly(vinyl siloxane) impression materials: Dimensional accuracy, wettability, and effect on gypsum hardness. *Int J Prosthodont* 1991;4:240.

28. Eames WB, Wallace SW, Suway NB, Rogers LB. Accuracy and dimensional stability of elastomeric impression materials. *J Prosthet Dent* 1979;42:159.

29. Hung SH, Purk JH, Tira DE, Eick JD. Accuracy of one-step versus two-step putty wash addition silicone impression technique. *J Prosthet Dent* 1992;67:583.

30. Gordon GE, Johnson GH, Drennon DG. The effect of tray selection on the accuracy of elastomeric impression materials. *J Prosthet Dent* 1990;63:12.

31. Wassell RW, Ibbetson RJ. The accuracy of polyvinyl siloxane impressions made with standard and reinforced stock trays. *J Prosthet Dent* 1991;65:748.

32. Campbell SD. Comparison of conventional paint-on die spacers and those used with all-ceramic restorations. *J Prosthet Dent* 1990;63:151.

33. Christensen GJ. Marginal fit of gold inlay castings. *J Prosthet Dent* 1966;16:297.

34. Davis SH, Kelly JR, Campbell SD. Use of an elastomeric material to improve the occlusal seat and marginal seal of cast restorations. *J Prosthet Dent* 1989;62:288.

35. Sorensen JA. Improving seating of ceramic inlays with a silicone fit-checking medium. *J Prosthet Dent* 1991;65:646.

36. White SN, Sorensen JA, Kang SK. Improved marginal seating of cast restorations using a silicone disclosing medium. *Int J Prosthodont* 1991;4:323.

37. Bomberg TJ, Hatch RA, Hoffman R. Impression material thickness in stock and custom trays. *J Prosthet Dent* 1985;54:170.

38. Gordon GE, Johnson GH, Drennon DG. The effect of tray selection on the accuracy of elastomeric impression materials. *J Prosthet Dent* 1990;63:12.

39. Tjan AHL, Nemetz H, Nguyen LTP, Contino R. Effect of tray space on the accuracy of monophasic polyvinylsiloxane impressions. *J Prosthet Dent* 1992;68:19.

40. De Araujo PA. Effect of material bulk and undercuts on the accuracy of impression materials. *J Prosthet Dent* 1985;54:791.

41. Johnson GH, Craig RG. Accuracy of addition silicones as a function of technique. *J Prosthet Dent* 1986;55:197.

42. McCabe JF, Storer R. Elastomeric impression materials: The measurement of some properties relevant to clinical practice. *Br Dent J* 1980;73:73.

43. Ciesco JN, Malone WFP, Sandrik JL, Mazur B. Comparison of elastomeric impression materials used in fixed prosthodontics. *J Prosthet Dent* 1989;45:89.

44. Eames WB, Sieweke JC, Wallace SW, Rogers LB. Elastomeric impression materials: Effect of bulk on accuracy. *J Prosthet Dent* 1979;41:304.

45. Tjan AHL, Whang SB. Comparing effects of tray treatment on the accuracy of dies. *J Prosthet Dent* 1987;58:175.

46. Bomberg TJ, Goldfogel MH, Hoffman W, Bomberg SE. Considerations for adhesion of impression materials to impression trays. *J Prosthet Dent* 1988;60:681.

47. Valderhaug J, Floystrand F. Dimensional stability of elastomeric impression materials in custom-made and stock trays. *J Prosthet Dent* 1984;52:514.

48. Chai JY, Jameson LM, Moser JB, Hesby RA. Adhesive properties of several impression material systems. *J Prosthet Dent* 1991;66:201.

49. Hogans WR, Agar JR. The bond strength of elastomer tray adhesives to thermoplastic and acrylic resin tray materials. *J Prosthet Dent* 1992;67:541.

50. Zainal Abidin Mohd Suolong M, Setchell DJ. Properties of the tray adhesive of an addition polymerizing silicone to impression tray materials. *J Prosthet Dent* 1991;66:743.

51. Garber DA, Goldstein RE, Feinman RA. *Porcelain Laminate Veneers*. Chicago: Quintessence, 1988.

52. Sheets CG, Taniguchi T. Advantages and limitations in the use of porcelain veneer restorations. *J Prosthet Dent* 1990;64:406.

53. Sorensen JA, Strutz JM, Avera SP, Materdomini D. Marginal fidelity and microleakage of porcelain veneers made by two techniques. *J Prosthet Dent* 1992;67:16.

54. Sheets C. Adjunctive laboratory procedures to optimize porcelain laminate veneer restorations. Presented at the Quintessence International Ceramics Symposium. New Orleans, LA, June 1, 1991.

55. Parel SM, Sullivan DY. *Esthetics and Osseointegration*. Osseointegration Seminars Inc. 1989.

56. *Technical Products Manual*. Carlsbad, Calif: Calcitek, 1990.

57. Parel SM, Lewis S (contributing ed): The SmiLine™ System. Stephen M. Parel. Osseointegration Seminars Incorporated, 1991.

58. Brånemark P-I, Zarb G, Abrektsson T. *Tissue-Integrated Prostheses: Osseointegration in Clinical Dentistry*. Chicago: Quintessence, 1985.

59. Spector MR, Donovan TE, Nicholls JI. An evaluation of impression techniques for osseointegrated implants. *J Prosthet Dent* 1990;63:444.

60. Assif D, Fenton A, Zarb G, Schmitt A. Comparative accuracy of implant impression procedures. *Int J Periodont Rest Dent* 1992;12:113.

61. Humphries RM, Yaman P, Bloem TJ. The accuracy of implant master casts constructed from transfer impressions. *Int J Oral Maxillofac Implants* 1990;5:331.

62. Ness EM, Nicholls JI, Rubenstein, JE, Smith DE. Accuracy of the acrylic resin pattern for the implant retained prosthesis. *Int J Prosthodont* 1992;5:542.

63. Leibowitch R. Soudure "secondaire" des éléments céramometalliques. *Acta Odontol Stomatol* 1969;85:259.

64. Perelmuter S, Ganzo F. Soudure secondaire à haute fusion des éléments céramo-metalliques. *RFOS* 1971;2:171.

65. Stade EH, Reisbick MH, Preston JD. Preceramic and postceramic solder joints. *J Prosthet Dent* 1975;34:527.

66. Leibowitch R. La soudure secondaire des constructions céramo-metalliques. *Acta Odontol Stomatol* 1979;126:351.

67. Staffanou RS, Radke RA, Jendresen MD. Strength properties of soldered joints. *J Prosthet Dent* 1980;43:31.

68. Sloan RM, Reisbick MH, Preston JD. Post-ceramic soldering of various alloys. *J Prosthet Dent* 1982;48:686.

69. Monday JL, Asgar K. Tensile strength comparison of presoldered and postsoldered joints. *J Prosthet Dent* 1986;55:23.

70. Ianzano JA, Johansen R, Shiu A. Postceramic soldering in fixed prosthodontics. *QDT Yearbook* 1989:69.

71. Bridger DV, Nicholls JI. Distortion of ceramometal fixed partial dentures. *J Prosthet Dent* 1981;45:507.

72. Fusayama T, Wakumoto S, Hosoda H. Accuracy of fixed partial dentures made by various soldering techniques and one-piece casting. *J Prosthet Dent* 1964;14:334.

73. Bruce W. Clinical applications of multiple castings for fixed prostheses. *J Prosthet Dent* 1967;18:359.

74. Huling JS, Clark RE. Comparative distortion in three-unit fixed prostheses joined by laser welding, conventional soldering, or casting in one piece. *J Dent Res* 1977;56:128.

75. Ziebert GJ, Hurtado A, Glapa C, Schliffleger BE. Accuracy of one-piece castings, preceramic and postceramic soldering. *J Prosthet Dent* 1986;55:312.

76. Garlapo DA, Lee SH, Choung CK, Sorensen SE. Spatial changes occurring in fixed partial dentures made as one-piece castings. *J Prosthet Dent* 1983;49:781.

77. Gegauff AG, Rosenstiel SF. The seating of one-piece and soldered fixed partial dentures. *J Prosthet Dent* 1989;62:292.

78. Sarfati E, Harter JC. Comparative accuracy of fixed partial dentures made as one-piece castings or joined by soldering. *Int J Prosthodont* 1992;5:377.

Chapter 9

Establishing an Esthetic Gingival Appearance

Richard Caudill and Gerard Chiche

Establishing an esthetic gingival appearance initially involves the restoration of gingival and periodontal health. Once the patient has demonstrated efficient plaque control, and once plaque, calculus, and deficient crowns have been eliminated, esthetic periodontal defects can be addressed. If provisional restorations are left in place for 2 to 6 weeks, soft tissue defects may become more apparent as gingival shrinkage occurs after the resolution of inflammation. Esthetic periodontal defects may include: (1) residual gingival/periodontal defects; (2) violations of proper biologic width; (3) gingival asymmetries; (4) inadequate keratinized gingiva; (5) localized gingival recessions; (6) deficient pontic areas; (7) frena impinging on the gingival margin; (8) excessive gingival display; and (9) deficient or absent interproximal papillae.

Residual gingival/periodontal defects

After periodontal scaling and root planing, gingival shrinkage of 1 to 2 mm may occur,[1] but suprabony or infrabony defects may still remain. These are detected by the periodontal probe and visualization of radiographs taken perpendicular to the long axis of the teeth. Usually, pockets greater than 3 mm cannot be rid of plaque by even the most conscientious patient.[2] Furthermore, clinicians cannot effectively accomplish subgingival scaling in pockets greater than 3 mm and especially in pockets of more than 5 mm.[3–5] Therefore, surgical reduction is generally indicated for pockets probing greater than 3 mm before definitive restorations.

Suprabony defects may be eliminated either by gingivectomy where there is an abundance of keratinized gingiva or by apically positioned flaps where less than 2 to 3 mm of attached keratinized gingiva would remain after resection of the pocket via simple gingivectomy. Buccolingual osseous defects are detected by sounding through anesthetized gingival tissues to the level of the crestal bone,[6] while interproximal vertical lesions are radiographically evident when bone contours are no longer parallel to a line connecting adjacent cementoenamel junctions.[7,8] Because the "biologic width" is reasonably consistent within the mouth, conventional probing depths coupled with accurate radiographs generally indicate the degree of underlying bony defects.

Bone defects

Shallower bony defects associated with gingival probing depths of 5 mm or less can usually be resolved by osseous resective techniques, assuming the removal of bone will not affect tooth mobility. Osseous recontouring may also be indicated for simultaneous crown lengthening or reestablishment of proper "biologic width." Therefore, root length relative to the amount of attachment loss is an important determinant. Especially suited to resective periodontal surgery are well-positioned teeth with long, straight, gently tapering roots and without significant mobility if single tooth restorations are planned. Osseous resection may not compromise the final esthetic result when crown restorations are expected to fill in interproximal embrasures enlarged after periodontal surgery for pocket elimination. If advanced mobility patterns already

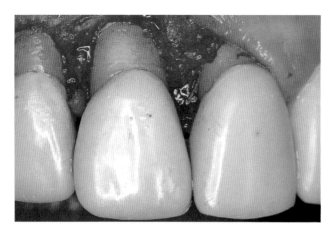

Fig. 9-1 Provisional restorations have been constructed before periodontal surgery. The desired gingival margin level, the biologic width requirements, and the amount of desired postoperative sulcus depth determine the amount of bone resection.

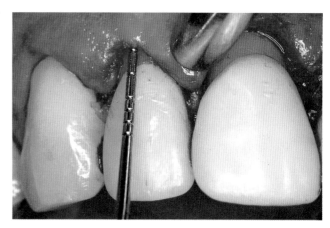

Fig. 9-2 A periodontal probe is used to ensure that the simulated position of the gingival margin has the osseous crest at least 3 mm apical for preservation of the biologic width.

exist but crowns can be splinted, resective periodontal surgery is still indicated, assuming tooth stability will be managed with splinting[9] and open interproximal embrasures can be compensated at least in part by the prosthetic contours.

Deeper intrabony defects (signified with gingival probing depths greater than 5 mm) may require regeneration of lost periodontal supporting structures with bone grafts and/or barriers for guided tissue regeneration. These procedures require 6 to 12 months for bone and connective tissues to mature to the degree that the healing result can be evaluated fairly. Strategic teeth in the prosthetic treatment plan may require this type of treatment; practically, however, nonstrategic teeth may have to be extracted to expedite the prosthetic treatment plan when required. Areas that have relatively shallow vertical defects may be difficult to maintain because of root flutes,[10] furcations,[11] or root proximity, and tooth preparation may reduce root concavities to the extent that they become maintainable by the patient.[12,13] Otherwise, minor tooth movement may be indicated to separate closely approximated roots to facilitate plaque control,[14] or strategic extractions may be ultimately necessary.

Reestablishing proper "biologic width"

Determining surgical methods

When conceptualizing the postsurgical result following osseous resection, the clinician should probe pockets and then superimpose the probe on the external facial gingiva apical to the gingival margin by the amount of pocket depth measured previously. If an

---

Considerations Before Bone Removal

- Adequate tooth length
- Adequate keratinized gingiva
- Minimal tooth mobility (unless splinted)
- Support requirements for planned prostheses
- Available tooth structure after caries excavation
- Symmetrical gingival form
- Adequate crown length for restoration

---

isolated deep pocket exists, it should be determined whether its surgical elimination would result in uneven gingival levels. If so, either regenerative techniques[15] or extraction of the tooth should be considered. If generalized shallow interproximal defects such as bony craters are present, osseous resection is usually required, and pocket elimination surgery involves recontouring the osseous margins to parallel a naturally scalloped gingival architecture.[16] Anatomic bone contours usually parallel the cementoenamel junctions.[7,8] In anticipation of subgingivally placed restorative margins, especially esthetic restorations in the maxillary anterior region, facial flap margins are best sutured no less than 3 mm coronal to the position of the recontoured osseous crest. This takes into consideration the dimensions for average "biologic width"[17] of the gingival unit, which includes approximately 1 mm

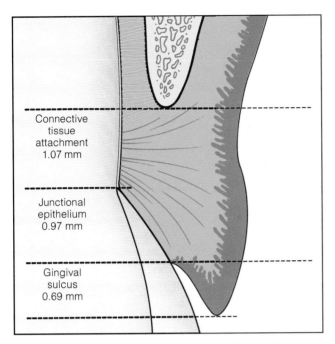

Fig. 9-3 Average physiologic dimensions of the periodontium. (Adapted from Wilson RD, Maynard G. Intracrevicular restorative dentistry. *Int J Periodont Rest Dent* 1981:1(4);35 and Garguilo AW, Wentz FM, Orban B. Dimensions and relations of the dento-gingival junction in humans. *J Periodont* 1961:32;261.)

for connective tissue attachment and 1 mm of junctional epithelium, plus at least 1 mm of sulcus upon healing (Figs. 9-1–9-3). The total dimension of this is enhanced by approximately 0.5 mm of bone resorption on the radicular aspects due to surgical trauma.[18,19] Generally, thinner bone with a thinner gingival covering is subject to greater amounts of post-operative bone resorption.

Determining bone quantity to be removed

Concurrent with bone removal for reestablishing proper "biologic width," several factors must be considered. More specifically, the clinician must consider the final locations of restorative margins, gingival margins, and crestal bone levels, in that order. The necessity for repositioning gingival units to control gingival crevice depths, conserve keratinized gingiva, or harmonize gingival margins must also be considered. The restorative dentist should have an understanding of what constitutes an esthetic gingival outline for proper communication with the surgeon (Figs. 9-4–9-7).

To assess the need for restoration of "biologic width," existing caries or demineralized margins should be excavated during preliminary tooth preparation. If the caries are so deep that surgery is needed for com-

plete excavation, aggressive bone removal may be necessary. In the absence of periodontal pockets, perfectly healthy bone must be resected to have the gingival margins properly located and the bone margins at least 3 mm apical to the level of tooth preparation.[17] Sometimes teeth to be surgically lengthened have only a long connective tissue attachment and therefore require no bone removal, only surgical removal of attached connective tissue fibers to the desired level. If only one tooth needs elongation and the clinician wants to avoid bone removal on an adjacent tooth, orthodontic extrusion with sequential fiberotomies should be considered as an alternative to flap surgery. Kozlovsky et al[20] reported that this technique could result in 1.5 to 5 mm of root exposure. Without single tooth extrusion or extraction, an entire group of teeth, such as the maxillary anterior teeth, might require surgical lengthening after the surgical elongation of one or more teeth for harmonization of gingival margins. The most apical gingival margin would dictate the position of the others for the sake of symmetry. This may be the treatment of choice where the initial treatment plan includes crowning or recrowning of the entire segment of teeth.

The position of the gingival margin is, therefore, surgically established according to the requirements dictated by tooth length and symmetry of gingival margins. Then the osseous level is adjusted to coincide with gingival levels, which assumes that bone removal will not result in an undue permanent increase in tooth mobility. Periosteal suturing may be helpful to ensure precise gingival margin placement,[21] especially when flaps are sutured apically. Usually, flaps reflected past the mucogingival junction are especially subject to apical movement of their gingival margins because of postoperative wound contracture. When there is an abundance of keratinized gingiva, flaps may only need to be reflected slightly past the alveolar crest to allow adequate resection of bone. Flap margins can then be sutured back precisely in apposition to the tooth, using simple interrupted sutures, without concern that the sulcus (planned for by relocating the osseous crest at least 3 mm from the gingival margin) will "shrink away." Holmes and Strem[22] showed that in routine apically positioned flaps for periodontal pocket elimination, the gingival margins are usually sutured approximately 2 mm coronal to the bone crest. However, suturing the margin of the flap that close to the osseous crest may result in a very shallow gingival sulcus in the early postoperative period, perhaps too shallow for the placement of a subgingival restorative margin.

The restorative dentist should communicate to the surgeon how much lengthening is desired and where

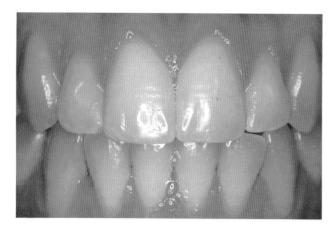

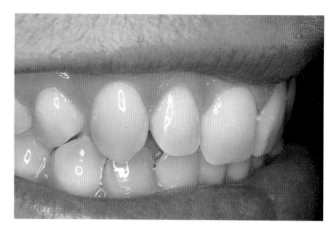

Fig. 9-4 and 9-5 Esthetic gingival outlines where the gingival margin of the lateral incisor is either situated below or along the tangent drawn from the gingival margin of the central incisor to that of the canine.

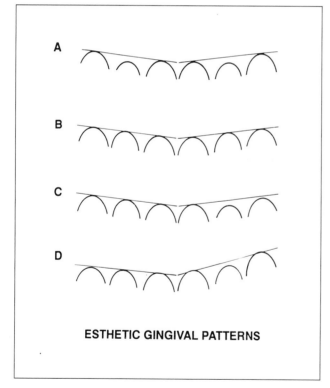

ESTHETIC GINGIVAL PATTERNS

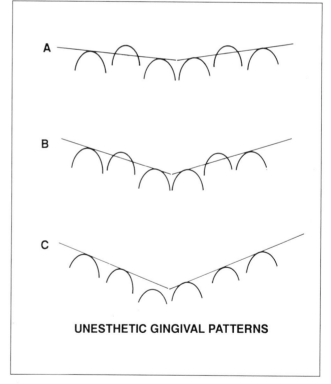

UNESTHETIC GINGIVAL PATTERNS

Fig. 9-6 **A,** The gingival margins of the lateral incisors are situated below the gingival margins of the central incisor and the canine bilaterally. **B,** The gingival margins of the lateral incisors are situated at the same level as the gingival margins of the central incisor and the canine bilaterally. **C,** The gingival margins of the lateral incisors are situated below the gingival margins of the central incisor and the canine on one side and are at the same level on the other side. **D,** Patterns **A, B,** or **C** are encountered with a steeper central incisor to canine progression on one side because the canine is in a higher position on that side.

Fig. 9-7 **A,** The gingival margins of the lateral incisors are situated above the gingival margins of the central incisor and the canine unilaterally or bilaterally. **B,** The gingival margins of the lateral incisors are situated above the gingival margins of the central incisors and the canines, but the central incisors have supra-erupted. The position of the lateral incisors is correct, and the central incisors must either be intruded or elongated surgically. **C,** Significant gingival asymmetry of the central incisor margins exists, requiring either orthodontic intrusion or surgical elongation.

restorative margins are to be placed in relation to the gingival margins. Although crown margins are seldom extended more than 0.5 mm into the gingival sulcus for cleansability, the sulcus must be deep enough to allow atraumatic tooth preparation and retraction procedures. The worst-case scenario would be to provide such a shallow sulcus postoperatively that subsequent tooth preparation would violate proper "biologic width," especially if the goal of the surgery was to remedy such a violation. After providing for 3 mm between gingival margin and osseous crest, any additional bone removal corresponds to the number of additional millimeters of sulcus depth desired in excess of 1 mm. For example, if a 2-mm sulcus is preferred postoperatively, the bone crest can be located 4 mm instead of 3 mm from the level of the sutured gingival margin, assuming an average gingival thickness.

Therefore, once the levels of the restorative margins have been established, gingival harmonization is secured in the initial surgical incisions, and bone is then resected to the same degree that gingival margins will be apically relocated, provided that the preoperative depth of the shallow, healthy sulcus coincides with the desired postoperative depth.

Impact of surgical healing on final tooth preparation

It is generally recommended that a minimum healing time of 6 to 12 weeks ensue after periodontal surgery to ensure that the position of the gingival margin is stabilized before final crown preparation and impressions. In most cases, changes will occur in the early postoperative healing stage. In cases of thin remaining facial bone, continued inflammation, and lack of sufficient facial attached gingiva, gingival recession or sulcular regrowth may occur many months, or even years, later.

Pennel et al[18] demonstrated a loss of crestal bone height averaging 0.63 mm up to 44 days after osseous surgery. Bragger et al[23] documented that 82% of sites undergoing periodontal flap procedures manifested osseous repair 1 to 6 months postoperatively. In the same study, 32% of the surgical sites showed a net loss in bone density 6 months after surgery as compared to the immediate postsurgical condition. Bragger et al[24] followed the results of clinical crown lengthening by osseous surgery over a 6-month period. Most sites had either no change in the immediately postoperative level of the gingival margin or 1 mm of gain or loss both at 6 weeks and 6 months postoperatively. Nevertheless, the same investigators reported that 12% of the sites undergoing the crown

lengthening procedure demonstrated 2 to 4 mm of gingival recession between 6 weeks and 6 postoperative months. It is unknown whether additional changes would have occurred beyond the 6-month time period of the study.

Especially in patients with prominent roots and/or thin gingiva, the clinician should keep the patient unrestored or in provisional restorations for longer postsurgical time periods to ensure the stability of surgically relocated gingival margins. A minimum wait of 3 months after surgery is recommended before initiating final restorations. Other types of periodontal surgery, such as gingival augmentation techniques using flaps or free mucosal grafts, are subject to long-term coronal "creeping" of gingiva over the grafted roots.[25] Clefts or irregularities in the marginal gingiva resulting from incisions or suture lines are usually self-correcting after 6 to 12 weeks of postsurgical healing.

Gingival asymmetries

The cause of gingival asymmetries of the maxillary incisors is varied and includes: altered passive eruption; trauma at an early age impeding normal tooth eruption; abnormal habits such as overzealous toothbrushing and fingernail biting; gingival hyperplasia due to chronic local irritants such as cement retained subgingivally on orthodontic bands; and tooth malposition or root prominence. The selection of appropriate corrective procedures for gingival asymmetries depends on several factors: adequacy of attached gingiva; localized excessive exposure of tooth root structure; the necessity for apically positioning existing bands of keratinized tissue; the nature of the gingival attachment and position of the cemento-enamel junction on any teeth whose crowns are to be lengthened; the type of restoration planned; and root angulation and form as determined by radiographs.

The surgeon should have a guideline furnished by the restorative dentist of the expected position of the gingival margins. This could be in the form of a written prescription of how much reduction is needed on certain aspects of the specified teeth, pencil lines on study casts, or an acrylic resin overlay provisional prosthesis fabricated from study casts and placed in the patient's mouth for final adjustment.[26] The clinician should attempt to locate the cementoenamel junction of any tooth to be lengthened by subgingival exploration with an explorer.

Preoperatively, the type of surgery needed for the correction can be determined by probing through the connective tissue at the base of the sulcus after anesthesia has been administered. Sounding more than 2 mm beyond the base of the sulcus indicates a long junctional or connective tissue attachment that can be rectified by simple gingivectomy or flap procedure without osseous resection. Otherwise, bone must be resected as is needed for crown elongation to preserve normal "biologic width" (Figs. 9-8 and 9-9). Surgical elongation should be avoided whenever it would result in unsightly root exposure, such as where no further crown is planned, or where enamel-bonded porcelain laminate veneers are desired. If, in the clinician's judgment, a predetermined width of 5 mm of keratinized gingival tissue is required around teeth to be restored with subgingival margins, 3 mm of which is attached,[27] the area may need preliminary gingival augmentation. After establishing the necessary width, keratinized gingiva can be subsequently relocated coronally, apically, or laterally to create symmetry of gingival margins. Only one or both central incisors may require surgical elongation to correct an asymmetry. If the level of only one gingival margin is to be adjusted, two vertical incisions can be made, one mesial and one distal to the same tooth. Two or more teeth may be adjusted simultaneously using segmental flaps with vertical incisions.

The correction of gingival asymmetries may involve single or multiple clinical goals (Fig. 9-10): simple elongation with no preexisting periodontal osseous defect; elongation with a preexisting bony defect; elongation in the presence of inadequate keratinized tissue; combination elongation/root coverage procedures—where one central incisor is elongated, the other central incisor root covered, or a more extensive procedure involving the whole anterior segment to correct the inclination of the gingival plane (Figs. 9-11–9-14); and combination elongation/ridge augmentation procedures—where one central incisor is elongated and the edentulous ridge of the adjacent missing tooth augmented.

Crown lengthening, by osseous resection, and gingival augmentation can be accomplished simultaneously. Subepithelial connective tissue grafts are especially well suited for this purpose. Multiple simultaneous procedures can also address deficient pontic areas contiguous to gingival recessions requiring root coverage procedures. Figure 9-15 depicts the interaction between these three modalities.

Precautions

When only the facial radicular aspect of a tooth needs to be elongated, with the requirement of gingival conservation, vertical or oblique incisions can be used to leave the interdental gingival papillae untouched. This safeguards against papillary loss or decrease in size, which would create a dark embra-

sure space between the teeth. Where papillae are bulky and well supported by interproximal bone at the outset, thinning incisions or gingivoplasty may be necessary to gain cosmetically acceptable gingival contours.

When planning a scalloped incision that will constitute the new, apically positioned gingival margin, periapical radiographs should be consulted to correctly match the root form, which is usually narrower, and follow any deviations from a vertical angulation either mesially or distally at the relocated position. Occasionally crowns are excessively tilted (eg, palatally) in reference to the long axis of the root. In such instances, the clinician will encounter an excessively thick periodontium as bone is removed more apically. Excessive elongation of these teeth may lead to a greater esthetic compromise than the preoperative condition, especially if facial bone is thinned faciolingually before apicocoronal resection. When gingival tissues are thicker faciolingually, submarginal scalloped incisions can be made safely, whereas with thinner tissues more coronal incisions are appropriate to prevent undue elongation of the clinical crown compared with those of the adjacent teeth. Thinner tissues are subject to greater amounts of apicocoronal, postoperative shrinkage, especially when inflammation is present.

Before final flap closure, the clinician should ensure that the maxillary anterior gingival margins are parallel to the interpupillary line. Unilaterally, gingival levels should be approximately the same on maxillary canines and central incisors and the lateral incisor may be coronal or at that line but not apical to it. Margins should be slightly more apical on the distofacial aspect of maxillary central incisors. This "distal semilunar effect" is often mentioned as a desired result, yet there are some limitations to obtaining it, such as root morphology, root position, and bone outline. "Distal semilunar effects" are most predictably maintained when ovoid roots are correctly aligned with no significant tooth rotations and where bone outlines mirror the desired gingival outline.

Complications

Even after the best surgical attempts, margins that were perfectly symmetrical at the time of suturing may sometimes heal with a slight asymmetry. This could be because of excessive flap shrinkage caused by inadequate preoperative tissue preparation; coronal "slippage" of the flap caused by premature suture loss or improper suturing technique; excessive postoperative swelling or hemorrhage causing a hematoma under the flap that subsequently organizes to thicken the gingival architecture; or shrinkage of the

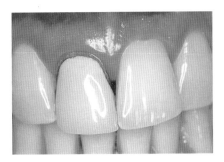

Fig. 9-8a Significant gingival asymmetry between the maxillary central incisors needs to be corrected before crown construction.

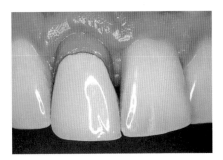

Fig. 9-8b Without any preexisting periodontal osseous defect, the flap surgery consisted of a simple elongation with the corresponding osseous resection to maintain biologic width.

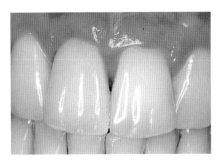

Fig. 9-8c Completed restoration. It is more critical to correctly match the shapes of the central incisors than to perfectly match their shade.

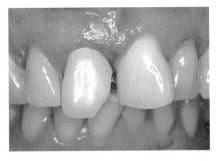

Fig. 9-9a Preoperative appearance with excessive gingival asymmetry between the central incisors. The broken crown was initially replaced with a provisional restoration.

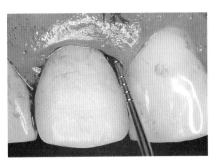

Fig. 9-9b Preoperative probing indicates a 5-mm pocket indicative of interproximal bone loss.

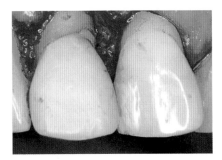

Fig. 9-9c Osseous resection is indicated to eradicate angular bony defect and provide proper biologic width.

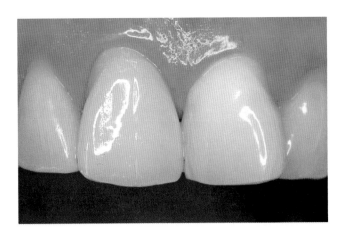

Fig. 9-9d Completed crown. To preserve the interdental papilla during surgery, the mesial crown margin was planned to be located at the base of the crevice. This requires proper plaque control by the patient and regular follow-up.

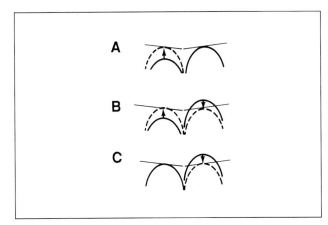

Fig. 9-10 Options for correction of gingival asymmetry of the maxillary central incisors are: **A**, elongation; **B**, combination elongation and root coverage; and **C**, root coverage.

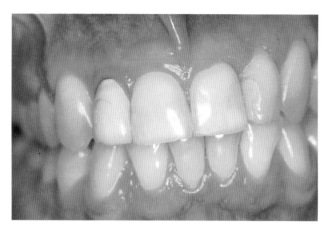

Fig. 9-11a Severe inclination of the maxilla in relation to the interpupillary line. The gingival and incisal planes follow the inclination of the maxilla. Orthodontics and/or orthognathic surgery should be considered with a defect of this severity when no crown restorations are planned.

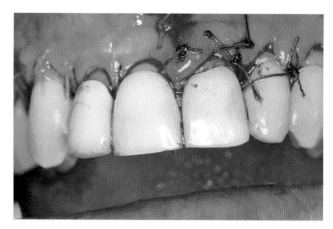

Fig. 9-11b In this situation, a combination procedure was used to realign the gingival plane with the interpupillary line: the lower aspect of the gingival plane was surgically elongated in combination with osseous resection, and the higher aspect was lowered through a root coverage procedure.

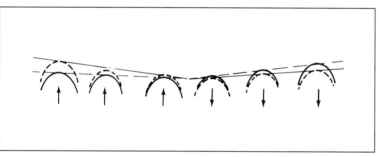

Fig. 9-12 Representation of the surgical procedure.

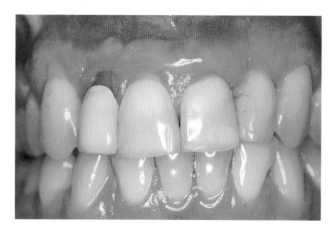

Fig. 9-13a Postoperative condition at 6 months. After realignment of the gingival plane, crown restorations were planned to shorten the incisal aspect of the longer teeth and lengthen the incisal aspect of the shorter teeth.

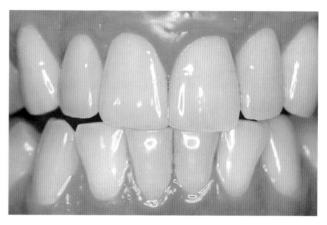

Fig. 9-13b Completed crowns 3 years postoperatively in protrusive relation. The incisal edges of the mandibular incisors were adjusted before crown reconstruction to partially correct the inclination of the mandibular incisal plane.

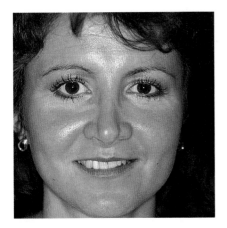
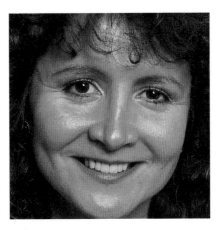

Fig. 9-14a and b   Preoperative and postoperative conditions.

Fig. 9-15   The three main procedures available for plastic periodontal surgery. Combination procedures between paired teeth and adjacent edentulous areas should be considered according to the situation.

flap due to ischemia from inadequate blood supply by surgical design or extraneous factors such as a tobacco smoking habit.[28]

If the flap margin migrates towards the osseous crest, then insufficient postoperative sulcus depth may be present for placement of a subgingival crown margin. Growing a new sulcus of adequate depth may take several months,[29,30] during which time the clinician should not place any restorative margin in the crevice. Postoperative aberrations in gingival contour, while unanticipated, may sometimes occur yet rarely require any surgical intervention. If bulbous contours are the result, a rubber tip stimulator can be used by the patient beginning at 2 weeks after the surgery to flatten the gingival architecture.

If aberrant contours are still present after the gingiva has undergone initial clinical healing 6 weeks after surgery, gingivoplasty is required, usually with a bur or scalpel.[31] If electrosurgery is used, special care must be taken to avoid contact between the electrode and the crestal bone, which can cause uncontrolled bone loss[32–34] and, in some cases, more exaggerated asymmetries. Impressions can be taken 2 to 4 weeks after simple gingivoplasty but must be delayed at least 12 weeks if resection of gingival height was necessary. Ideally, provisional restorations should be worn for several additional weeks to confirm that asymmetries will not recur.

Inadequate keratinized gingiva

In the unrestored dentition, marked recession is not uncommon and may be related to plaque,[35] overaggressive toothbrushing,[36] smokeless tobacco habits,[37] and facial malpositioning.[38] These factors should be cor-

rected before determining the need for augmenting narrow bands of keratinized gingiva or replacing marginal alveolar mucosa with gingiva. In intact dentitions with excellent plaque control, gingival recession usually does not progress over time, even when gingival units are narrow. When plaque is allowed to accumulate, however, areas lacking keratinized gingiva may be more predisposed to gingival recession.[35] The apicocoronal width of attached gingiva in the maxillary anterior area can vary widely from approximately 2 to 8 mm.[39] In the authors' opinion, a 3-mm width of keratinized gingiva may be sufficient when subgingival crown margins are planned, but at least 1 mm should be attached.

There is some evidence that teeth with subgingival crown margins may exhibit greater gingival inflammation than their unrestored counterparts.[40] The labiolingual dimension of gingival tissue is approximately 1.5 mm at the base of the gingival sulcus.[41] Maynard and Wilson[27] suggested that when facial marginal gingiva is so thin that the outline of a periodontal probe placed intrasulcularly can be seen, it may be too thin for placement of subgingival crown margins. Areas with inadequate bands of keratinized gingiva that require crown lengthening can have gingival grafts placed at the time of lengthening. Connective tissue grafts provide better color matching than free gingival grafts containing intact epithelium because the latter can be more or less pigmented than the recipient site. For the same reasons, subepithelial connective tissue grafts,[42] which will be subsequently discussed, can also be placed simultaneously during crown lengthening. Occasionally the augmented gingiva may have to be coronally positioned approximately 6 weeks after its placement to provide adequate sulcus depth for crown margin placement or to cover denuded roots for cosmetic reasons.

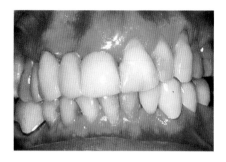

Fig. 9-16a The significant asymmetry between the central incisors is caused by gingival recession and a short clinical crown on the opposing side.

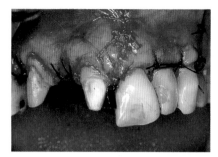
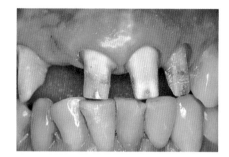

Fig. 9-16b and c Correction with a combination procedure where one central incisor was elongated and the adjacent root was covered. The root coverage procedure was performed according to the technique described by Langer and Langer[42]: a palatal connective tissue graft was placed over the denuded roots and the recipient connective tissue bed. The overlying gingival flap was sutured over the connective tissue graft for secondary blood supply.

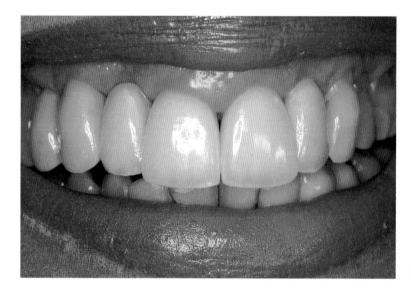

Fig. 9-16d Completed crown and bridge restorations.

Localized gingival recessions

Prominent teeth with a thin periodontium are subject to gingival recession, especially where there is gingival inflammation.[43] Exposed roots may cause hypersensitivity as well as esthetic problems and can be covered using a variety of periodontal mucogingival procedures. The feasibility of successful root coverage is dictated by the presence of ample interproximal bone height and width.[44] If roots to be covered contain restorations or contaminants, these must first be removed and the roots flattened.

Where ample gingival tissue exists adjacent to the root to be covered, a laterally positioned flap[45] may be used and usually provides approximately 70% root coverage.[46,47] Mlinek,[25] using free gingival grafting, reported root coverage success according to the configuration of the defect to be treated. He found 59% root coverage for narrow shallow defects, 39% for deep narrow defects, and 13% for wide defects (greater than 3 mm). The success of free gingival grafts has also been enhanced by using thicker grafts, butt joints on recipient papillary sites, mattress sutures over the graft, vigorous root preparation, and by burnishing roots with citric acid.[48–50] Miller[50] claimed 100% root coverage 90% of the time treating deep wide recessions. Bertrand[51] reported 74% root coverage using citric acid and 66% without it.

To enhance the success of connective tissue grafts, Langer and Langer[42] demonstrated the concept of a subepithelial connective tissue graft placed over the root yet secondarily vascularized by the overlying gingival flap (Figs. 9-16 and 9-17). This technique is especially useful where the situation dictates healing of the donor site mostly by primary intention. Variations of this technique include the "subpedicle connec-

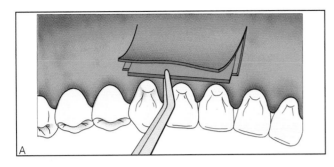

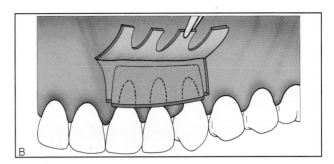

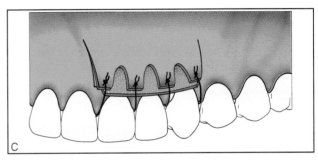

Fig. 9-17 Subepithelial connective tissue graft. **A,** Palatal flap elevated with removal of underlying connective tissue and an island of epithelium that will serve as donor tissue. **B,** Placement of the donor tissue directly over the denuded roots. Extension of the graft on the periosteum of the nondenuded portion of these teeth in order to help supply circulation to the donor tissue. **C,** The donor connective tissue and epithelium are sutured to the underlying connective tissue interproximally. The recipient flap is then sutured directly over the graft. (Adapted from Langer B, Langer L. Subepithelial connective tissue graft technique for root coverage. *J Periodont* 1985:56;715–720.)

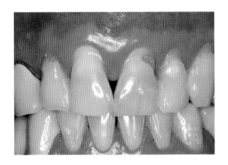

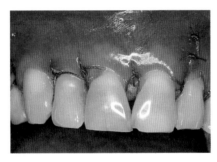

Fig. 9-18a and b A coronally sutured flap via vertical releasing incisions was made in an attempt to correct gingival recessions and elongated teeth before crown restorations. The prognosis is very guarded because some interproximal bone has been lost as a result of periodontitis.

tive tissue graft,"[52] which achieved 88% root coverage, and the "envelope" technique, which averaged 80% coverage.[53] The histologic method of healing may entail a connective tissue attachment, a long junctional epithelium, or a combination of the two.[54–57] Unfortunately, little or no gingival sulcus may be present after healing for placement of a crown margin. Therefore, in some cases the increased band of keratinized gingiva may have to be coronally positioned approximately 6 weeks after the initial surgical procedure, especially when additional root coverage is desired. Depending on the amount of available keratinized gingiva at the outset, the coronally positioned flap may either be planned as a one-stage[53,58] or two-stage procedure.[59,60] Coronally positioned flaps produce about the same amount of root coverage (65% to 70%) as lateral sliding flaps but with minimal recession at the donor site as compared with approximately 1 mm for the lateral sliding flap.[61] Free gingival mucosal grafts taken from the palate may heal with a

distinct color contrast to the adjacent gingiva, especially if the gingiva is well-pigmented. Therefore, as stated previously, this problem may be circumvented by using subepithelial connective tissue grafts.

If one-step mucogingival procedures are undertaken for root coverage, it is advisable to wait at least 3 months to assess the healing result. Coverage of multiple adjacent roots may demonstrate remarkable gains initially but may regress to further recession during late-stage wound contracture, especially where roots are prominent and interproximal bone has been previously lost as a result of periodontitis (Fig. 9-18). It is advisable to alert the patient at the outset of therapy that more than one surgical procedure may be required to obtain the desired esthetic result. When a patient presents with severe facial alveolar bone loss or a dehiscence with an associated infrabony defect, there is also growing evidence that facial gingival tissues may be predictably restored through barriers for guided tissue regeneration.[62,63]

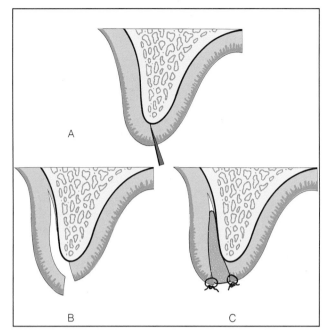

Fig. 9-19 Inlay-onlay or wedge procedure. **A**, Crestal incision. **B**, Elevated pouch-like flap. **C**, A wedge-shaped section of connective tissue with its overlying epithelium is removed from the palate and inserted like a wedge between the flap and the ridge. (Adapted from Seibert JS, Cohen DW. Periodontal considerations in preparation for fixed and removable prosthodontics. *Dent Clin North Amer* 1987:31:529.)

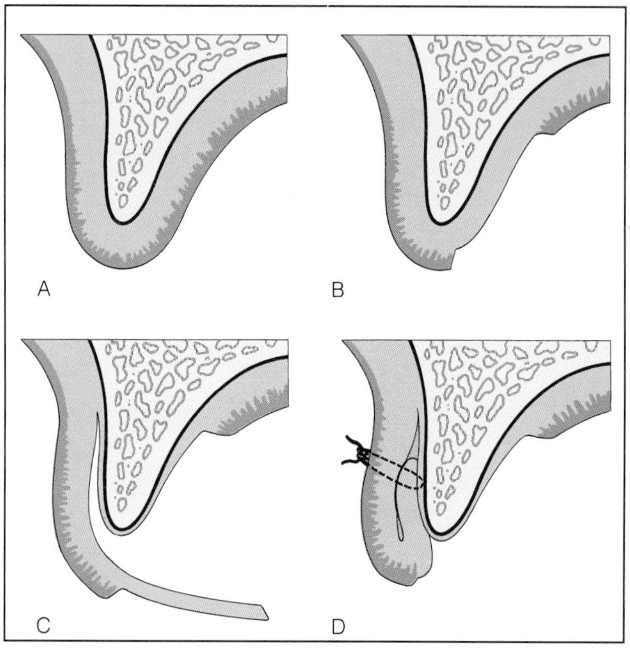

Fig. 9-20 De-epithelialized connective tissue pedicle graft for residual ridge augmentation ("roll technique"). **A**, Edentulous ridge before the procedure. **B**, The ridge is first de-epithelialized. **C**, Elevation of a triangular flap involving the de-epithelialized area and creation of a pouch anterior to the alveolar ridge. **D**, Flap secured by sutures placed in the mucogingival junction. (Adapted from Abrams L. Augmentation of the deformed residual edentulous ridge for fixed prosthesis. *Compend Cont Educ Gen Dent* 1980:1; 205–214.)

Deficient pontic areas

Several surgical techniques have been devised for restoring the contour of edentulous ridges that have been altered by disease or trauma before the adaptation of pontics.[64,65] Reel[66] has suggested the application of these various techniques according to defect severity. Allen[67] has classified edentulous ridge defects as A, B, or C (see page 193).

Buccolingual edentulous ridge defects

Surgical procedures such as the interpositional graft or "wedge procedure"[64] (Fig. 9-19) or the de-epithelialized connective tissue pedicle graft or "roll technique"[65] (Fig. 9-20) are appropriate for augmentation of Allen type B buccolingual edentulous ridge defects. Vertical incisions can be made lateral to the buccolingual deficiency and either grafts of connective tissue[68] or hydroxyapatite[69] are placed into the pouch created by subperiosteal tunneling (Fig. 9-21). For connective tissue grafting, the donor site selected is usually the one with the thickest available connective tissue, such as the maxillary tuberosity. Submerging the donor wedge of tissue under the flap of the

recipient site ensures a double blood supply to the graft and usually does not change the color of the overlying tissues (Fig. 9-22). Augmenting the edentulous ridge at the time of surgery slightly more than appears necessary will compensate for the shrinkage that occurs during surgical healing.

Loss of an anterior tooth generally requires a provisional fixed partial denture that can limit the amount of pontic space available for augmentation. Preoperatively, a removable provisional partial denture or pontic on a provisional fixed partial denture can be hollowed out to act as a guide for ridge augmentation. The restorative dentist should execute a trial wax-up of the expected final prosthetic result to convey specific guidelines to the surgeon with two main objectives: to have enough soft tissue bulk so that an ovate pontic mimics the emergence profile of a natural tooth, and to preserve the height of the interdental soft tissues to create the illusion of papillae in the final restoration.

Once unsalvageable teeth are extracted, significant edentulous ridge defects can occur. If endosseous implants are not planned for the foreseeable future, a nonresorbable alloplastic material such as

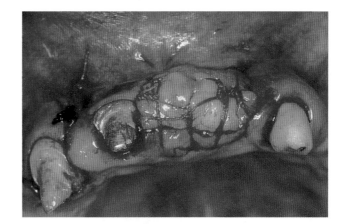

Fig. 9-21 Buccolingual ridge augmentation with an interpositional graft combined with surgical elongation of the left canine and central incisor. Vertical incisions were made lateral to the buccolingual deficiency, and a connective tissue graft was placed into the pouch created by subperiosteal tunneling. The edentulous ridge was augmented more than appears necessary to compensate for the shrinkage that occurs during surgical healing.

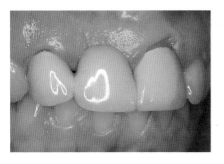
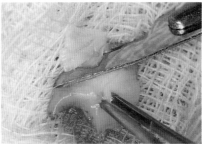
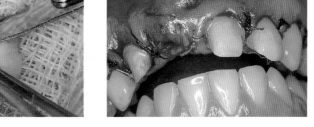

Fig. 9-22a A buccolingual edentulous ridge defect (Allen type B). The patient requested a natural emergence of the pontic from the edentulous ridge as well as the narrowest possible incisors.

Fig. 9-22b and c The surgical procedure consisted of an interpositional graft or "wedge procedure." The donor site selected for connective tissue grafting was the maxillary tuberosity. Submerging the donor wedge of tissue under the flap of the recipient site ensures a double blood supply to the graft. The incisors and canines were also elongated to enhance the required length.

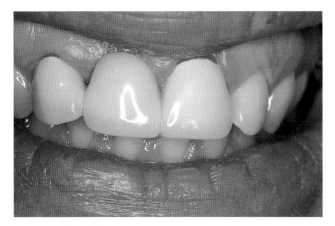
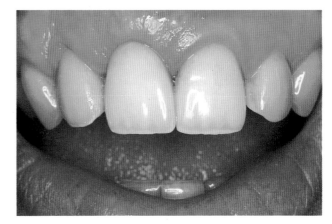

Fig. 9-22d and e Preoperative and postoperative conditions.

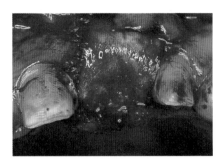

Fig. 9-23 Buccolingual ridge augmentation: the facial bone plate was lost because of endodontic failure with a fistula. A freeze-dried bone allograft was applied to the prepared extraction site, and a type I bovine collagen membrane (Collatec, Plainsboro, NJ) was applied over the bone graft before suturing the flap coronally over the bone graft and the membrane.

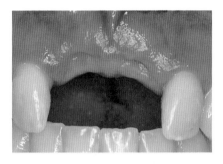
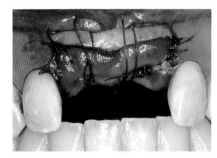

Fig. 9-24a Interpositional graft required after extraction of the central incisors to correct a severe apicocoronal defect. Appearance of site preoperatively.

Fig. 9-24b Graft from tuberosity sutured in place (note apicocoronal augmentation). (Surgery performed by Dr Gerald H Evans.)

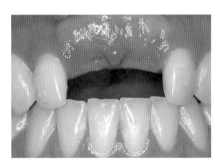
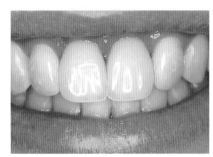

Fig. 9-24c Three months postoperatively, the graft was recontoured with electrosurgery to create recipient beds for the pontics. The midline area was left untouched to create the appearance of an interdental papilla.

Fig. 9-24d Completed restoration.

hydroxyapatite or an autogenous or allogeneic bone grafting material can be placed in the socket to maintain the buccolingual dimension, which may be covered with a collagen membrane to secure the particles in place (Fig. 9-23). Allen type B buccolingual ridge deficiencies are the easiest to augment after initial extraction site healing. Allen et al[67] compared moderate type B defects, treated with connective tissue grafts, with nonresorbable hydroxyapatite under facially reflected flaps. They found less shrinkage where hydroxyapatite was implanted. Alternatively, when the facial aspect of a tooth scheduled for extraction is largely devoid of bone because of periodontal disease or endodontic failure, a decision must be made whether to surgically attempt regeneration of bone in the extraction socket at the time of tooth removal or to wait until initial soft tissue healing has occurred before attempting gingival augmentation procedures.

Apicocoronal edentulous ridge defects

Allen type A apicocoronal edentulous ridge defects are more difficult to treat (Fig. 9-24). Although slight defects in any plane of space can be treated with any of the aforementioned procedures, usually in one stage, moderate-to-severe type A defects often require multiple procedures, and the patient should be duly informed (Fig. 9-25). Usually, the buccolingual dimension is preliminarily grafted to provide a broader base for the apicocoronal augmentation. This initial procedure consists of a connective tissue graft, full-thickness onlay graft, or de-epithelialized connective tissue pedicle graft. Hydroxyapatite grafts are not recommended before successive gingival grafts because hydroxyapatite tends to cause fibrosis and diminished vasculature in the area of the graft.

Two main objectives in repeated onlay grafting are to fully de-epithelialize the recipient site and to provide an adequate vascular bed in the recipient site. Seibert[70] recommended making several parallel incisions down to the osseous level for the latter purpose. Also, the graft should be sutured firmly in place, ensuring that it will not be displaced if a relieved prosthesis must be worn (Fig. 9-26). Any pontics impinging on the graft should be shortened appropriately.

Seibert[70] has fully described the use of full-thickness onlay grafts, which are usually taken from the anterior palate in the area of the first molar and premolars. The entire soft tissue dimension down to bone can be donated, yielding grafts several millimeters thick. Unless the patient wears a denture to cover the donor site, an acrylic stent should be fabricated to provide patient comfort and protect the blood clot during initial wound healing. A hemostatic agent such as Collacote or Collatape (Colla-Tec, Plainsboro, NJ) can be applied directly over the wound and under the stent to control hemorrhage. While thick onlay grafts might be expected to swell considerably,[70] their actual shrinkage is usually minimal. If shrinkage occurs, it takes place in the first 6 to 8 postoperative weeks. Therefore, when subsequent grafting procedures are planned, the clinician should wait at least 6 to 8 weeks after the most recent augmentation procedure before undertaking additional surgery.

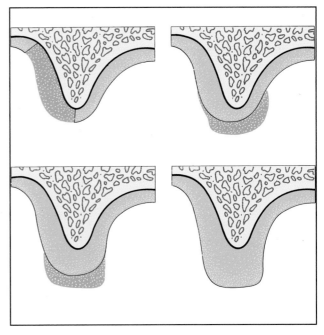

Fig. 9-25 Progressive ridge augmentation according to Seibert.[70] The buccolingual dimension is preliminarily grafted to provide a broader base. Multiple onlay grafts are then performed for apicocoronal augmentation.

Fig. 9-26a and b Combination procedure where one central incisor was elongated and the edentulous ridge of the adjacent missing central incisor was augmented. This mild apicocoronal defect was augmented with an onlay graft from the maxillary tuberosity in one procedure. The combination of the two procedures allows sufficient latitude in the laboratory for proper pontic construction.

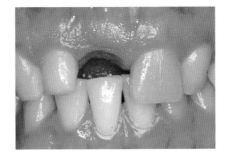
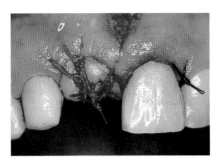

Fig. 9-26c and d Final aspect of the restored pontic area 3 years postoperatively. Plaque control must be satisfactory in the interproximal areas because the grafting procedure increased the probing depth.

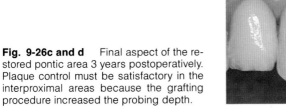
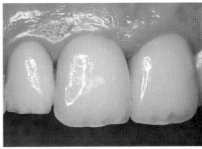
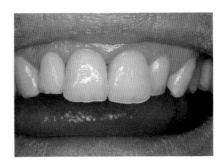

Combination edentulous ridge defects

The most difficult edentulous ridges to augment adequately are those in Allen's type C category, which have moderate-to-severe buccolingual and apicocoronal deformities. Because they often require multiple procedures, the availability of ample donor tissue and tolerance of the patient will determine the rapidity with which the deformity can be resolved. Palatal donor sites should be totally filled in within 4 to 8 weeks and can again serve as donor sites if necessary. Sometimes an interpositional graft can provide initial augmentation in both buccolingual and apicocoronal dimensions and is a reasonable first-stage choice if ample tissue is available. Hydroxyapatite grafts should be reserved for buccolingual augmentation only after adequate thicknesses of keratinized mucosa have been established with which to cover and mask the implanted hydroxyapatite particles or blocks.

When ridge augmentation can be accomplished predictably by mucogingival procedures alone, it may be impractical to use guided tissue regeneration techniques. The latter are used to restore bone, usually for the purpose of placing endosseous implants and are indicated with moderate-to-large defects of all types. Bone grafts and alloplastic materials have been successfully used to make space under barriers for guided bone regeneration of edentulous ridges. The advantage of guided tissue regenerative techniques using a barrier is the possibility of regenerating lost alveolar bone. The disadvantage is the potential for infection and the loss of regenerating tissues under the barrier. The techniques are contraindicated when there is insufficient mucosa to cover the barrier. Seibert[71] demonstrated in dogs that bone could be regenerated under GORE-TEX expanded polytetrafluoroethylene (e-PTFE) membranes (WL Gore and Associates, Flagstaff, Ariz) by creating space using blocks of porous hydroxyapatite (Interpore International, Irvine, Calif). Caudill and Meffert[72] also demonstrated bone apposition on edentulous canine ridges using the e-PTFE material alone. Nyman et al[73] and Buser et al[74] have presented human cases of successful jawbone enlargement using GORE-TEX e-PTFE barriers preceding the placement of endosseous implants. Nevins and Mellonig[75] utilized bone allografts to create space for regeneration under GORE-TEX membranes.

Although such regeneration is possible, the surgical technique is exacting and care must be taken not only to create space for regeneration, but also to gain primary mucosal closure over the barrier and prevent infection in the newly regenerating tissues under the barrier. Patient management considerations include weekly or biweekly follow-up and going without esthetic provisional prostheses during the early wound-healing phases of therapy. The e-PTFE barriers often become exposed to the oral cavity, and patients must be followed closely to ensure that the barrier remains in place for the 4- to 6-week period required for initial tissue regeneration to occur. Recent literature suggests that Type I xenografts may also serve as an adequate barrier for guided bone regeneration.[76]

Correction of aberrant frena

The maxillary anterior frenum may require resection (frenectomy) or repositioning (frenotomy) during any surgery of the maxillary anterior area. These alterations are indicated when: the frenum pulls on the gingival margin; the patient reports frequent toothbrush trauma to the frenum due to its proximity to the gingival margin; orthodontic relapse is probably caused by the frenum's presence; the maxillary anterior frenum is unsightly because of an unusually high lip line; or the position of the gingival margin is changed by progressive recession or surgery. The last two indications are the most frequent reasons for surgical manipulation of the frenum for cosmetic reasons.

During a crown lengthening procedure or with a flap procedure to harmonize gingival margins, a submarginal incision is frequently made. This can reduce the width of the existing band of keratinized gingiva and in effect make the frenum closer to the gingival margin and more vulnerable to abrasion by oral hygiene devices. In such instances the frenum and any associated fibers should be totally resected.

Surgical displacement or elimination of the frenum is especially applicable when facial gingiva is to be relocated at a more apical or coronal position utilizing flap procedures.[77] Scarring does not occur in the keratinized gingiva, and if the void left by the frenum has to heal by granulation from underlying bone it may do so without scarring. Some return of alveolar mucosa in the same site is possible, especially if mobile underlying fibers were left behind.

Ridge Augmentation Procedures*

Technique	Indications	Contraindications	Advantages	Disadvantages
Re-epithelialized connective tissue pedicle graft (roll technique)	Mild deformities	Thin alveolar ridge; insufficient palatal tissue thickness	One surgical site	Limited tissue available
Subepithelial connective tissue graft	Mild-to-moderate Allen type A, B, C		Preserves recipient site tissue color; donor tissue can be layered; subsequent augmentations are possible; stable after shrinkage	Requires remote surgical site; limited amount of donor tissue; shrinkage first 4–6 weeks postoperatively
Full-thickness onlay graft	Moderate-to-large Allen type B and C		Stable after initial shrinkage; permits sequential augmentations; permits subsequent use of implant procedures; can be placed over clefts	Requires remote surgical site; limited amount of donor tissue; color difference of donor/recipient tissue (especially in patients with moderate-to-dark pigmentation)
Hydroxyapatite	All defects supported by bone	Lack of bone support (clefts)	One surgical site; unlimited implant material; nonresorbable, moldable, sterilizable, inert	Sequestration of particles; requires primary closure; elasticity of tissue limits degree of build-up; color change if overlying tissue is thin

*Adapted from Reel.[66]

To expedite surgical healing and smooth any deep alveolar "sluices," a free masticatory mucosal graft can be used to cover any large voids previously occupied by the frenum. A connective tissue graft without overlying epithelium will provide the best color match with the adjacent tissues. Occasionally the contiguous gingiva has enough width to allow suturing one or two pedicle flaps at the midline to close the area that the frenum occupied previously. When minimal keratinized gingiva is present and gingival margins must be relocated apically, the frenum may be repositioned along with the flap, both assuming a new, more apical position. Unless there is frenum pull on the gingival margin when the lip is manually distended, or the frenum is especially prominent when the patient smiles, the frenotomy is usually used.

Guided Tissue Regeneration Techniques Using a Barrier				
Technique	**Indications**	**Contraindications**	**Advantages**	**Disadvantages**
Guided tissue regeneration barriers (with/without bone graft)	Moderate to large ridge defects of all types	Inadequate mucosa to cover the barrier	Possibility of regenerating lost alveolar bone	Potential for infection and loss of regenerating tissues under the barrier

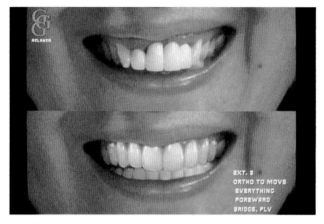 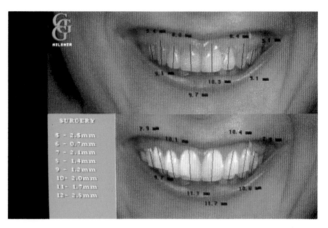

Fig. 9-27a and b   Computer imaging for visualizing final result of periodontal restorative procedures. This useful tool communicates to the patient the restorative and periodontal treatment objectives. (Courtesy of Dr D Garber.) 9-27a, Patient shows gummy smile, irregular gingival margins, and asymmetry of the anterior teeth. The lower half shows the projected widening of the arch and gingival relocation procedures, as well as four new restorations. 9-27b, The upper image shows the patient with dark tetracycline-stained teeth, as well as a gummy smile and lack of gingival harmony between the form of the upper lip and the gingival margin. The lower image shows the surgical prescription on gingival relocation, as well as incisal reduction to develop dentofacial harmony and a more pleasing smile.

Excessive gingival display

Displaying more than 3 mm of gingiva in the maxillary anterior region during a relaxed smile may be indicative of a "gummy smile." If bands of keratinized gingiva are ample and the teeth exhibit pseudopockets due to altered passive eruption, excessive unsightly gingiva can be resected with a simple gingivectomy, producing shallow sulcus depths and teeth of normal length. Planning for surgical elongation (Figs. 9-27–9-31) should take into consideration the location of the cementoenamel junction, width of keratinized gingiva, and root length, form, and position. When root exposure will result from surgical elongation, it may lead to tooth hypersensitivity and poor esthetics. It is critical, therefore, to know preoperatively whether any type of esthetic restorations such as full veneer crowns or porcelain laminate veneers are planned postoperatively for the teeth to be elongated. A trial wax-up and presurgical template will help to determine if too much of a biologic compromise will ensue after surgical correction of a "gummy smile." Operating maxillary incisors with existing diastemata and widely diverging roots would only enlarge the interproximal embrasures and accentuate the dark spaces. Teeth with large crowns and spindly roots are especially contraindicated for surgical elongation, as are postorthodontic cases of severe root resorption, where unfavorable crown-root ratios would contraindicate the removal of any periodontium before single crown construction.

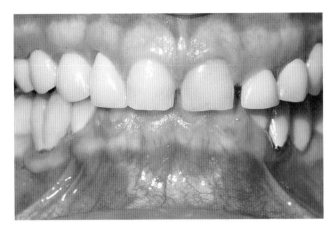 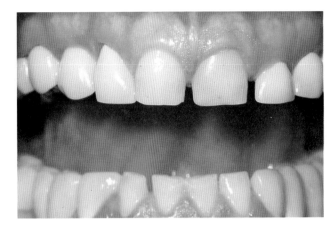

Fig. 9-28a and b Preoperative condition. The patient desired improvement of the esthetic appearance of her teeth, including correction of the diastemas and gummy smile. Closure of the diastemas would result in short square teeth of unesthetic proportions, therefore surgical elongation was required with widening of the central incisors prosthetically. The shape and gingival outline of the central incisors are not conducive to pleasing tooth-to-tooth proportion from central to lateral incisors, thus extraction of the primary lateral incisors was indicated. The mandibular anterior teeth also need surgical elongation.

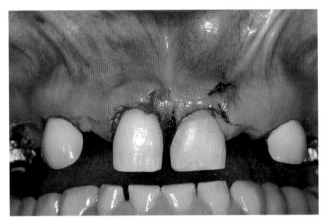 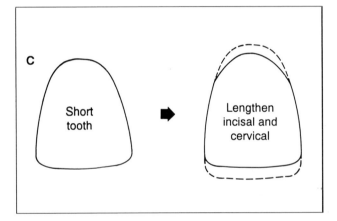

Fig. 9-29 Surgical elongation of the central incisors was performed several weeks after the lateral incisors were extracted. The canines were not involved in the procedure because they are primary.

Fig. 9-30 Representation of the alteration in morphology of the central incisors.

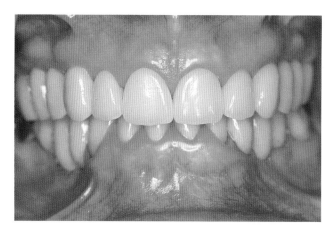

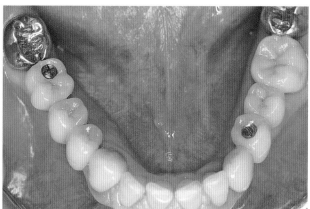

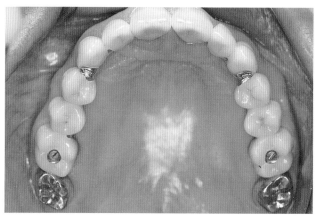

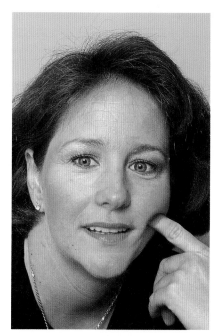

Fig. 9-31a–d   Completed full-mouth rehabilitation and occlusal views. The proportions of the central incisors as well as the tooth-to-tooth progression are consistent with the treatment objectives. The gingival outlines corrected by extraction of the lateral incisors and subsequent ridge augmentation are now satisfactory. The incisal length was increased by 1 mm over the initial situation to optimize the shape and proportion of the central incisor. This elongation was well accommodated by the face. Incisal display is in harmony with the outline of the lips and the face.

References

1. Proye M, Caton J, Polson A. Initial healing of periodontal pockets after a single episode of root planing monitored by controlled probing forces. *J Periodontol* 1982;53:296–301.

2. Waerhaug J. Effect of toothbrushing on subgingival plaque formation. *J Periodontol* 1981;52:30–34.

3. Waerhaug J. Healing of the dento-epithelia junction following subgingival plaque control. II. As observed on extracted teeth. *J Periodontol* 1978;49:119.

4. Staubaugh R, Dragoo M, et al. The limits of subgingival scaling. *Int J Periodont Rest Dent* 1981;1(5):31–41.

5. Rabbani G, Ash MM, Caffesse R. The effectiveness of subgingival scaling and root planing in calculus removal. *J Periodontol* 1981;52:119.

6. Greenberg J, Laster L, Listgarten MA. Transgingival probing as a potential estimator of alveolar bone level. *J Periodontol* 1976;47:514.

7. Ritchey B, Orban B. The crests of the interdental alveolar septa. *J Periodontol* 1953;24:75–87.

8. O'Connor TW, Biggs NL. Interproximal bony contours. *J Periodontol* 1964;35:326–330.

9. Nyman S, et al. The role of occlusion for the stability of fixed bridges in patients with reduced periodontal tissue. *J Clin Periodontol* 1975;2:53–66.

10. Gher ME, Vernino AR. Root morphology—clinical significance in pathogenesis and treatment of periodontal disease. *J Am Dent Assoc* 1980;101:627–633.

11. Matia JI, et al. Efficiency of scaling the molar furcation area with and without surgical access. *Int J Periodont Rest Dent* 1986;6(6):25–35.

12. Ross S, Gargiulo A. The concepts, contours and cosmetics of periodontics and restorative dentistry for the general practitioner. *CDS Rev* 1983;76(8):26.

13. Hamp SE, Nyman S, Lindhe J. Periodontal treatment of multirooted teeth. Results after 5 years. *J Clin Periodontol* 1975;2:126–135.

14. Carnevale G, DiFebo G, Tonelli MP, Marin C, Fuzzi M. A retrospective analysis of the periodontal-prosthetic treatment of molars with interradicular lesions. *Int J Periodont Rest Dent* 1991;11:189–205.

15. Kramer GM. Surgical alternatives in regenerative therapy of the periodontium. *Int J Periodont Rest Dent* 1992;12:11–31.

16. Ochsenbein C. Osseous resection in periodontal surgery. *J Periodontol* 1958;29:15–26.

17. Ingber FJS, Rose LF, Coslet JG. The "biologic width"—a concept in periodontics and restorative dentistry. *Alpha Omegan* 1977;10:62–65.

18. Pennel BM, King KO, Wildernman M, et al. Repair of the alveolar process following osseous surgery. *J Periodontol* 1967;38:426–431.

19. Tavtigian R. The height of the facial radicular alveolar crest following apically positioned flap operations. *J Periodontol* 1970;41:412–418.

20. Kozlovsky A, Tal H, Lieberman M. Forced eruption combined with a gingival fiberotomy. A technique for clinical crown lengthening. *J Clin Periodontol* 1988;15:534–538.

21. Kramer GM, Nevins M, Kohn JD. The utilization of periosteal suturing in periodontal surgical procedures. *J Periodontol* 1970;41:457.

22. Holmes CH, Strem BE. Location of flap margin after suturing. *J Periodontol* 1976;47:674–675.

23. Bragger U, Pasquali L, Kornman KS. Remodeling of interdental alveolar bone after periodontal flap procedures assessed by means of computer assisted-densitometric-image-analysis. *J Clin Periodontol* 1988;15:558–564.

24. Bragger U, Lauchenauer D, Lang NP. Surgical lengthening of the clinical crown. *J Clin Periodontol* 1992;19:58–63.

25. Mlinek A. The use of free gingival grafts for coverage of denuded roots. *J Periodontol* 1973;44:248–254.

26. Spear F, Townsend C. Esthetics: A multidisciplinary approach. Presented at the American Academy of Periodontology, 77th Annual Meeting, Vancouver, October 2, 1991.

27. Maynard JG, Wilson RDK. Physiologic dimensions of the periodontium significant to the restorative dentist. *J Periodontol* 1979;50:170.

28. Miller PD. Root coverage with the free gingival graft. Factors associated with incomplete coverage. *J Periodontol* 1987;58:674–681.

29. Lindhe J, Nyman S. Alterations in the position of the marginal soft tissue following periodontal surgery. *J Clin Periodontol* 1980;7:525–530.

30. Afshar-Mohajer K, Stahl SS. The remodeling of human gingival tissues following gingivectomy. *J Periodontol* 1976;48:136–139.

31. Goldman HM. The development of physiologic gingival contours by gingivoplasty. *Oral Surg Oral Med Oral Pathol* 1950;3:879–888.

32. Wilhelmsen H, Ramfjord S, Blankenship J. Effects of electrosurgery on the gingival attachement in rhesus monkeys. *J Periodontol* 1976;47:160–170.

33. Glickman I, Imber TR. Comparison of gingival resection with electrosurgery and periodontal knives—a biometric and histologic study. *J Periodontol* 1970;41:142–148.

34. Nixon DC, Adkins KFD, Keys DW. Histological evaluation of effects produced in alveolar bone following gingival incision with an electrosurgical scalpel. *J Periodontol* 1975;46:40–44.

35. Kennedy J, Bird W, Palcanis K, Dorfman H. A longitudinal evaluation of varying widths of attached gingiva. *J Clin Periodontol* 1985;12:667–675.

36. O'Leary TJ, Drake RB, Crump PP, Allen MF. The incidence of recession in young males: A further study. *J Periodontol* 1971;42:264–267.

37. Robertson PB, Walsh M, Greene J, et al. Periodontal effects associated with the use of smokeless tobacco. *J Periodontol* 1990;61:438–443.

38. Batenhorst KF, Bowers GM, Williams JE. Tissue changes resulting from facial tipping and extrusion of incisors in monkeys. *J Periodontol* 1974;45:660–668.

39. Bowers GM. A study of the width of attached gingiva. *J Periodontol* 1963;34:201–209.

40. Stetler KJ, Bissada NE. Significance of the width of keratinized gingiva on the periodontal status of teeth with submarginal restorations. *J Periodontol* 1987;58:697–700.

41. Goaslind GD, Robertson PB, Mahan CJ, et al. Thickness of facial gingiva. *J Periodontol* 1977;48:768–771.

42. Langer B, Langer L. Subepithelial connective tissue graft technique for root coverage. *J Periodontol* 1985;56:715–720.

43. Novaes AB, Ruben MP, Kon S, et al. The development of the periodontal cleft. A clinical and histopathologic study. *J Periodontol* 1975;46:701–709.

44. Miller PD. A classification of marginal tissue recession. *Int J Periodont Rest Dent* 1985;5:9–13.

45. Grupe HE, Warren RE. Repair of gingival defects by a sliding flap operation. *J Periodontol* 1956;27:92–95.

46. Smukler H. Laterally positioned mucoperiosteal pedicle flaps in the treatment of denuded roots—a clinical and statistical study. *J Periodontol* 1976;47:590–595.

47. Espinel MC, Caffesse RG. Lateral positioned pedicle sliding flap—revised technique in the treatment of localized gingival recessions. *Int J Periodont Rest Dent* 1981;1(5):23–51.

48. Miller PD. Root coverage using a free soft tissue autograft following citric acid application. I. Technique. *Int J Periodont Rest Dent* 1982;2(1):65.

49. Holbrook T, Ochsenbein C. Complete coverage of denuded root surface with a one stage gingival graft. *Int J Periodont Rest Dent* 1983;3(3):8.

50. Miller PD. Root coverage using the free soft tissue autograft following citric acid application. III. A successful and predictable procedure in areas of deep-wide recession. *Int J Periodont Rest Dent* 1985;5(2):15–36.

51. Bertrand PM, Dunlap RM. Coverage of deep, wide gingival clefts with free gingival autografts: Root planing with and without citric acid demineralization. *Int J Periodont Rest Dent* 1988;8(1):65–67.

52. Nelson SW. The subpedicle connective tissue graft. A bilaminar reconstructive procedure for the coverage of denuded root surfaces. *J Periodontol* 1987;58:95–102.

53. Raetzke PB. Covering localized areas of root exposure employing the "envelope" technique. *J Periodontol* 1985;56:397–407.

54. Wilderman M, Wentz F. Repair of a dentogingival defect with a pedicle flap. *J Periodontol* 1965;36:218–231.

55. Sugarman EF. A clinical and histologic study of the attachment of grafted tissue to bone and teeth. *J Periodontol* 1969;40:381–387.

56. Pfeifer JS, Heller J. Histologic evaluation of full and partial thickness lateral repositioned flaps: A pilot study. *J Periodontol* 1971;42:331–333.

57. Caffesse RG, Kon S, Castelli WA, Nasjleti CE. Revascularization following the lateral sliding flap procedure. *J Periodontol* 1984;55:352–358.

58. Tarnow DP. Semilunar coronally repositioned flap. *J Clin Periodontol* 1986;13:182–185.

59. Bernimoulin JP, Luscher B, Muhlemann HR. Coronally repositioned periodontal flaps. *J Clin Periodontol* 1975;2:1–13.

60. Maynard JG. Coronal positioning of a previously placed autogenous gingival graft. *J Periodontol* 1977;48:151–155.

61. Caffesse RG, Guinard EA. Treatment of localized gingival recessions. Part IV. *J Periodontol* 1980;51:167.

62. Gottlow J, Karring T, Nyman S. Guided tissue regeneration following treatment of recession-type defects in the monkey. *J Periodontol* 1990;61:680–685.

63. Pini Prato G, Tinti C, Vincenzi G, Magnani C, Cortellini P, Clauser C. Guided tissue regeneration versus mucogingival surgery in the treatment of human buccal recession. *J Periodontal* 1992;63:919–928.

64. Seibert JS, Cohen DW. Periodontal considerations in preparation for fixed and removable prosthodontics. *Dent Clin North Am* 1987;31:529–555.

65. Abrams L. Augmentation of the deformed residual edentulous ridge for fixed prosthesis. *Compend Cont Educ Dent* 1980;1:205–214.

66. Reel DC. Establishing esthetic contours of the partially edentulous ridge. *Quintessence Int* 1988;19:301–310.

67. Allen EP, Gainza CS, Farthing GG, Newbold DA. Improved technique for localized ridge augmentation. A report of 21 cases. *J Periodontol* 1985;56:195–199.

68. Garber DA, Rosenberg ES. The edentulous ridge in fixed prosthodontics. *Compend Contin Educ Dent* 1981;2:212–233.

69. Gray JL, Quattlebaum JB. Correction of localized alveolar ridge defects utilizing hydroxyapatite and a "tunneling" approach: A case report. *Int J Periodont Rest Dent* 1988;3:73–78.

70. Seibert JS. Reconstruction of deformed, partially edentulous ridges, using full thickness onlay grafts. Part I. Technique and wound healing. *Compend Cont Educ Dent* 1983;4:437.

71. Seibert JS, Nyman S. Localized ridge augmentation in dogs: A pilot study using membranes and hydroxylapatite. *J Periodontol* 1990;61:157–165.

72. Caudill RF, Meffert RM. Histologic analysis of the osseointegration of endosseous implants in simulated extraction sockets with and without e-PTFE barriers. Part I. Preliminary findings. *Int J Periodont Rest Dent* 1991;11:207–215.

73. Nyman S, Lang NP, Buser D, Brägger U. Bone regeneration adjacent to titanium dental implants using guided tissue regeneration: A report of two cases. *Int J Oral Maxillofac Implants* 1990;5:9–14.

74. Buser D, Brägger U, Lang NP, Nyman S. Regeneration and enlargement of jaw bone using guided tissue regeneration. *Clin Oral Implants Res* 1990;1:22–32.

75. Nevins M, Mellonig J. Enhancement of the damaged edentulous ridge to receive dental implants: A combination of allograft and the GORE-TEX membrane. *Int J Periodont Rest Dent* 1992;12:97–111.

76. Sevor JJ, Meffert RM, Cassingham RJ. Regeneration of dehisced alveolar bone adjacent to endosseous dental implants utilizing a resorbable collagen membrane: Clinical and histologic results. *Int J Periodont Rest Dent* 1993;13:71–83.

77. Miller PD, Binkley LH. Root coverage and ridge augmentation in class IV recession using a coronally positioned free gingival graft. *J Periodontol* 1986;57:360–363.

Index